Obstetrics
and Gynecology
in Low-Resource Settings

BMA

Obstetrics *and* Gynecology

in Low-Resource Settings

A PRACTICAL GUIDE

Edited by

Nawal M. Nour

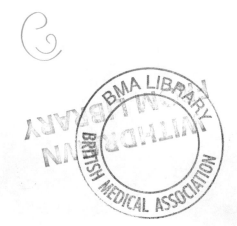

Harvard University Press

Cambridge, Massachusetts
London, England
2016

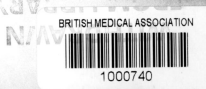

First printing

Library of Congress Cataloging-in-Publication Data

Names: Nour, Nawal M., editor.

Title: Obstetrics and gynecology in low-resource settings :
a practical guide / edited by Nawal M. Nour.

Description: Cambridge, Massachusetts : Harvard University
Press, 2016. | Includes index.

Identifiers: LCCN 2016017748 | ISBN 9780674731240
(pbk. : alk. paper)

Subjects: LCSH: Obstetrics—Developing countries—Handbooks,
manuals, etc. | Gynecology—Developing countries—Handbooks,
manuals, etc. | Reproductive health—Developing countries—
Handbooks, manuals, etc. | Women—Health and hygiene—
Developing countries—Handbooks, manuals, etc. | Maternal
health services—Developing countries—Handbooks, manuals, etc.

Classification: LCC RG101 .O28 2016 | DDC 618.2009172/4—dc23

LC record available at https://lccn.loc.gov/2016017748

To my parents

Contents

Introduction

Nawal M. Nour

The worldwide state of women's and girls' health is a matter of great concern. Approximately 800 women die every day from labor and delivery; 99% of these deaths occur in resource-poor nations. Cervical cancer—which is a preventable disease—is responsible for over 270,000 deaths per year; 85% of them occur in resource-poor nations. In countries with high HIV prevalence, 25% of pregnancy-related deaths are caused by HIV; women's access to adequate HIV treatment is limited by cost, logistics, and education. Obstetric fistula, unsafe abortions, malaria, poor-quality anesthesia, female genital cutting, violence against women: these issues form a terrible synergy, producing the devastating morbidity and mortality rate among women in resource-poor settings. It is time to mobilize practitioners interested in global health to help decrease these numbers and prevent unnecessary deaths.

Interest in global health is steadily increasing. More medical schools are creating global-health courses, medical residencies now offer international elective rotations, and numerous practitioners choose to practice for a year or two in low-resource settings after retirement.

Working in low-resource settings will challenge the most seasoned health provider. Even diseases and conditions found in more developed parts of the world require different approaches. Issues of hygiene, lack of equipment, supplies, and facilities all make it more difficult to practice high-quality medicine. Traveling abroad to work specifically in women's health poses particular challenges—but offers exceptional rewards.

This book was designed to provide an accurate, up-to-date picture of the overall state of women's reproductive health care in low-resource areas, along with practical advice for providing high-quality care in such settings. The hope is to inform, educate, and inspire medical students to enter the field of global obstetrics and gynecology; to train the next generation of ob-gyns providing care to women in low-resource areas; and to offer a practical resource for physicians, midwives, and nurses at any career stage choosing to practice in low-resource areas. Though many of us may have expertise in one area of obstetrics and gynecology, given the very real possibility of finding ourselves the only health practitioner in the village, we may need refreshers in other areas. Although this volume focuses on obstetric and gynecologic issues, its eventual audience is intended to also include midwives, nurse-practitioners, and physician assistants who are interested in improving the medical care of women in the low-resource settings.

This guide is organized into five broad sections: introductory material; challenges in obstetrics; the interaction of infectious diseases and pregnancy; gynecologic challenges; and what we have called "teamwork" challenges.

The contributors to this volume were chosen thoughtfully to reflect both state-of-the art medical expertise and on-the-ground experience in providing ethical, respectful, and high-quality health care to women and girls in the world's resource-limited areas. Some authors are well-established educators, clinicians, and policy makers with national and international reputations; other "next-generation" contributors have already demonstrated their commitment to improving the global health of girls and women through recent on-the-ground work as well as excellent scholarship.

All the chapters are designed to present an epidemiologic picture of their subject as well as practical approaches to treating real-world patients, derived from direct experience and careful research.

In Chapter 1, I suggest how this text might be used by the widest possible range of health-care professionals, in terms of years and range of expertise as well as their relative independence or team-based contributions: final-year medical school students, residents, and ob-gyns already in practice. However, I hope that the volume will also be helpful to attending physicians, midwives, nurse-practitioners, and physician assistants interested in working in women's health care in low-resource areas. Then I offer a discussion of the logistical aspects of approaching work in women's global health: how to prepare, what kind of differences an institutional affiliation might make, and some links to resources you may find useful. One caveat: because of the rapidly growing interest in global health, such organizations and sources of information will have proliferated enormously by the time this volume is printed and distributed; but we will have made a start.

OBSTETRIC CHALLENGES

Chapter 2 presents an important overview of maternal mortality by two eminent health practitioners in the field, Andre B. Lalonde of McGill University in Montréal and Suellen Miller of the UC Berkeley School of Public Health. The chapter discusses the epidemiology of maternal mortality, its multiple etiologies, and approaches to prevention and reduction of mortality.

In Chapter 3, Zulfiqar Ahmed Bhutta and Jai K. Das of Toronto's Hospital for Sick Children and Pakistan's Aga Khan University collaborate on a global perspective of the causes and approaches to reducing the incidence of stillbirths.

In Chapter 4, L. Lewis Wall of Washington University in St. Louis and Mekelle University in Ethiopia presents a sensitive and comprehensive discussion of obstetric fistula: its etiology and what can be done to treat this stigmatizing—and indirectly, life-threatening—condition.

INFECTIOUS DISEASES AND PREGNANCY

Chapter 5 is an overview of the sexually transmitted infections encountered by female patients in low-resource settings, by Khady Diouf of Brigham and Women's Hospital and the Harvard Medical School in Boston, including current approaches to management and treatment options.

In Chapter 6 on HIV and pregnancy, Christin Price and Sigal Yawetz, two other clinician-researchers from Brigham and Women's and Harvard Medical School, discuss primary considerations in the care of pregnant women with HIV, including treatment of coinfections and the use of retroviral therapy in the prevention of mother-to-child transmission.

Chapter 7 presents important insights into the effects of malaria on pregnancy, by Johanna Daily of the Albert Einstein College of Medicine in New York and Blair Wylie of Massachusetts General Hospital and

Harvard Medical School in Boston. Topics include the elevated risk of severe disease in pregnancy, the need for rapid treatment, and the dangers associated with parasitic infection of the placenta as well as the central role of prevention and effective treatment strategies to improve both maternal and child health.

GYNECOLOGIC CHALLENGES

In Chapter 8, Maria I. Rodriguez of the Oregon Health and Science University in Portland provides crucial information on the central role of contraception in women's health worldwide, including important findings from the WHO on key elements for the safe and effective provision of contraception and a call to integrate contraceptive services into any existing health care system.

Chapter 9's discussion of cervical cancer was contributed by Rengaswamy Sankaranarayanan of the International Agency for Research on Cancer in Lyon, France. In addition to epidemiological data on the fourth most common cancer worldwide, the author guides the reader through the central issues: from screening and prevention (including vaccination), through to diagnosis, staging, and treatment.

Gender-based violence is presented in Chapter 10 by Rose Leonard Molina and Jennifer Scott of Beth Israel Deaconess Medical Center and Harvard Medical School. They clearly demonstrate the underlying role of pervasive gender inequality and point out that health providers can be instrumental in helping women: through education outreach, confidential and compassionate screening, treating both acute and chronic injuries, and effecting changes in policy through nongovernmental organizations and professional societies, and supporting local champions of gender equality in the community.

In Chapter 11, I offer historical and epidemiologic information about female genital cutting, gained from my own experience in caring for women who have experienced it, both in their countries of origin and at the African Women's Health Center at Brigham and Women's Hospital and Harvard Medical School.

Chapter 12 is a practical look at performing obstetric-gynecologic surgery in low-resource settings, with special consideration of issues surrounding blood loss and blood supply, by Julianna Schantz-Dunn, also of Brigham and Women's Hospital and Harvard Medical School.

TEAMWORK CHALLENGES

In Chapter 13, Dinesh Kumar Jagannathan and Bhavani Shankar Kodali, both anesthesiologists at Brigham and Women's Hospital and Harvard Medical School, provide crucial information on obstetric anesthesia, focusing on its potential to greatly reduce maternal mortality and the need for better-trained practitioners in resource-limited areas.

In Chapter 14, Sadath Ali Sayeed of Boston Children's Hospital and Harvard Medical School offers a careful evaluation of the incidence of neonatal death in low-resource areas and the central role of resuscitation in saving newborns. After presenting the epidemiology involved, he closes the volume on an optimistic note, suggesting that deliberate approaches to improving newborn-care practices are already beginning to improve survival, even where resources are scarcest.

As you approach this book, I suggest that you try to acquire a kind of dual perspective. First, improving global women's health is critical to advancing human equality on all fronts, across cultures, religions, and ethnicities, socioeconomic levels, and of course between genders—all truly worthwhile goals.

However, at the same time you must be aware that both the medical and cultural context in which you find yourself will differ dramatically from your training. For that reason, it is wise to approach this work with great humility. Your goal is true collaboration with medical colleagues, and if you are open-minded enough, you will learn as least as much as you teach. For example, you may find that your in-country colleagues practice medicine that may be outdated. You must understand first that they are continuously practicing medicine under very difficult conditions and are in all likelihood getting the best result possible under the circumstances. Though you are eager to help—and why else would you have chosen this work?—make sure to listen deeply and understand the reasons behind the practices you find, and let that inform your efforts to make positive change.

1

Preparing for Global Women's Health Work

NAWAL M. NOUR

Women in lower-resource countries are at elevated risk for many health problems, including obstetric fistulas, infectious diseases, cervical cancer, and even maternal death. Exacerbating these risks are the need for better facilities, inadequate supplies of medication and functioning equipment, and lack of well-trained staff. To address these disparities, in 2000 the United Nations included among its eight Millennium Development Goals (MDG) four objectives that were directly applicable to maternal health:

- to promote gender equality and empower women
- to reduce child mortality
- to improve maternal health, and
- to combat HIV/AIDS, malaria, and other diseases

A publication from the World Health Organization, the United Nations Children's Emergency Fund, the United Nations Population Fund, the World Bank Group, and the United Nations Population Division (World Health Organization et al. 2015) focused on maternal mortality. While no MDG region managed to achieve the identified target of a 75% reduction in maternal mortality, all the regions did show "substantial progress, particularly after announcement of the MDGs in 2000," indicating that such goals have substantial effects in stimulating improvement. The UN's new Sustainable Development Goals (SDGs) call for "an acceleration of current progress in order to achieve a global maternal mortality rate of 70 maternal deaths per 100,000 live births, or less, by 2030, working towards a vision of ending all preventable maternal mortality" (World Health Organization et al. 2015, 38).

In addition, a policy statement by the American College of Obstetricians and Gynecologists (ACOG 2012) has acknowledged the direct connection between women's health and human rights worldwide. There is a genuine desire among health-care professionals to become involved in global women's health, but recognizing the best way to help can be challenging.

A SHORT HISTORY OF GLOBAL HEALTH

Historically, most international medical or health aid has been provided by nongovernmental organizations (often religious in nature) or the United Nations. The International Committee of the Red Cross, formed in 1863 to aid the victims of war atrocities, was one of the first. Organizations such as Save the Children and Oxfam focused on particular populations or issues. The impartial humanitarian organization Médecins sans Frontières (Doctors without Borders) was established in 1971 to assist high-risk populations; it received the Nobel Peace Prize in 1999.

Though many physicians have accepted the challenge of working in low-resource areas, a few individual practitioners have become well known for such work. Albert Schweitzer's (1924) book *On the Edge of the Primeval Forest* and the much more recent description of Paul Farmer's work in Haiti in *Mountains beyond Mountains* (Kidder 2003) showcase passionate physicians dedicated to improving health care in resource-poor nations. In addition, actors and artists have directed the attention of the world to famines, wars, natural disasters, and political injustice not only through U.S. congressional testimony but also via fundraising concerts and songs such as "We Are the World" and "Do They Know It's Christmas?" (see Levs 2012). Such projects highlight disparities in health and justice and have motivated many health workers to participate in global health.

Between 1984 and 2011, the proportion of graduates of U.S. medical schools who took part in global health experiences rose from 6% to 31% (Nelson et al. 2012). Even more recently, data from the Association of American Medical Colleges suggest that over 65% of students entering medical school would like to pursue global learning (Krisberg 2015).

The acronym *MCH*, for "maternal and child health," was coined to encompass the allied health concerns of mothers and children. In 1985, the

Lancet published a pivotal editorial, "Maternal Mortality, a Neglected Tragedy: Where Is the M in MCH?" (Rosenfield and Maine 1985). The authors' main point was that maternal health—and, in particular, maternal mortality—has been largely ignored and that "obstetricians are particularly neglectful of their duty in this regard." Another thrust of the article was the fallacy of the axiom "whatever is good for the child is good for the mother," since family planning is in fact one of the best ways to reduce maternal mortality. Rosenfield and Maine's article managed to broaden the spotlight on the child to include the mother.

Reflecting the steadily increasing interest of obstetricians, gynecologists, midwives, and nurse-practitioners in global health, ACOG has created a Global Operations Advisory Group to assist fellows of the college, existing university programs in global women's health, and residency programs in developing and implementing more meaningful international maternal health interventions. Additionally, ACOG has joined the American College of Nurse-Midwives and the American Academy of Pediatrics in a Global Development Alliance with other public-private enterprises under the umbrella of the United States Agency for International Development, under the name Survive & Thrive.

WHO IS THE AUDIENCE FOR THIS BOOK?

My intention in preparing this book is to create a resource usable by the widest possible range of health practitioners interested in providing obstetric and gynecologic care in areas of the world where resources are scarce and the infrastructure for health care is inconsistent or even absent. Thus it was designed to be helpful to individuals just beginning medical training, those with many years of practice behind them, and everyone in between.

Even before receiving any clinical training, first- and second-year medical students, midwives, and nurse-practitioners interested in global health will find this volume useful in approaching research or educational projects in low-resource countries. (Of course, ethical considerations prevent all physicians from engaging in any type of care, procedure, or other activity for which they are unlicensed or untrained in their home country; this point is touched upon below.) Third- and fourth-year medical students, who have usually completed some clinical training, can consider becoming involved in direct patient care; this book offers a wealth of information to help young clinicians get the most from a field placement in what might become their most demanding teaching hospital.

Residents will be able to function at a higher level, given their clinical training. For those in the first or second year of residency, the book can be part of their curriculum, global-health journal clubs, conference presentations, and so on. The chapters on aspects of obstetric practice should provide rich sources of hands-on tips and practical advice about providing quality care in the absence of many technological resources that could be taken for granted in a Western hospital. Third- and fourth-year residents, who are more likely to be able to travel, might make more use of the chapters on hands-on work, prevention of maternal mortality, postpartum hemorrhage, and more involved gynecologic surgery, including fistula repair.

For physicians or midwives who already have considerable obstetric and gynecologic experience under their belt, my hope is that the information on cultural and political considerations, creative solutions to logistical problems, and the many implied opportunities to educate other physicians and help create much-needed infrastructure will be appreciated and bring their own rewards. In addition, practitioners with research backgrounds may discover new avenues for inquiry by delving more deeply into the links offered with each chapter.

IS GLOBAL HEALTH RIGHT FOR YOU?

All health practitioners—whether physicians, midwives, or nurse-practitioners—who consider committing themselves to a global-health mission must honestly ask whether they are well suited to this kind of work. Despite enthusiasm and the best of intentions, a number of pitfalls await the first-time health-care provider in the low-resource setting. One is the likelihood of facing a new language and unfamiliar climate and food, and the culture shock may be amplified by witnessing extreme poverty and being forced to work with limited resources. A competent practitioner in a data-driven U.S. hospital will not necessarily succeed in a rural health center.

In addition, it is difficult to predict how individuals will react in challenging and unfamiliar settings. Some candidates who seem unsuitably rigid and inflexible have flourished, finding creative solutions to stressful conditions. Other physicians who planned on a global-health career have become overwhelmed and forced to conclude that the best way for them to help is through donating to organizations doing this difficult work. However, good mentorship by experienced practitioners or local advisers, along with thoughtful preparation, increases the chances of success.

ARE YOU DOING THIS FOR THE RIGHT REASONS?

We consider global health travel for a variety of reasons. In discussing her students' and her own motivations for working in low-resource areas, Jane Philpott (2010) writes that such impulses run the gamut from those she would rather suppress, to those she finds tolerable, to those to which she herself aspires. The most problematic of these border on neocolonialism or simply a fascination with the exotic; she cites the dangers of exploitation and condescension. There is also the temptation of a kind of reverse glamour, derived from having worked in a dangerous, terrible place.

Some may feel moved to introduce relatively advanced surgical techniques such as laparoscopy or hysteroscopy; others might want to learn procedures uncommon in resource-rich countries, such as fistula repair. Both these approaches are also problematic. Unless you plan to return to the country on a regular basis to perform "advanced" procedures (including helping to establish them by teaching), you would simply be enriching your own medical training, not bringing about lasting improvements to women's health. And if your genuine goal is to educate local physicians, you should commit to remaining in-country until all your patients have completely recovered. Risk of morbidity or even mortality would be created if local surgeons were later required to manage unfamiliar complications.

The desire to learn unfamiliar techniques on the job should never figure into a decision to work in low-resource settings. Though some such countries lack medicolegal systems altogether, such an absence of enforcement should not be taken as carte blanche to practice outside your area of expertise (Philpott 2010, 8). In fact, it is likely that your medical liability and malpractice insurance will not cover you if you practice outside the scope of your training.

It is also important to consider research suggesting that medical missions rarely create permanent solutions and may actually do more harm than good; they often fail to meet the goals of sustainability and commitment to the region (Leow et al. 2010; Wall 2006). The American College of Obstetricians and Gynecologists (ACOG 2010) published a seminal and practical set of guidelines in *Ethical Considerations for Performing Gynecologic Surgery in Low-Resource Settings*. Included in fundamental standards of ethical practice for traveling clinicians are adequate medical resources, surgical competence, continuity of postoperative care, protection of human subjects in research, and sustainability of humanitarian efforts (Wall et al. 2006).

HOW DO YOU FIT INTO THE PICTURE OF GLOBAL WOMEN'S HEALTH?

Philpott's (2010) article concludes, "The finest motivation for global health education is the recognition of our common humanity, our shared destiny, and the interconnected determinants of health" and describes the doctors who have the best outcomes at the end of this process as "excellent physicians with a global state of mind." If this image is one to which you aspire, it may be time to think about finding your own place in global women's health. Providers considering working with women in low-resource areas are well served to determine the overall goal of such a trip, any particular medical interest, and the type of facility in which they would like to work.

Of course, medical interests are diverse: from pure obstetric care to gynecologic surgery and cervical cancer screening or treatment of HIV-infected persons to gathering data for research. Some providers prefer to focus on public health or community work. The possible practice settings vary widely, from the relative familiarity of direct inpatient hospital care and rural outpatient clinics to the challenging environment of refugee camps.

The decision about where to work should be informed by learning all you can about the local culture, religion, language, and politics. Other practical considerations are how long the travel itself will take, the best time of year to travel, the weather, and any endemic diseases and their associated seasons (for example, malaria during rainy seasons).

The net effect and sustainability of your trip will depend directly on how long you stay. Imagine the difference in the scope of helpful change possible in a week versus a month or in six months versus several years.

ORGANIZATIONAL AFFILIATIONS

At this writing, the number and types of organizations sponsoring global health work are greater than ever before and still growing. This has the happy effect of increasing the range of experiences one might choose for a global health-care experience. Of course, any work in women's health in a low-resource setting helps those who need it the most and is thus an opportunity for service. However, global health work also offers possibilities for providing education (to both patients and colleagues), opportunities for giving much-needed clinical care while helping to train local physicians or midwives, and a platform for carrying out research that may have worldwide applicability.

Many universities and medical schools have created global health concentrations or even departments dedicated to this type of training and offering field placement opportunities not only for medical students and residents but also for obstetrician-gynecologists (ob-gyns) already in practice. Even if an institution does not have its own program, it is likely to have some type of official link to another global health program. Medical societies often have some affiliation or even their own programs for placing members in low-resource areas for varying periods of time. Many health-based nongovernmental organizations place physicians and other health practitioners, offering not only clinical services but also work in policy and education; religious organizations (whose work in low-resource areas may include a missionary component); and programs that exist solely to match students or practitioners to a placement, though this service may require a fee.

The choice of an institutional affiliation is not one to be made lightly. The kind of work you will be doing, the type of facility you will work in, and even which patients you may provide care for will depend upon the objectives of your sponsoring organization and your interactions with that organization. The experiential material in the chapters of this book should help you envision the type of work you want to do, the clinical setting, and the patient population you seek to serve. The hope is that, regardless of where you are in your medical training, you will find a place in women's global health work that fits your needs.

PRACTICAL CONSIDERATIONS

In considering various programs, it is vital to identify an enthusiastic and reliable contact person in-country. A good contact can help you find a place to live, assist in obtaining a medical license, or even make personal introductions in the hospital or health center. Programs run by academic centers usually have established contacts both in the United States and overseas. One example of training programs in the northeastern United States is the prestigious Massachusetts General Hospital's School of Nursing, which offers a certificate in global health nursing. In the Northwest, Oregon Health Science University's Global Health Center features a broad selection of international opportunities.

At the professional level, the U.S.-based Society for Maternal-Fetal Medicine offers not only a Global Health Group for its members but also a useful list of maternal, neonatal, and child health resources on the web. In addition, ACOG has a well-developed Office on Global Women's Health that lists four areas of service: improving clinical competencies and quality of care (for doctors, clinical officers, nurses, and midwives); professional association strengthening; a Global Health Resource Center; and an exchange program called Global Health Scholars, a collaboration among ACOG, a U.S. university, and an obstetrics and gynecology department or residency program in a resource-limited country.

The American College of Nurse-Midwives has a Division of Global Health, which offers, among other important resources, guidance for "students seeking an international exchange during their midwifery school (i.e. contracts, models, guidelines)" and maintains lists of sponsoring organizations for medical missions. Finally, websites evaluate and rate nongovernmental organizations in their effectiveness and use of funding.

Of course, your own safety is paramount; the U.S. State Department's website offers reliable information in this regard. Your institution may employ a travel risk-management company that can assist you in planning international travel. For example, Partners HealthCare in Massachusetts employs iJET to support employees working abroad.

You should check with your own institution regarding preparations for international work; you may be required to obtain some type of consent, and your institution may already have made arrangements for protecting its employees' health and safety while working internationally. Many organizations use International SOS, a medical evacuation and security company; in the event of an emergency, typically the company should be alerted first, then a series of contacts made at the home institution. It is critical to have emergency contact numbers with you at all times, preferably programmed into your phone or computer; and you should provide your in-country contact and emergency contacts at home with all information necessary to communicate with the security company and your home institution.

Before departure, your institution will most likely require you to provide documentation, such as a consent to contact your primary-case physician and emergency medical information. Below is a sample list of information to include in each communication in case of emergency:

- your exact current location
- your plans for possible movement from your current location, and the route you will take
- the best way to contact you or those traveling with you, in case of emergency, including telephone country code
- when you next expect to contact your home institution
- information about your medical emergency or security situation
- your specific most urgent need right now
- whether you wish your home institution to inform your emergency contact of your situation

Despite various types of specific support and insurance coverage that may be offered by your home institution while you work abroad, it is important to keep in mind that such travel is generally undertaken at your own risk.

Once you decide to become involved in global health travel, practical preparations begin. Your checklist might include the following:

- Learn all you can about the culture, language, and politics of the region.
- Find a reliable in-country mentor.
- Purchase a round-trip ticket.
- Obtain a visa and consider registering with the U.S. State Department. Make sure you have up-to-date contact information for the nearest U.S. embassy or consulate.
- Check the U.S. State Department's website for safety information.

- Identify endemic diseases in the region.
- Make an appointment with a travel clinic for immunizations (and possibly a supply of postexposure prophylaxis).
- Obtain international health insurance.
- Confirm international medical and emergency evacuation coverage.
- Inform yourself about the need for medical licensing in the country, which is most likely granted through the local ministry of health and may be facilitated by your local sponsor.
- Determine whether your home malpractice insurance covers you abroad or whether you will need to make other arrangements.
- Ensure contact will greet you at airport or meet you at a well-known address.
- Buy or rent a cell phone in-country.

NATURAL DISASTERS

At this writing, multiple natural disasters are playing out on the global stage—and the affected populations will be recovering for some time to come. In 2015 alone, there was a tsunami in Nepal and a typhoon in the Philippines. The 2014 Ebola outbreak in West Africa consisted of more than 28,000 cases and had nearly a 40% fatality rate (Centers for Disease Control and Prevention 2015). Though that outbreak has nominally ended, survivors continue to require follow-up care and surveillance. Even the 2010 earthquake in Haiti is still having repercussions. Each event of this scale requires qualified maternal health-care providers and may serve as a catalyst for someone who has considered global health work to pursue placement in a disaster-affected area.

However, such a decision is not to be approached without careful thought and preparation. A visiting doctor will quite likely be exposed to scenes and injuries much more shocking than nearly anything he or she could possibly witness in an emergency room in a high-resource nation. Preparatory courses are highly recommended before undertaking such a trip.

Disasters in low-resource areas affect women most strongly. Internationally, women are more likely than men to be poor and malnourished and less likely than men to be educated, and they make up the vast majority of displaced persons. Having lost most of their access to support and resources in the disaster, women still have family responsibilities, which are probably even greater than those before the incident. They are still charged with caring for their children and the elderly, to which the injured and sick are now added. In addition to the effects of the disaster itself, women become more likely to suffer from reproductive and sexual health problems and to be at greater risk of physical and sexual violence. All this means that a visiting ob-gyn will be called upon to help women who are enduring not only extreme privation but also a constantly life-threatening level of danger and risk.

Practitioners must carefully consider whether they have the dedication and fortitude to be helpful in such an extreme environment. It is a rare practioner who is not deeply affected—and whose abilities quite likely compromised—by this extreme set of stressors.

EMERGING FIELDS WITHIN GLOBAL HEALTH

Respectful Maternal Care

Among the multifaceted aspects of women's global health is a new, or perhaps renewed, focus on respectful maternal care. In fact, research over three decades has documented the mistreatment of this vulnerable population in every region of the world. A recent publication by Jewkes and Penn-Kekana (2015) divides the problem into two broad areas: the purposeful use of violence, including physical and verbal abuse, and "negligent withholding of care"; and "structural disrespect," a term that encompasses not only departures from normal use of medical staff, equipment, and supplies but also nonnecessary interventions, extortion, and even holding women against their will until their bills are paid. These authors find parallels between such systemic abuse and broader issues of gender inequality and violence against women in general.

In a recent systematic review, Bohren et al. (2015) offer a system to type and categorize violence and other abuse of women in childbirth, laying the foundation for much more detailed multicountry research, analysis of the problem, and creation of effective interventions and eventually large-scale changes in health policy. For a health-care worker interested in global women's health experience—from physicians and midwives to nurse-practitioners and medical students—helping to reverse such systemic abuse would be a complex but potentially deeply rewarding area in which to work.

Capacity Building

Another issue of increasing interest among all stakeholders in global health is capacity building. With particular reference to sub-Saharan Africa, Anderson and Johnson (2015) point out that the previous model for improving obstetric and gynecologic care in a low-resource area was to temporarily import clinicians and trainers from higher-resource countries via nongovernmental organizations or other entities, often to instruct local providers on a very specific task. However, this approach had notably limited and localized effects on the overall level of care in-country. Among doctors who left their low-resource country to obtain superior training elsewhere, another well-known phenomenon was a brain drain: relatively few of them returned, with the majority opting for the economic rewards of practicing abroad.

In contrast, the goal of capacity building in low-resource areas is not just to improve patient care but also to build permanent in-country structures for training new generations of excellent skilled clinicians and to create a supportive environment for research. For example, capacity for epidemiologic research was strengthened in response to the HIV epidemic in the worst-affected African countries. In the area of training, Anderson and Johnson (2015) point out newer approaches that are based on partnerships between medical schools in high-resource countries and low-resource areas. One success story is that of Ghana, where the ministry of health and two university-based obstetrics and gynecology departments teamed up with ACOG, the United Kingdom's Royal College of Obstetricians and Gynaecologists, and obstetrics and gynecology departments in universities in the United States and the United Kingdom. This five-year postgrad program includes three months' rotation in the two countries, six months in a district medical facility in Ghana, and three months of business management study. As of late 2012, 142 doctors had completed the program, and only one was practicing outside Ghana, an excellent retention rate that bodes well for similar partnerships.

A holistic view of global health work holds that students, residents, and trained ob-gyns who practice in-country must approach their work and its legacy with an eye toward improving the long-term capacity for obstetric and gynecologic training and related research. Perhaps the ideal to strive for would be this: Everything you do should reduce the need for someone like you in the future.

Implementation Science

Translational science aims to put the findings of bench research into clinical practice. A parallel discipline is implementation science, which studies the successful enactment of evidence-based health-care interventions in diverse locations with varying resources and infrastructure. This discipline seeks to find common problems, create and test solutions, and determine the best ways to fit new solutions into existing health-care systems. As participants in any engagement and experience in global obstetrics and gynecology, readers of this volume will be putting into practice evidence-based approaches that address not just patient care but changes in policy, practice, and organizational structures as well.

For example, decades of research have taught us why, where, and how maternal and neonatal deaths occur. In response, we have created effective interventions to prevent such deaths, and in higher-resource countries we have built the infrastructure to make sure these interventions are carried out correctly and consistently. However, in low-resource areas much work remains in implementation and scaling up.

Peterson et al. (2012) suggest that enactment of such vital initiatives as the UN secretary general's Global Strategy for Women's and Children's Health will require vigorous financial commitment from the governments of both low- and high-resource countries. That strategy is broken down into six components: "1) country-led health plans; 2) a comprehensive, integrated package of essential interventions and services; 3) integrated care; 4) health systems strengthening; 5) health workforce capacity building; and 6) coordinated research and innovation." (United Nations Secretary-General 2010)

Furthermore, the authors present their recommendations as a standard for emergency obstetric services: a minimum of ten emergency obstetric centers, including at least two comprehensive facilities, for every million in population. However, they point out that the challenge of implementation (that is, the work facing those who are active in global obstetrics and gynecology care) will relate to strengthening weak health-care systems not just at the local level but also in "their larger contexts, including social, cultural, political, and economic factors" (Peterson et al.

2012). Scientific approaches to leveraging what we already know about making an intervention successful are crucial if we are to maximize hard-won funding; few programs will continue to receive support—from any source—without being able to show cost-effectiveness.

Among the most promising avenues for improving both direct care and infrastructure is a platform we all use daily: mobile technologies. Certainly, the widespread availability and use of mobile phones, even in resource-poor areas, will facilitate scaling up, or the purposeful dissemination of interventions already proved successful in a particular geographic area. Healthcare workers seeking to provide care in the area of global obstetrics and gynecology are likely to find themselves involved in projects whose goal is broadening the scale of approaches already proved valuable elsewhere: intervention science in action.

CONCLUSION

Working on the ground in global health offers rich rewards, but there is also great potential for frustration. Compared with caring for women in resource-rich countries, providing excellent care in low-resource areas will continually challenge your creativity. There will be miraculous successes and heartbreaking losses. However, the goal of improving the health and well-being of women worldwide is worth the effort.

USEFUL WEBSITES

American College of Nurse-Midwives. Provides a page of guidance for those interested in global women's health. Accessed May 23, 2016. http://www.midwife.org/Getting-Started-in-International-Health.

American College of Obstetricians and Gynecologists. Provides a list of organizations that work in developing nations. https://www.acog.org/-/media/Departments/International-Activities/organizationdatabase.pdf?dmc=1&ts=20160523T1714339109.

American College of Obstetricians and Gynecologists, Office of Global Women's Health. Accessed May 23, 2016. http://www.acog.org/About-ACOG/ACOG-Departments/Global-Womens-Health.

Charity Navigator. An independent charity evaluator that works to advance a more efficient and responsive philanthropic marketplace by assessing the financial health, accountability, and transparency of 6,000 of America's largest charities. Accessed May 23, 2016. www.charitynavigator.org.

Charity Watch. A nationally prominent charity evaluator and rater that is dedicated to helping donors make informed giving decisions. Accessed May 23, 201. www.charitywatch.org.

Society for Maternal-Fetal Medicine, Global Health section. Accessed May 23, 2016. https://www.smfm.org/society/global-health.

U.S. State Department Travel. Provides useful travel information and services, including travel warnings, travel alerts, passports, and visas. Accessed May 23, 2016. http://travel.state.gov.

REFERENCES

(ACOG) American College of Obstetricians and Gynecologists. 2010. Ethical considerations for performing gynecology surgery in low-resource settings. ACOG Committee Opinion 466. *Obstetrics and Gynecology* 116:793–799.

———. 2012. "ACOG Statement of Policy on Global Women's Health." http://www .acog.org/~/media/Statements%20of%20Policy/Public/2012GlobalWmHlth Rights.pdf.

Anderson, F. W., and T. R. Johnson. 2015. Capacity building in obstetrics and gynaecology through academic partnerships to improve global women's health beyond 2015. *BJOG* 122:170–173. doi:10.1111/1471-0528.13176. Epub 2014 Nov 13.

Bohren, M. A., J. P. Vogel, E. C. Hunter, O. Lutsiv, S. K. Makh, J. P. Souza, C. Agular, et al. 2015. The mistreatment of women during childbirth in health facilities globally: A mixed-methods systematic review. *PLoS Med* 12 (6): e1001847. doi:10.1371/journal.pmed.1001847.

Centers for Disease Control and Prevention. 2015. "Outbreaks chronology: Ebola virus disease." Updated October 23, 2015. http://www.cdc.gov/vhf/ebola /outbreaks/history/chronology.html.

Jewkes, R., and L. Penn-Kekana. 2015. Mistreatment of women in childbirth: Time for action on this important dimension of violence against women. *PLoS Med* 12 (6): e1001849. doi:10.1371/journal.pmed.1001849.

Kidder, T. 2003. *Mountains beyond Mountains: The Quest of Dr. Paul Farmer, a Man Who Would Cure the World.* New York: Random House.

Krisberg, Kim. 2015. "Global community: Medical schools meet student desire for international learning experiences." *Association of American Medical Colleges Reporter.* https://www.aamc.org/newsroom/reporter/september2015/442220 /global-community.html.

Leow, J., P. Kingham, K. Casey, and A. Kushner. 2010. Global surgery: Thoughts on an emerging surgical subspecialty for students and residents. *J Surg Educ* 67 (3): 143–148.

Levs, Josh. 2012. "Clooney testifies on 'constant drip of fear' in Sudan." *CNN World.* Updated March 14, 2012. http://www.cnn.com/2012/03/14/world/africa/sudan -clooney.

Nelson, B. D., J. Kasper, P. L. Hibberd, D. M. Thea, and J. M. Herlihy. 2012. Developing a career in Global Health: Considerations for physicians-in-training and academic mentors. *J Grad Med Educ* 4 (3): 301–306. doi:http://dx.doi.org/10.4300/JGME-D-11-00299.1.

Peterson, H. B., J. Haidar, M. Merialdi, L. Say, A. M. Guülmezoglu, P. J. Fajans, M. T. Mbizvo, et al. 2012. Preventing maternal and newborn deaths globally: Using innovation and science to address challenges in implementing life-saving interventions. *Obstet Gynecol* 120 (September): 636–642.

Philpott, J. 2010. Training for a global state of mind. *Virtual Mentor/AMA J Ethics* 12:231–236. http://journalofethics.ama-assn.org/2010/03/mnar1-1003.html.

Rosenfield, A., and D. Maine. 1985. Maternal mortality, a neglected tragedy: Where is the M in MCH? *Lancet* 2: 83–85.

Schweitzer, A. 1924. *On the Edge of the Primeval Forest: Experiences and Observations of a Doctor in Equatorial Africa.* London: A&C Black/Bloomsbury Publishing.

United Nations Secretary-General. 2010. Global Strategy for Women's and Children's Health. New York: The Partnership for Maternal, Newborn and Child Health. http://www.who.int/pmnch/knowledge/publications/fulldocument_global strategy/en/index3.html.

Wall, L. L. 2006. Obstetric vesicovaginal fistula as an international public-health problem. *Lancet* 368:1201–1209.

Wall, L. L., S. D. Arrowsmith, A. T. Lassey, and K. Danso. 2006. Humanitarian ventures or "fistula tourism"? The ethical perils of pelvic surgery in the developing world. *Int Urogynecol J Pelvic Floor Dysfunct* 17:559–562. PMID: 16391881.

World Health Organization, United Nations Children's Emergency Fund, the United Nations Population Fund, the World Bank Group, and the United Nations Population Division. 2015. "Trends in Maternal Mortality: 1990 to 2015." Geneva: World Health Organization.

PART ONE

Obstetric Challenges

2

Maternal Mortality in Low-Resource Countries

ANDRE B. LALONDE AND SUELLEN MILLER

During the 1980s and 1990s, over half a million women died annually from pregnancy-related causes—99% in low- and middle-income countries, where complications of pregnancy and childbirth are often the leading cause of death among women and girls of reproductive age. The 2015 Maternal Mortality Interagency Report and the United Nations Interagency Report have reported a dramatic improvement in the maternal mortality ratio (MMR), the rate of maternal deaths per 100,000 live births. In the past twenty-five years the global MMR decreased from an estimated 380 per 100,000 to 210 in 2015, a 45% reduction. However, most of this reduction has occurred since 2000, and there are disparities between regions. Southeast Asia showed a 64% reduction in MMR, whereas sub-Saharan Africa decreased by only 49%. Global births attended by skilled health personnel increased from 59% in 1990 to 71% in 2014 (United Nations 2015).

One of the factors behind the improving trends is the Millennium Development Goals (MDGs), which have placed maternal health at the core of the struggle against poverty and gender inequality. While MDG 5, to reduce maternal mortality by 75% by 2015, was not reached, there has been some progress. To reach the 75% reduction would have entailed a decrease of approximately 5.5% per year from 2000 to 2015; recent evidence shows a decline of only 3.1% (United Nations 2015). As reflected in Figure 2.1, maternal mortality varies among both regions and countries.

Though the 2015 goal of a 75% reduction in maternal mortality has not been reached, there is significant progress in many regions. Tables 2.1 and 2.2 demonstrate the reductions and how close or far regions have been

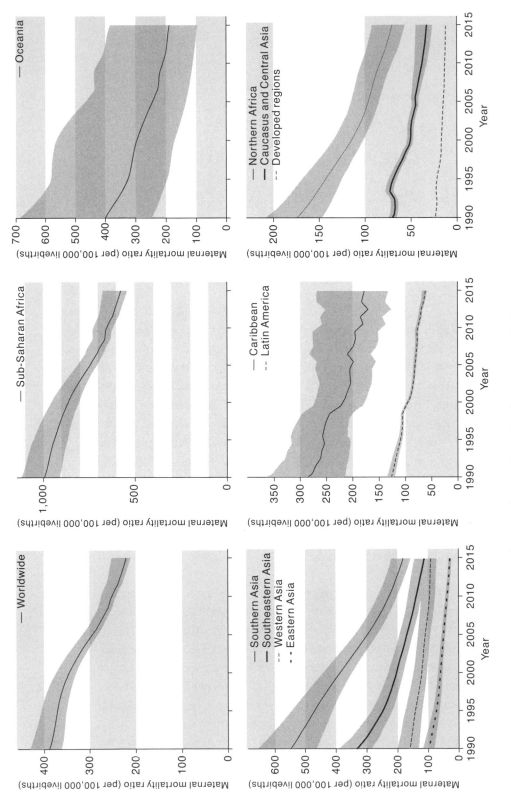

FIGURE 2.1. Global and regional estimates of maternal mortality ration from 1990 to 2015.

to reducing the 1990 rates by the goal of 5.5%. Definitions of maternal death are given in Tables 2.3 and 2.4.

APPROACHES TO MEASURING MATERNAL MORTALITY

Five main methods have been used for reporting statistics on maternal mortality: civil registration systems, household surveys, census, reproductive-age mortality studies, and verbal autopsy. Each method has its own advantages and disadvantages. Whatever the method used, maternal mortality is difficult to measure, and many countries in low-resource areas do not have reliable reporting systems.

Sub-Saharan Africa (56%) and Southeast Asia (29%) account for 85% of the global burden of maternal deaths (287,000 in 2010). Two countries account for a third of global maternal deaths: India at 19% (56,000) and Nigeria at 14% (40,000). The global maternal mortality ratio in 2015 as reported in *Lancet* was 210 maternal deaths per 100,000 live births, down from 400 maternal deaths per 100,000 live births in 1990 (Lozano et al. 2011). However, the maternal mortality ratio in developing regions was fifteen times higher than in developed regions (240 versus 16 per 100,000). Regionally, sub-Saharan Africa has the highest maternal mortality ratio at 500 per 100,000 live births, while Eastern Asia has the lowest among MDG developing regions at 37 per 100,000 live births. In contrast, the developed regions report 16 deaths per 100,000 live births (2.5%). In 2010, forty countries had high maternal mortality ratios (more than 300 maternal deaths per 100,000 live births). Although most sub-Saharan African countries have very high maternal mortality ratios (500 MMR), Mauritius, Sao Tome, Principe, and Cape Verde have low maternal mortality ratios (20–99 per 100,000 live births).

Sub-Saharan Africa has the largest proportion of maternal deaths attributed to HIV, at 10%, while the Caribbean has the second largest, at 6%. Of the 19,000 maternal deaths owing to HIV/AIDS worldwide, 17,000 (91%) are in sub-Saharan Africa, while 920 (5%) occur in Southeast Asia.

The Final Report for the Countdown to 2015 states that "the global maternal mortality ratio has fallen around 45% over the past two decades, and the number of maternal deaths has dropped from around 523,000 a year to 289,000. Although the reduction in mortality appears to have accelerated—75% of Countdown countries reduced maternal mortality

Table 2.1 Estimates of maternal mortality ratio, number of maternal deaths, and lifetime risk, by United Nations Millennium Development Goal region, 2015[a]

Region	MMR	Range of MMR uncertainty (80% UI)[b]		Number of maternal deaths[c]	Lifetime risk of maternal death in:[d]
		Lower estimate	Upper estimate		
World	216	207	249	303,000	180
Developed regions[e]	12	11	14	1,700	4,900
Developing regions	239	229	275	302,000	150
Northern Africa[f]	70	56	92	3,100	450
Sub-Saharan Africa[g]	546	511	652	201,000	36
Eastern Asia[h]	27	23	33	4,800	2,300
Eastern Asia excluding China	43	24	86	378	1,500
Southern Asia[i]	176	153	216	66,000	210
Southern Asia excluding India	180	147	249	21,000	190
Southeastern Asia[j]	110	95	142	13,000	380
Western Asia[k]	91	73	125	4,700	360
Caucasus and Central Asia[l]	33	27	45	610	1,100
Latin America and the Caribbean	67	64	77	7,300	670
Latin America[m]	60	57	66	6,600	760
Caribbean[n]	175	130	265	1,300	250
Oceania[o]	187	95	381	500	150

Source: Reprinted from World Health Organization. 2015. Trends in maternal mortality: 1990 to 2015: estimates by WHO, UNICEF, UNFPA, World Bank Group and the United Nations Population Division. Table 3.1. © World Health Organization 2015.

a. MMR (maternal mortality ratio = maternal deaths per 100,000 births) estimates have been rounded according to the following scheme: less than 100 rounded to nearest 1; 100 to 999 rounded to nearest 10; and greater than 1,000 rounded to nearest 100.

b. UI: uncertainty interval.

c. Numbers of maternal deaths have been rounded according to the following scheme: less than 100 rounded to nearest 1; 100 to 999 rounded to nearest 10; 1,000 to 9,999 rounded to nearest 100; and greater than 10,000 rounded to nearest 1,000.

d. Lifetime risk numbers have been rounded according to the following scheme: less than 100 rounded to nearest 1; 100–999 rounded to nearest 10; and greater than 1,000 rounded to nearest 100.

e. Albania, Australia, Austria, Belarus, Belgium, Bosnia and Herzegovina, Bulgaria, Canada, Croatia, Cyprus, Czech Republic, Denmark, Estonia, Finland, France, Germany, Greece, Hungary, Iceland, Ireland, Israel, Italy, Japan, Latvia, Lithuania, Luxembourg, Malta, Montenegro, Netherlands, New Zealand, Norway, Poland, Portugal, Republic of Moldova, Romania, Russian Federation, Serbia, Slovakia. Slovenia, Spain, Sweden Switzerland, The former Yugoslav Republic of Macedonia, Ukraine, United Kingdom, United States of America.

f. Algeria, Egypt, Libya, Morocco, Tunisia.

g. Angola, Benin, Botswana, Burkina Faso, Burundi, Cameroon, Cabo Verde, Central African Republic, Chad, Comoros Congo, Côte d'Ivoire, Democratic Republic of the Congo, Djibouti, Equatorial Guinea, Eritrea, Ethiopia, Gabon, Gambia, Ghana, Guinea, Guinea-Bissau, Kenya, Lesotho, Liberia, Madagascar, Malawi, Mali, Mauritania, Mauritius, Mozambique, Namibia, Niger, Nigeria, Rwanda, Sao Tome and Principe, Senegal, Sierra Leone, Somalia, South Africa, South Sudan, Sudan, Swaziland, Togo, Uganda, United Republic of Tanzania, Zambia, Zimbabwe.

h. China, Democratic People's Republic of Korea, Mongolia, Republic of Korea.

i. Afghanistan, Bangladesh, Bhutan, India, Iran (Islamic Republic of), Maldives, Nepal, Pakistan, Sri Lanka.

j. Brunei Darussalam, Cambodia, Indonesia, Lao People's Democratic Republic, Malaysia, Myanmar, Philippines, Singapore, Thailand, Timor-Leste, Viet Nam.

k. Bahrain, Iraq, Jordan, Kuwait, Lebanon, Oman, Palestine (State of), Qatar, Saudi Arabia, Syrian Arab Republic, Turkey, United Arab Emirates, Yemen.

l. Armenia, Azerbaijan, Georgia, Kazakhstan, Kyrgyzstan, Tajikistan, Turkmenistan, Uzbekistan.

m. Argentina, Belize, Bolivia (Plurinational State of), Brazil, Chile, Colombia, Costa Rica, Ecuador, El Salvador, Guatemala, Guyana, Honduras, Mexico, Nicaragua, Panama, Paraguay, Peru, Suriname, Uruguay, Venezuela (Bolivarian Republic of).

n. Bahamas, Barbados, Cuba, Dominican Republic, Grenada, Haiti, Jamaica, Puerto Rico, Saint Lucia, Saint Vincent and the Grenadines, Trinidad and Tobago.

o. Fiji, Kiribati, Micronesia (Federated States of), Papua New Guinea, Samoa, Solomon Islands, Tonga, Vanuatu.

Table 2.2 Maternal mortality ratio (MMR) and number of maternal deaths, by United Nations Millennium Development Goal Region, 1990 and 2015[a]

Region	1990		2015		% change in MMR between 1990 and 2015[d]	Average annual % change in MMR between 1990 and 2015	Average annual % change in MMR between 1990 and 2000	Average annual % change in MMR between 2000 and 2015
	MMR[b]	Maternal deaths[c]	MMR	Maternal deaths				
World	385	532,000	216	303,000	44	2.3	1.2	3.0
Developed regions[e]	23	3,500	12	1,700	48	2.6	3.3	2.2
Developing regions	430	529,000	239	302,000	44	2.4	1.3	3.1
Northern Africa[f]	171	6,400	70	3,100	59	3.6	4.1	3.2
Sub-Saharan Africa[g]	987	223,000	546	201,000	45	2.4	1.5	2.9
Eastern Asia[h]	95	26,000	27	4,800	72	5.0	4.8	5.0
Eastern Asia excluding China	51	590	43	380	16	0.7	-3.0	3.1
Southern Asia[i]	538	210,000	176	66,000	67	4.5	3.6	5.1
Southern Asia excluding India	495	57,800	180	21,000	64	4.1	2.5	5.1
Southeastern Asia[j]	320	39,000	110	13,000	66	4.3	4.7	4.0
Western Asia[k]	160	6,700	91	4,700	43	2.2	2.7	1.9
Caucasus and Central Asia[l]	69	1,300	33	610	52	3.0	3.1	2.9
Latin America and the Caribbean	135	16,000	67	7,300	50	2.8	3.1	2.6

Latin America[m]	124	14,000	60	6,000	52	2.9	3.1	2.8
Caribbean[n]	276	2,300	175	1,300	37	1.8	2.5	1.4
Oceania[o]	391	780	187	500	52	3.0	2.9	3.0

Source: Reprinted from World Health Organization. 2015. Trends in maternal mortality: 1990 to 2015: estimates by WHO, UNICEF, UNFPA, World Bank Group and the United Nations Population Division. Table 3.3. © World Health Organization 2015.

a. MMR=maternal deaths per 100,000 live births.

b. MMR estimates have been rounded according to the following scheme: less than 100 rounded to nearest 1; 100–999 rounded to nearest 10; and greater than 1,000 rounded to nearest 100.

c. Numbers of maternal deaths have been rounded according to the following scheme: less than 100 rounded to nearest 1; 100–999 rounded to nearest 10; 1,000–9,999 rounded to nearest 100; and greater than 10,000 rounded to nearest 1,000.

d. Overall change.

e. Albania, Australia, Austria, Belarus, Belgium, Bosnia and Herzegovina, Bulgaria, Canada, Croatia, Cyprus, Czech Republic, Denmark, Estonia, Finland, France, Germany, Greece, Hungary, Iceland, Ireland, Israel, Italy, Japan, Latvia, Lithuania, Luxembourg, Malta, Montenegro, Netherlands, New Zealand, Norway, Poland, Portugal, Republic of Moldova, Romania, Russian Federation, Serbia, Slovakia, Slovenia, Spain, Sweden, Switzerland, The former Yugoslav Republic of Macedonia, Ukraine, United Kingdom, United States of America.

f. Algeria, Egypt, Libya, Morocco, Tunisia.

g. Angola, Benin, Botswana, Burkina Faso, Burundi, Cameroon, Cabo Verde, Central African Republic, Chad, Comoros Congo, Côte d'Ivoire, Democratic Republic of the Congo, Djibouti, Equatorial Guinea, Eritrea, Ethiopia, Gabon, Gambia, Ghana, Guinea, Guinea-Bissau, Kenya, Lesotho, Liberia, Madagascar, Malawi, Mali, Mauritania, Mauritius, Mozambique, Namibia, Niger, Nigeria, Rwanda, Sao Tome and Principe, Senegal, Sierra Leone, Somalia, South Africa, South Sudan, Sudan, Swaziland, Togo, Uganda, United Republic of Tanzania, Zambia, Zimbabwe.

h. China, Democratic People's Republic of Korea, Mongolia, Republic of Korea.

i. Afghanistan, Bangladesh, Bhutan, India, Iran (Islamic Republic of), Maldives, Nepal, Pakistan, Sri Lanka.

j. Brunei Darussalam, Cambodia, Indonesia, Lao People's Democratic Republic, Malaysia, Myanmar, Philippines, Singapore, Thailand, Timor-Leste, Viet Nam.

k. Bahrain, Iraq, Jordan, Kuwait, Lebanon, Oman, Palestine (State of), Qatar, Saudi Arabia, Syrian Arab Republic, Turkey, United Arab Emirates, Yemen.

l. Armenia, Azerbaijan, Georgia, Kazakhstan, Kyrgyzstan, Tajikistan, Turkmenistan, Uzbekistan.

m. Argentina, Belize, Bolivia (Plurinational State of), Brazil, Chile, Colombia, Costa Rica, Ecuador, El Salvador, Guatemala, Guyana, Honduras, Mexico, Nicaragua, Panama, Paraguay, Peru, Suriname, Uruguay, Venezuela (Bolivarian Republic of).

n. Bahamas, Barbados, Cuba, Dominican Republic, Grenada, Haiti, Jamaica, Puerto Rico, Saint Lucia, Saint Vincent and the Grenadines, Trinidad and Tobago.

o. Fiji, Kiribati, Micronesia (Federated States of), Papua New Guinea, Samoa, Solomon Islands, Tonga, Vanuatu.

Table 2.3   Definitions related to maternal death in ICD-10

Maternal death
Death of a woman while pregnant or within forty-two days of termination of pregnancy, irrespective of the duration and site of the pregnancy, from any cause related to or aggravated by the pregnancy or its management but not from accidental or incidental causes

Pregnancy-related death
Death of a woman while pregnant or within forty-two days of termination of pregnancy, irrespective of the cause of death

Late maternal death
Death of a woman from direct or indirect obstetric causes, more than forty-two days but less than one year after termination of pregnancy

Data source: Hogan et al. (2010), © World Health Organization 2010. Published by Elsevier Ltd/Inc/BV.

Table 2.4   Statistical measures of maternal mortality

Maternal mortality ratio (MMR)
Number of maternal deaths during a given time period per 100,000 live births during the same time period

Maternal mortality rate (MMRate)
Number of maternal deaths in a given period per 100,000 women of reproductive age during the same time period

Adult lifetime risk of maternal death
The probability that a fifteen-year-old woman will eventually die from a maternal cause

The proportion of maternal deaths among deaths of women of reproductive age (PM)
Number of maternal deaths in a given time period divided by the total deaths among women aged fifteen to forty-nine years

Data source: Hogan et al. (2010), © World Health Organization 2010. Published by Elsevier Ltd/Inc/BV.

faster over 2000–13 than over 1990–2000—very few Countdown countries will achieve Millennium Development Goal 5." Further, their evidence shows that "only six countries achieved the 5.5% annual rate of reduction in maternal mortality needed to achieve Millennium Development Goal 5. Four countries—Cambodia, Eritrea, Nepal and Rwanda—achieved the required annual rate of reductions for both goals" (Countdown to 2015).

WHAT FACTORS ACCOUNT
FOR THE DECREASE IN MMR?

There have been four powerful drivers for maternal mortality reductions. The first is a drop in total fertility rates, from 3.7 in 1980 to 3.26 in 1990 and to 2.56 in 2008. Contraceptive prevalence among women aged fifteen to forty-nine, married or in a union, increased from 55% in 1990 to 64% in 2015.

The second improvement is increased income in low-resource countries. Many women have started small businesses and with their partners have been able to increase their level of income, obtaining better nutrition and housing. Evidence points to greater power in decision making on health issues associated with women's income generation.

The third factor is maternal education, which is strongly associated with decreased maternal mortality. The average years of schooling for women aged twenty-five to forty-four years in sub-Saharan Africa rose from 1.5 in 1980 to 4.4 in 2008. Finally, the fourth factor is the proportion of women giving birth with a skilled attendant, which has increased in Egypt, Romania, Bangladesh, India, and China.

BACKGROUND SUMMARY

Despite reductions in global maternal mortality over the past two decades, too many women still die in childbirth. For countries to reach MDG goal 5, there need to be annual 5.5% declines in maternal mortality. Few low-resource countries achieve such levels, and some countries have actually seen a small increase in maternal mortality during the past twenty years. Such countries often suffer conflicts such as civil wars or external wars (for example, Sierra Leone, Afghanistan) or with political and economic instability, such as Zimbabwe.

We describe the major causes of maternal deaths with an emphasis on developing countries, then outline the evidence-based strategies and technologies proved to reduce maternal mortality. We conclude with a discussion of the delays that contribute to women's dying of direct causes and what needs to be done to help protect mothers in low-resource settings.

WORLDWIDE CAUSES OF MATERNAL MORTALITY

The majority of maternal deaths are a result of a few major direct causes: hemorrhage, hypertensive diseases of pregnancy (preeclampsia and eclampsia), complications resulting from abortion, obstructed labor, infection (sepsis), and HIV/AIDS. Among indirect causes are infectious diseases (malaria, tuberculosis, hepatitis) and chronic conditions (such as heart disease, anemia, or asthma). Below we describe each direct cause of maternal death, some of the technological advances that may reduce these deaths, and clinical tips for health-care providers. We also touch on the social, economic, political, and gender inequities that contribute to maternal mortality in low-resource settings.

Postpartum Hemorrhage

Obstetric hemorrhage, including postpartum hemorrhage (PPH), is the leading cause of maternal mortality worldwide. Rates vary by region, but 24 to 45% of direct maternal deaths result from hemorrhage, the majority of which occur postpartum (Khan et al. 2006). Postpartum hemorrhage, defined as blood loss exceeding 500 mL in the first twenty-four hours after delivery, occurs in 6 to 18% of births; severe hemorrhage, defined as blood loss exceeding 1,000 mL, occurs in less than 2% of births (Carroli et al. 2008; Devine and Wright 2009).

Women in low-resource settings are at elevated risk of death from PPH (Carroli et al. 2008). This is can result not only from the lack of infrastructure, equipment, and human resources but also because of social, gender, and economic inequities that lead to delays in recognizing hemorrhage, in obtaining transport and care during transport, and in receiving quality emergency obstetrical care (Ransom and Yinger 2002). Therefore, a continuum-of-care approach is critical for saving lives, whether hemorrhage occurs at home or in a facility (Kapungu et al. 2012).

Causes of PPH are traditionally referred to as the 4-Ts: *tone,* for atony, that is, failure of the uterus to contract, is responsible for approximately 70% of PPH; *trauma,* for injury to the uterus, cervix, or vagina (20% of cases); *tissue,* for retained placenta, membranes, or clots (10%); and *thrombin,* for coagulopathies (1%) (Oyelese and Ananth 2010; Anderson and Etches 2007; Bauer and Bonanno 2009; Benedetto et al. 2010). Any uncontrolled PPH can lead to hypovolemic shock, which requires blood transfusions; intractable PPH may require conservative surgery or emergency hysterectomy.

Although risk factors for PPH have been identified, such as multiple gestation, induction or augmentation of labor, macrosomia, prolonged labor, and retained placenta, most PPH is unexpected (Sosa et al. 2009).

The incidence of uterine atony can be decreased by implementing the active management of the third stage of labor (AMTSL) (Lalonde 2012), which recommends a uterotonic within five minutes of delivery, which can decrease the risk of blood loss of more than 500 milliliters by 24 to 60% (World Health Organization 2012; Richard J. Derman et al. 2006; N. Mobeen et al. 2010). This step promotes uterine contractions and a shorter third stage. The uterotonics approved for prevention of PPH are oxytocin (intramuscularly), ergometrine (intramuscularly), and oral misoprostol, when oxytocin is not available or cannot be safely used (World Health Organization 2007). Other steps of AMTSL—delivering the placenta by controlled cord traction (only by a skilled attendant) and uterine massage after delivery of the placenta—have lower levels of evidence for independent contribution to reduction of risk (World Health Organization 2007). Cord traction by an unskilled provider and without uterotonics may actually increase PPH (Lalonde 2012).

Even with AMTSL, women may still die from intractable uterine atony. The other etiologies of PPH (retained tissue, lacerations, uterine rupture, and so on) do not respond to uterotonics. Therefore, learning to recognize excessive bleeding, diagnose the etiology, and manage PPH is as important as learning to prevent it. For out-of-hospital deliveries or community-based deliveries, early recognition and complication readiness (having a plan, obtaining transportation, having funds for transport to, and care in the facility) are essential (Kapungu et al. 2012).

Accurate recognition of excessive bleeding is largely dependent on visual estimation (Duthie et al. 1991). Attendants can learn to recognize amounts of blood absorbed by common supplies (such as gauze or perineal pads) (Bose, Regan, and Paterson-Brown 2006). Commonly used items, like the wrapper that women wear in Tanzania called a kanga, may become saturated with blood, and attendants can be trained to recognize that if a certain number of kangas are saturated, that equals PPH (Prata et al. 2005). This concept is being operationalized globally by the use of a blood mat. Developed in Bangladesh, this low-cost, low-technology, absorbent mat holds a maximum of 500 milliliters blood and has been used by traditional birth attendants to recognize when to transport a woman from home to a facility (Prata et al. 2012). See Chapter 12 for more information on assessing approaches to blood loss.

Once PPH is recognized, action must be taken. Even at a home birth, some obstetric first aid can be administered; however, the first line of management for PPH resulting from uterine atony is medical. Uterine massage will help determine whether the bleeding is from atony or another source. If the uterus is not contracted and does not stay contracted with massage, a uterotonic such as oxytocin, misoprostol, or methergine should be the next step. If bleeding continues, and the birth is at a facility, intravenous fluids should be started and more uterotonics can be given intravenously, as well as rapid infusion of fluids to prevent hypovolemia.

Other treatments to resolve uterine atony include bimanual uterine compression, insertion of a hydrostatic intrauterine balloon (IUB), manual aortic pressure, and circumferential counter-pressure with a nonpneumatic antishock garment (NASG). The cost of balloon tamponade may be prohibitive in lower-resource areas (Bakri, Amri, and Jabbar 2001). Therefore, improvised IUBs such as sterile exam gloves or even condoms attached to a urinary catheter have been used successfully (Akhter, Begum, and Kabir 2005). Once inflated with saline and inserted using aseptic techniques, the balloon presses against the walls of the uterus to stop bleeding (Georgiou 2009). The IUB is also diagnostic: if inflation does not stop bleeding, another source may be indicated.

Two methods to stop pelvic, uterine, or vaginal bleeding regardless of etiology are manual aortic compression and the NASG. Exerting downward pressure on the aorta decreases blood flow to the lower body. While it can be easily learned and does not require any specialized equipment, it is not easy to maintain over a long time period or during difficult transports. The NASG, a low-cost, easy-to-use, first-aid compression device, is particularly applicable to low-resource settings, where there are long delays in transport or before definitive care in referral facilities. A simple neoprene and Velcro "suit," wrapped tightly around a woman's abdomen, pelvis, and lower extremities, was shown to reduce blood loss and increase survival rates by more than 50% (Miller et al. 2012; Stenson, Miller, and Lester 2012).

Continued bleeding may require surgery. If uterine-sparing surgical procedures such as compression sutures (B-Lynch) and stepwise ligation of the uterine blood supply do not succeed, or the surgeon is not adept at them, a hysterectomy may be the only way to stop the bleeding and save the woman's life.

Clinical education and skills training need to be conducted regularly for all health care workers—from community and lay workers through the surgical team—who may encounter a woman with hemorrhage. Listed below are some clinical practices that should prove useful to women's health workers at all levels.

Clinical Tips

1. Attention must be paid to the patient's vital signs, level of consciousness and skin color as well as the estimated blood loss to recognize shock in its earliest phases.
2. All staff should be able to perform uterine massage to expel clots and to help keep the uterus firm.
3. A uterotonic agent should be used immediately after birth to prevent PPH.
4. All staff should learn and regularly practice both manual aortic compression and how to apply the NASG for intractable PPH.
5. Crystalloid fluids are the first choice for intravenous fluid replacement for women in shock secondary to PPH.
6. Professional staff should learn how to insert balloon tamponade.
7. Uterine-sparing techniques for surgical management must be learned by all.

Conclusion: Postpartum Hemorrhage

The use of prophylactic uterotonics and oral uterotonics and better management are all helping to decrease the global incidence of PPH. New technologies and strategies such as balloon tamponade, NASG, and compression sutures are helping to decrease mortality and severe morbidity from PPH. The last decade has seen remarkable changes in the prevention, early recognition, and management of PPH, all of which should improve maternal health outcomes. Figure 2.2 illustrates current recommendations in the prevention and treatment of PPH.

Hypertensive Disorders in Pregnancy: The Impact of Preeclampsia and Eclampsia

Preeclampsia-eclampsia is one of the three leading causes of maternal morbidity and mortality worldwide (Duley 2009). Hypertensive disorders of pregnancy account for 14 to 20% of maternal mortality in developing countries (Magee 2008). During the past fifty years there has been a significant reduction in the rates of eclampsia, maternal mortality, and morbidity in developed countries. In contrast, mortality associated with eclampsia and

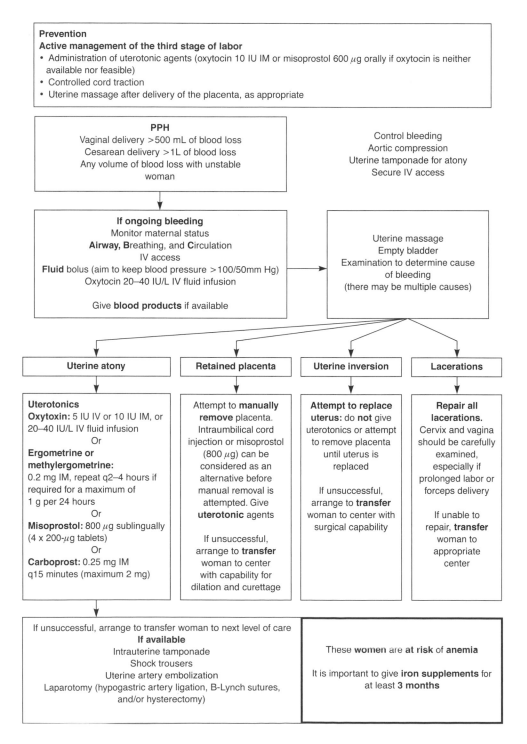

FIGURE 2.2. FIGO recommendations for prevention and treatment of PPH.

hypertensive disorders of pregnancy remains high in developing countries. Most maternal deaths and complications in developing countries are the result of a lack of prenatal care, lack of access to emergency obstetric care facilities, lack of resources, and inappropriate diagnosis and management of preeclampsia and eclampsia (Ghulmiyyah and Sibai 2012).

Preeclampsia

Preeclampsia is a condition characterized by high blood pressure and proteinuria in a pregnant woman. If left untreated, it can progress rapidly to eclampsia, a life-threatening disease characterized by seizures. Though preeclampsia may develop at any time after twenty weeks of gestation, it is considered early onset before thirty-two weeks and is associated with increased morbidity. Symptoms may develop during later pregnancy, in labor, or up to six weeks postdelivery. Preeclampsia-eclampsia is doubly deadly, as it affects both the mother and the fetus. Maternal problems include liver, kidney, brain, and circulatory system (clotting) disorders; risks for the baby include poor growth and prematurity. In severe eclampsia both mother and baby may die.

CRITERIA AND SYMPTOMS

Preeclampsia is diagnosed by blood pressure greater than 140 systolic and/or greater than 90 diastolic (two separate readings taken at least six hours apart) as well as greater than or equal to 0.3 grams protein in a twenty-four-hour urine sample (proteinuria). In low-resource countries, dipstick urine measurement is used rather than a twenty-four-hour urine sample (Ghulmiyyah and Sibai 2012). A rise in baseline blood pressure of 30 mmHg systolic or 15 mmHg diastolic is still considered important to note but is not considered diagnostic. Severe preeclampsia involves blood pressure over 160/110, proteinuria of more than five grams per twenty-four hours, and signs of end-organ dysfunction with symptoms such as headache, difficulty breathing, renal dysfunction, oliguria, and increased levels of creatinine.

RISK FACTORS

Risk factors for preeclampsia include nulliparity, diabetes mellitus, renal disease, chronic hypertension, a prior history of preeclampsia, extreme age (younger than fifteen or older than thirty-five years of age), obesity, antiphospholipid antibody syndrome, and multiple gestation (Ghulmiyyah and Sibai 2012).

PATHOGENESIS

Though its exact pathogenesis remains uncertain, many different causes have been suggested for preeclampsia. It appears likely that substances from the placenta can cause endothelial dysfunction in the maternal blood vessels.

DIFFERENTIAL DIAGNOSIS

Preeclampsia can be confused with many other diseases, including chronic renal disease, chronic hypertension, primary fever disorders, gallbladder and pancreatic disease, immune thrombotic purpura, antiphospholipid syndrome, and hemolytic-uremic syndrome. Preeclampsia should always be considered a possibility in any pregnant woman beyond twenty weeks of gestation with elevated blood pressure, edema (especially of the face), and proteinuria.

COMPLICATIONS

Preeclampsia and eclampsia affect both mother and baby. For the baby, risks are increased of having a preterm birth or a baby who is too small at birth, has acidosis, or is dying. Maternal complications include kidney or liver damage, blood clotting problems, and pulmonary edema. The most serious complication for the mother is eclampsia, that is, elevated blood pressure to the brain resulting in seizures, culminating in stroke, disability, or death.

PREVENTION

Antiplatelet agents, low-dose aspirin, and calcium supplementation have shown evidence of prevention in high-risk pregnancy. The Pre-eclampsia Integrated Estimate of RiSk model (PIERS) has strong predictive value in the management of women at risk in higher-resource areas, while the Mini-PIERS is being developed for lower-resourced settings (von Dadelszen et al. 2011).

TREATMENT

The only definite treatment is delivery, either by labor induction or cesarean section (Sibai 2002). Patients with severe hypertension, severe preeclampsia, or eclampsia must be carefully monitored and rapidly transferred to a referral hospital. To prevent and control seizures, magnesium sulfate is the drug of choice in higher-resource areas. Labetalol, hydralazine, and nifedipine are often the antihypertensives of choice; labetalol in particular is less likely to cross the placenta and affect the fetus. While using magnesium sulfate to control or prevent convulsions, fetal assessment must be undertaken, and corticosteroids may be administered to promote fetal lung maturity when labor before thirty-seven weeks' gestation is considered. It is important to note that though it is recommended by the International Federation of Gynecology and Obstetrics (FIGO) and the World Health Organization, magnesium sulfate is suboptimal in many developing countries for the following reasons (Langer et al. 2008):

1. Most low-resource countries do not have guidelines mandating its use, and many do not include it on a national essential drug list.
2. Even with national guidelines, health professionals may not know how to use it correctly.
3. Many clinicians working at level-1 and level-2 hospitals are not trained in its use and believe that magnesium sulfate should be used only at level-3 referral hospitals.
4. Because this low-cost drug is not promoted by the pharmaceutical industry, it is unavailable in many countries.

Research

Pioneering research is being conducted on hypertensive diseases in pregnancy. Notable is the PRE-Eclampsia and Eclampsia Monitoring, Prevention and Treatment Program (PRE-EMPT), a large research program of global partners created to develop new knowledge related to preeclampsia. Information is available on the web site, https://pre-empt.cfri.ca.

Clinical Tips

1. Monitor the blood pressure of women during antenatal care, labor, and delivery, and postpartum.
2. Keep urine dipsticks to test for proteinuria.
3. When preeclampsia becomes severe (blood pressure 160/110), immediately administer magnesium sulfate and transfer to the appropriate level of care.
4. Keep magnesium sulfate and labetalol on hand.
5. All health-care professionals should receive training in the diagnosis and management of preeclampsia and eclampsia.

Conclusion: Preeclampsia and Eclampsia

Although etiologies remain unknown, mortality is preventable by early rec-ognition, monitoring of blood pressure and other symptoms, the wide-spread use of magnesium sulfate ($MgSO_4$) and labetalol, and access to rapid delivery. Early diagnosis and aggressive management can reduce mor-tality and morbidity for mothers and infants.

Unsafe Abortions

Unsafe abortions are those performed by unskilled providers under un-hygienic conditions, those that are self-induced by a woman inserting a foreign object into her uterus or consuming toxic products, and those instigated by physical trauma. A woman may die from an unsafe abor-tion usually secondary to severe bleeding, infection, or organ damage. Unsafe abortion is one of the major causes of maternal mortality and morbidity in low-resource countries. It accounts for 8 to 14% of maternal mortality, but those rates could be 20% or higher in countries where abor-tion is illegal, as it is difficult to obtain accurate statistics (WHO et al. 2012a; Barot 2011).

The Guttmacher Institute (2012) and the World Health Organization (WHO 2011b; Singh and Darroch 2012) report that deaths from unsafe abortion worldwide dropped from 69,000 to 47,000 by 2008, paralleling the worldwide reduction in maternal mortality. However, the proportion of women dying from unsafe abortions has remained stagnant at approx-imately 13% of maternal deaths. The number of unsafe abortions world-wide increased from 19.7 million in 2003 to 21.6 million in 2008, following a growth in the overall population of women of childbearing age.

Prevention of Abortion-Related Mortality

Family planning empowers women to plan their childbearing for when they are healthiest and most able to care for children, forgo contraception altogether for those who wish it, and select the safest and most effective method for their personal circumstances. It is estimated that 215 million women—mostly in developing countries—cannot access modern voluntary family planning.

Dramatic improvement in contraceptive quality and access in Eastern Europe reduced abortion rates 25 to 50%. Similar effects have been seen in Bangladesh and in certain African countries such as Rwanda (Basinga et al. 2012). Satisfying unmet needs for contraception could reduce maternal mortality by 29%, preventing more than 100,000 maternal deaths each year (WHO et al. 2012a) and making effective modern contraception (including the availability of contraceptive implants) not only a family planning and health issue but a maternal mortality and morbidity issue.

Access to contraception and safer abortion services has a huge impact on unsafe abortion rates. Four out of five unintended pregnancies are the result of unmet need for contraceptives (Singh and Darroch 2012). In 2012, 645 million women in the developing world were using modern methods of contraception, 42 million more than in 2008. See Chapter 8 for detailed information on contraception. Worldwide, these levels of contraceptive currently prevent:

- 218 million unintended pregnancies
- 55 million unplanned births
- 138 million abortions (40 million of which are unsafe)
- 25 million miscarriages
- 118,000 maternal deaths

If all needs for contraception were met, a further 26 million abortions and 79,000 maternal deaths would be prevented (WHO 2011b; Singh and Darroch 2012).

Restrictive Abortion Laws

Most countries today have some legislation on provision of abortion services, although the majority of countries have some restrictions, except in western and eastern Europe and North America, including Mexico. Abortion, even to save a woman's life, is currently illegal in Chile, El Salvador, Nicaragua, the Dominican Republic, and Malta. Although abortion is illegal in many countries, it is well known that abortion can be obtained in private practice.

Studies have shown that abortion rates in countries that have highly restrictive abortion laws are as high in those where abortion is legal. However, illegal and unsafe abortions confer greater risk of maternal morbidities and mortality. As with other causes, maternal mortality from illegal abortion is more likely among poor women.

In 2008, nearly half of all abortions worldwide were unsafe, and nearly all unsafe abortions occur in developing countries. For example, 50% of all abortions are unsafe in developing countries, compared with 6% in developed countries. As noted above, highly restrictive abortions laws are

Table 2.5   Global and regional estimates of induced abortion, 1995, 2003, and 2008

Region	Number of abortions (millions)			Abortion rate (%)[a]		
	1995	2003	2008	1995	2003	2008
World	45.6	41.6	43.8	35	29	28
Developed countries	10.0	6.6	6.0	39	25	24
Excluding Eastern Europe	3.8	3.5	3.2	20	19	17
Developing countries	35.5	35.0	37.8	34	29	29
Excluding China	24.9	26.4	28.6	33	30	29
Africa	5.0	5.6	6.4	33	29	29
Asia	26.8	25.9	27.3	33	29	28
Europe	7.7	4.3	4.2	48	28	27
Latin America	4.2	4.1	4.4	37	31	32
North America	1.5	1.5	1.4	22	21	19
Oceania	0.1	0.1	0.1	21	18	17

Source: Reprinted from Guttmacher Institute (2012).
a. Abortions per 1,000 women aged fifteen to forty-four.

not associated with lower abortion rates. For example, the abortion rate is high among women of childbearing age in Africa and Latin America (29 and 32 abortions per 1,000 women, respectively), regions where abortion is illegal under most circumstances. In western Europe, where abortion is generally permitted on broad grounds, the abortion rate is 12 per 1,000 (see Table 2.5).

Medical and Surgical Abortions

Three types of abortifacient drugs are used in early pregnancy: mifepristone (an antiprogestational steroid) taken with misoprostol (a prostaglandin analog), or methotrexate (an antimetabolite or cancer drug) taken with misoprostol, or misoprostol alone. Surgical procedures to provoke abortion include suction-aspiration (also called vacuum aspiration). This can be performed with a manual tool, known as manual vacuum aspiration, or electrically with electric vacuum aspiration. Dilatation and curettage involves scraping the uterine wall with a sharp curette.

Many initiatives have been proposed and implemented in regards to reducing unsafe abortion. The Guttmacher Institute (http://www.gutt macher.org/sections/abortion.php), International Pregnancy Advisory Service (http://www.ipas.org/en/What-We-Do/Comprehensive-Abortion -Care.aspx), and other agencies offer many resources for abortion and postabortion care. Media kits, fact sheets, state policies, policy articles, research articles, reports, and videos are freely available at these websites. United States Agency for International Development produced and implemented a postabortion care program in many counties under its Post-Abortion Care-Family Planning (PAC-FP) Program with Engender Health (https:// www.usaid.gov/what-we-do/global-health/maternal-and-child-health/post -abortion-care-%E2%80%93-family-planning). It addressed emergency treatment for complications of spontaneous and induced abortion, postabortion family planning and counseling, and the crucial links between emergency care and other reproductive health services such as management of sexually transmitted diseases.

Clinical Tips

1. All health-care professionals including midwives and trained birth attendants should receive education on the safe use of misoprostol alone or with mifepristone. Provide access to oral misoprostol and mifepristone. Use misoprostol for termination of pregnancy up to ten weeks when misoprostol oral can be used alone or with mifepristone. Provide access to oral misoprostol and mifepristone. Use misoprostol with mifepristone up to thirteen to fourteen weeks.

2. All health-care professionals, including general physicians, midwives, and nurses should be trained in postabortion care, which is legal in all countries, as promoted by the NGO Ipas. Training in and guidelines for postabortion care are also important for the treatment of incomplete abortions, which may lead to septic abortion. More widespread use of misoprostol for early arrested pregnancy or incomplete abortion would significantly reduce maternal morbidity and mortality.

3. Providers should be active in supporting advocacy programs for donor countries and in-country professionals to promote safe abortion in all countries.

Conclusion: Unsafe Abortion

Unsafe abortion is a major cause of maternal morbidity and mortality. Increased family planning can decrease maternal mortality associated with unsafe abortion. However, because unplanned pregnancies do occur even with consistent contraception, all women should have access to safe abortion services and postabortion care. Medical abortion gives more women access to safe abortion services. Postabortion family planning is also crucial.

Obstructed Labor

Obstructed labor is defined as a failure to progress through labor owing to a disproportion between the fetal head or presenting part and the maternal pelvis (also called cephalopelvic disproportion, CPD). Obstructed labor is responsible for 8% of maternal mortality and may be the leading cause of short-term morbidity (infection) and long-term, severe maternal morbidity (fistula).

Types of Obstructed Labor

Obstructed labor has two main patterns. In primiparous women the main etiology is CPD, mainly owing to inadequate pelvic size, with an arrest of labor, often after several days. This can result in a dead fetus and chorioamnionitis from prolonged ruptured membranes. For the mother, the outcome could be a fistula or even death from sepsis. For multiparous women, the main cause is malpresentation, particularly transverse presentation, in which the uterus continues contracting and the woman may die from a ruptured uterus. Deaths from obstructed labor may be underestimated, because the proximal cause of death is either sepsis or hemorrhage from a ruptured uterus (Hofmeyr 2004).

Prevention

Because obstructed labor can occur because of a lack of skilled attendance, lack of knowledge of normal labor, and lack of access to cesarean delivery, it can also be prevented by improving the continuum of care during the pregnancy as follows (Hofmeyr 2004; Neilson et al. 2003):

1. Antepartum: Look for risk factors and arrange for facility delivery. Risk factors include
   a. young age (girls' pelvises do not mature until at least two years after menarche)
   b. primigravid status
   c. small stature compared with others in the community (owing to poor nutrition or disease)
   d. rickets, osteomalacia, or pelvic deformities (congenital or owing to accidents)

  e. grand multiparity

  f. malpresentation, especially shoulder presentation or other transverse lie

2. Late pregnancy: Procedures include

  a. moving women at risk who live far from Comprehensive Emergency Obstetric Care (CEmOC) facilities or any care to maternity homes during the last trimester

  b. monitoring for external cephalic version of transverse or oblique lie at term or in early labor

3. Labor and delivery: Procedures and responses include

  a. partogram/partograph or systematic monitoring length of labor, cervical dilation, and descent of fetal presenting part

  b. assisted vaginal delivery (vacuum extractor or forceps)

  c. access to cesarean delivery with antibiotic coverage

  d. transport accessibility and funding for hospitalization

  e. symphysiotomy where there is no access to cesarean

However, it must be kept in mind that evidence for most of these recommendations is both sparse and inconsistent. A systematic review found vacuum extractor to be associated with less maternal trauma and fewer cesarean sections than forceps (Hofmeyr 2004). Cochrane reviews of the partogram/partograph (in any of its many forms) have failed to show any decrease in mortality (Lavender, Hart, and Smyth 2008). The Odon device, a plastic bag that is inflated and fixes around the baby's head, and is one of the Saving Lives at Birth Grand Challenges winners, is a new technology currently being tested, which may decrease the risk of instrumental delivery (Odon device n.d.). Similarly, maternity homes, facilities established where women who are at risk or women who live far from CEmOC facilities to spend the last weeks of their pregnancy to improve access, have been the subject of reviews, with no definitive finding for improving maternal outcomes (van Lonkhuijzen, Stekelburg, and Roosmalen 2012).

  Symphysiotomy, the surgical separation of the symphysis pubis to increase pelvic diameter, has long been conducted in low-resource settings. There are no experimental data on efficacy or harmful effects, though expert opinion is to perform based on lack of access to surgical or assisted vaginal delivery on a case-by-case basis (van Lonkhuijzen, Stekelburg, and Roosmalen 2012, 46). However, the contribution of cesarean delivery in saving the lives of both mothers and babies suffering obstructed labor seems quite reliable, and lack of access to cesarean delivery is associated with elevated rates of mortality from obstructed labor (Hofmeyr 2004).

Severe Morbidity from Fistula

Obstructed labor, particularly fistula, also causes maternal morbidity. An estimated 2 million to 3.5 million women suffer from obstetric fistula worldwide, with 50,000 to 100,000 new cases each year, primarily in sub-Saharan Africa and South Asia (WHO 2006a). For further information, please refer to Chapter 4 on fistula.

Clinical Tips

1. Continuous training in labor management, not just preservice but also drills on how to manage normal labor and what constitutes early signs of prolonged or obstructed labor
2. Morbidity and mortality reviews (see below) so that all providers can learn from adverse maternal outcomes, including monthly review of partograms/partographs
3. Training in instrumental delivery, whether forceps or lower-risk vacuum methods
4. Potential for using new Odon device to eliminate risk of instrumental delivery

Conclusion: Obstructed Labor

Maternal mortality and morbidity owing to obstructed labor can be prevented through improving nutrition, education, and access to family planning; reduction in the number of child brides or delay of first birth after marriage; education of all community members about the risks to fetal and maternal health; and wider access to skilled antenatal and childbirth attendance and cesarean deliveries and the empowerment of women.

Sepsis

Puerperal sepsis (infection) accounts for approximately 15% of maternal deaths annually (WHO et al. 2012b; Hussein et al. 2011). Experts estimate that infection rates can be reduced by 32% using optimal infection control measures, which suggests that the lives of 17,000 women could be saved each year. Millions of women suffering from maternal sepsis and its long-term consequences would also benefit.

Good access to care and the safety and quality of care are crucial when considering infections resulting from childbirth. Improving and maintaining infection control requires an efficiently functioning health-care system. Life-threatening infections can be introduced into the mother and baby's organs and bloodstream and lead to maternal, fetal, and neonatal death. The World Health Organization ranks maternal sepsis as the sixth leading cause of disease burden for women aged fifteen to forty-four years. Over 5.2 million new cases of maternal sepsis occur annually, leading to an estimated 62,000 maternal deaths (Hussein et al. 2011).

Epidemiology

The World Health Organization defines puerperal sepsis as infection of the genital tract at any time between the onset of rupture of membranes or labor and the forty-second day postpartum in which fever and one or more of the following are present: pelvic pain, abnormal vaginal discharge, abnormal smell, foul odor, foul discharge, and delay in the rate of reduction of the size of the uterus. Though infections can be contracted during childbirth in any setting, campaigns to have more women deliver in health facilities will require close monitoring. Evidence on effective infection-control measures during labor and delivery in low-resource settings is limited (Hussein et al. 2011).

Regional Variations in Incidence

In industrialized countries, puerperal sepsis is rare, causing 2.1% of maternal deaths. In Latin America and the Caribbean, its contribution to maternal mortality is 7.7%, coming in just after hypertensive disorders and abortion. In Africa and Asia, infections are the second most common cause of maternal mortality after hemorrhage, causing 9.7% and 11.6% of deaths, respectively (Khan et al. 2006).

Pathogenesis

Infection in obstetrical patients can be classified into pregnancy-related infections (chorioamnionitis, endometritis, mastitis), non-pregnancy-related infections (urinary tract infections, malaria, hepatitis), and infections incidental to pregnancy (HIV, appendicitis, nosocomial infections, urinary tract infections) (van Dillen et al. 2010). The most important causes of septic shock in pregnancy are pyelonephritis, chorioamnionitis, and endometritis. The most common cause of puerperal sepsis is beta-hemolytic streptococci group A followed by *E. coli*, beta-hemolytic strep, group B, G and *Streptococcus aureus* as well as *Staphylococcus aureus,* Citrobacter, and Fusobacterium. Beta-hemolytic streptococci group A produces pyrogenic exotoxin and increases the activity of the immune system, precipitating a cascade of events that is the major cause of the high virulence and mortality rate in pregnant women.

Risk Factors

Risk factors for the development of maternal sepsis include unhygienic conditions, low socioeconomic status, poor nutrition, primiparity, anemia, prolonged rupture of membranes, prolonged labor, multiple vaginal examinations in labor (more than five), cesarean section, multiple pregnancies, artificial reproductive techniques, maternal obesity, and obstetrical maneuvers. The single most important risk factor for postpartum infection is cesarean section, with an average for a nonelective case of 28.6% of infections compared with 9.2% for elective cesarean sections (Acosta and Knight 2013).

Puerperal Sepsis Prevention

The three main prevention strategies are hand hygiene, intravaginal application of antiseptic, and prophylactic antibiotics (WHO 2008). Recent concurrent systematic review identified eighty-six randomized controlled trials comparing antibiotic prophylaxis with no treatment for both elective and nonelective cesarean sections. Prophylactic antibiotics in women undergoing cesarean sections, both elective and emergency, substantially reduce the risk of febrile morbidity. Another concurrent systemic review studied prophylactic antibiotics in prelabor rupture of membranes at or near term and found that antibiotics reduced the rates of maternal infection and morbidity.

The World Health Organization has spearheaded the powerful Your Five Moments for Hand Hygiene campaign (WHO 2006b) (Table 2.6). In most low-income countries the root cause of puerperal sepsis is health-system failure, for example, noncompliance with long-established infection prevention control and management procedures, rather than the lack of appropriate technologies.

Infection Prevention at Home Deliveries

Prevention of infection at home births in the community is important for obstetrical care. The campaign to have trained birth attendants present at all deliveries could decrease maternal infections with the use of clean

Table 2.6 Your five moments for hand hygiene

1. Before touching a patient	WHEN? Clean your hands before touching a patient when approaching him or her. WHY? To protect the patient against harmful germs carried on your hands.
2. Before clean or aseptic procedure	WHEN? Clean your hands immediately before performing a clean or aseptic procedure. WHY? To protect the patient against harmful germs, including the patient's own, from entering his or her body.
3. After body fluid exposure risk	WHEN? Clean your hands immediately after an exposure risk to body fluids (and after glove removal). WHY? To protect yourself and the health-care environment from harmful patient germs.
4. After touching a patient	WHEN? Clean your hands after touching a patient and his or her immediate surroundings, when leaving the patient's side. WHY? To protect yourself and the health-care environment from harmful patient germs.
5. After touching patient surroundings	WHEN? Clean your hands after touching any object or furniture in the patient's immediate surroundings, when leaving, even if the patient has not been touched. WHY? To protect yourself and the health-care environment from harmful patient germs.

Source: Reprinted from WHO (2009). © World Health Organization 2009.

practices and both sterile gloves and instruments. Distribution of clean birthing kits to mothers during antenatal care or by community outreach workers, along with attention to hand hygiene at home, could help reduce the incidence of infection at home births.

Clinical Tips

Practices to protect against puerperal sepsis include

1. Aggressive treatment of prolonged rupture of membranes
2. Staff procedures for hand hygiene
3. Limit vaginal exams
4. Multidisciplinary infectious disease committee at each hospital that monitors and reports monthly on infection rate
5. Antibiotic prophylaxis for cesarean section

Conclusion: Sepsis

Despite limited evidence regarding effective measures to control infection during labor and delivery, continuing education, surveillance, organizational change, and quality improvement interventions need to be established in maternity units. We also need to improve our understanding of organizational and behavioral change to effectively implement infection-control measures. Clean birthing kits and hand hygiene need to be implemented for home deliveries. Finally, globalized targeted health policies or initiatives have the potential to bring attention to puerperal sepsis, an important but neglected cause of maternal mortality.

HIV/AIDS IN PREGNANCY

In countries with high HIV prevalence, the most common causes of maternal death among HIV-positive women are non-pregnancy-related infections, including AIDS, pneumonia, tuberculosis, and meningitis. HIV/AIDS has also an effect on anemia and sepsis (Moran and Moodley 2012). For more information, please see Chapter 6 on HIV.

REDUCING MATERNAL MORTALITY

Addressing Major Direct Causes of Maternal Mortality

In this chapter we have touched on certain technologies and strategies to reduce maternal mortality in low-resource settings. Figure 2.3 shows not only the major direct causes of maternal mortality but also some of the evidence-based strategies to address them.

Implementing and maintaining these practices (and improving them as new evidence comes along) requires an enabling environment, including functioning health systems, health infrastructure, clinician training and supervision, accountability of health systems and individual clinicians, attention to quality of care, and donor aid for countries with very few resources:

1. Improvement in the health system. Little can be accomplished without investment in physical structures, personnel, equipment, and medical supplies.

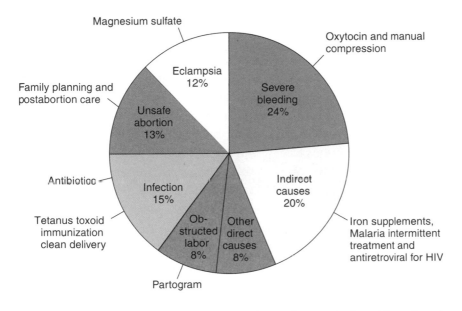

FIGURE 2.3. Major causes of maternal mortality and strategies for evidence-based treatment and management.

2. Health-care provider-training, monitoring, and supervision at all levels. Maternal mortality cannot be reduced without continuous training and evaluation of diagnostic and therapeutic skills of health-care personnel, from village community workers through nurses, midwives, doctors, and specialists. Training is not a one-time occurrence but needs to be repeated at regular intervals. Practical and interactive sessions need to be incorporated into all training, and multidisciplinary training is essential.

3. Quality-of-care initiatives. Overall quality-of-care initiatives are central to improving maternal health and decreasing maternal mortality. Currently the International Federal of Gynecology and Obstetrics (FIGO), in partnership with the World Health Organization (WHO), the International Confederation of Midwives (ICM), and the White Ribbon Alliance, is developing a certification program, the Mother-Friendly Facility Initiative, to promote respectful and dignified care during labor in line with best clinical practices.

4. Maternal death surveillance response. Understanding the major causes of maternal mortality and the underlying factors leading

to death are critical to preventing mortality. FIGO and WHO have proposed the use of a protocol called the maternal death surveillance response (MDSR), a form of continuous surveillance that links health information and quality improvement processes at local, regional, and national levels. The protocol includes routine identification, notification, calculation, and determination of causes of maternal mortality. It allows for discussion of avoidable actions to reduce maternal mortality and improve the responses of the entire birthing system. All maternal deaths in health facilities should be identified, reported on, and reviewed. Based on what was learned in the MDSR process, a plan is implemented to prevent future maternal death. It is important that a no-blame philosophy be at the core of this process, as the goal is to learn what was done or not done at each step of a woman's progress through a complication that led to morbidity or mortality. The major professional associations should take leadership vis-à-vis their member national societies to implement this process globally. United Nations agencies could partner with the national professional organizations to facilitate the implementation of MDSR.

5. International donor aid. In 2010 the United Nations secretary-general Ban Ki-moon launched a campaign called Every Woman, Every Child to mobilize the world toward addressing and working to reach Millennium Goals 4 and 5. The most active donor countries were the United States, the United Kingdom, Canada, Australia, Sweden, Norway, Holland, and France, with the involvement of many international organizations such as FIGO, ICM, and the International Pediatric Association (IPA) as well as major contributions from the Bill and Melinda Gates Foundation.

Multisectorial Efforts

Substantially decreasing maternal mortality requires more than individual technologies; it calls for the political will to make changes in gender inequities as well as a health-care system that is responsive to the twenty-four-hour medical needs of women in labor and delivery and the ability to transport a woman to a site where she can access that system, with possible surgical intervention when needed.

Multisectorial efforts must be undertaken to address the three delays that affect most women in developing countries, especially in very low resource areas. The first delay is the delay in seeking care, which is a socioeconomic, cultural, and gender problem. Many women do not have the power and authority to seek care without the decision of their husband, mother-in-law, or relative. Furthermore, owing to lack of education, neither the laboring woman nor her family or community may realize when labor is not progressing normally, when postpartum bleeding becomes excessive, or when, how, and why to seek care. These factors alone and in combination result in delays that may exacerbate complications, raising the risk of their becoming fatal.

The second delay is in transport. Some low-resource countries have no or very poor ambulance services. Women must reach the first level of care on their own, often with no motorized transport. In some places, villagers must use local trucks or other means of transport. Many women who believe the first level of care is inadequate must travel many hours to reach a higher level of care.

The third delay is the delay in provision of high-quality, appropriate emergency obstetric care at the referral facility. Staff must be trained to make women feel welcome when they reach the center, provide evidence-based care, and strive to eliminate financial barriers.

The Continuum of Care

The most integrated approach to maternal mortality reduction is sometimes called the continuum of care (WHO 2011a), which starts at the community level and extends through the highest-level referral facility. It incorporates multiple strategies to address the full spectrum of clinical, social, and systems factors, as well as medical factors and health services inefficiencies, related to maternal mortality. Starting at the community level with mobilization and raising awareness of complications and the need for developing emergency communications, transport, and referral plans before complications arise, if complications arise, the next stage of the continuum would be to administer emergency obstetric or midwifery first aid. If complications continue, the next step would be to alert transport systems and prepare for a referral. The referral level in turn must offer emergency preparedness, the highest possible level of trained staff, adequate supplies and blood, the full range of evidence-based medical and midwifery practices, and access to cesarean delivery and anesthesia.

CONCLUSION

Mothers' lives cannot be saved by single medical interventions. Mortality reduction requires health system solutions that start with access to family planning and include addressing the social, economic, education, and gender inequities that produce the stark disparities between high and low maternal-mortality rates in lower- and higher-resource countries, respectively. A multisectorial approach may be the way forward to reduce maternal mortality in the coming decade: maintenance and improvement of health system infrastructure; an emphasis on training, monitoring, and supervision; adoption of a system of accountability; implementation of evidence-based medical interventions; and political will, attention to gender inequities, and a continuum of care that involves community education and mobilization.

ACKNOWLEDGMENTS

The authors acknowledge the contributions of Ruwani Ekanayake and Christiane Menard.

REFERENCES

Acosta, C. D., and M. Knight. 2013. Sepsis and maternal mortality. *Curr Opin Obstet Gynecol* 25 (2): 109–116.

Akhter S., M. R. Begum, and J. Kabir. 2005. Condom hydrostatic tamponade for massive postpartum hemorrhage. *Int J Gynaecol Obstet* 90 (2): 134–135.

Alkema L., D. Chou, D. Hogan, S. Zhang, A. B. Moller, A. Gemmill, D. M. Fat, et al. 2015. Global, regional, and national levels and trends in maternal mortality between 1990 and 2015, with scenario-based projections to 2030: A systematic analysis by the UN Maternal Mortality Estimation Inter-Agency Group. *Lancet* 387:462–474. pii:S0140–6736(15)00838-7. doi:10.1016/S0140-6736(15)00838-7. [Epub ahead of print] PMID: 26584737.

Bakri, Y. N., A. Amri, and F. Abdul Jabbar. 2001. Tamponade-balloon for obstetrical bleeding. *Int J Gynaecol Obstet* 74 (2): 139–142.

Barot, S. 2011. Unsafe abortion: The missing link in global efforts to improve maternal health. *Guttmacher Policy Review* 14 (2): 24–28.

Basinga, P., A. M. Moore, S. Singh, L. Remez, F. Birungi, and L. Nyirazinyoye. 2012. "Unintended pregnancy and induced abortion in Rwanda: Causes and consequences." Washington, DC, and New York, NY: Guttmacher Institute. Accessed

June 5, 2016. https://www.guttmacher.org/report/unintended-pregnancy-and
-induced-abortion-rwanda.

Bauer, S. T., and C. Bonanno. 2009. Abnormal placentation. *Semin Perinatol* 33 (2):
88–96.

Benedetto, C., L. Marozio, A. M. Tavella, L. Salton, S. Grivon, and F. Di Giampalolo.
2010. Coagulation disorders in pregnancy: Acquired and inherited thrombo-
philias. *Ann N Y Acad Sci* 1205:106–117.

Bose, P., F. Regan, and S. Paterson-Brown. 2006. Improving the accuracy of estimated blood loss at obstetric haemorrhage using clinical reconstructions. *BJOG*
113 (8): 919–924.

Carroli, G., C. Cuesta, E. Abalos, and A. M. Gulmezoglu. 2008. Epidemiology of
postpartum haemorrhage: A systematic review. *Best Pract Res Clin Obstet Gynaecol*
22 (6): 999–1012.

Countdown to 2015: Maternal Newborn & Child Survival. 2015. *A Decade of Tracking
Progress for Maternal, Newborn and Child Survival: The 2015 Report.* Geneva:
UNICEF and the World Health Organization.

Derman, R. J., B. S. Kodkany, S. S. Goudar, S. E. Geller, V. A. Naik, M. B. Bellad,
S. S. Patted, et al. 2006. Oral misoprostol in preventing postpartum haemorrhage in resource-poor communities: A randomised controlled trial. *Lancet*
368:1248–1253.

Devine, P. C., and J. D. Wright. 2009. Obstetric hemorrhage: Introduction. *Semin
Perinatol* 33 (2): 75.

Duley, L. 2009. The global impact of pre-eclampsia and eclampsia. *Semin Perinatol*
33 (3): 130–137.

Duthie, S. J., D. Ven, G. L. Yung, D. Z. Guang, S. Y. Chan, and H. K. Ma. 1991.
Discrepancy between laboratory determination and visual estimation of
blood loss during normal delivery. *Eur J Obstet Gynecol Reprod Biol* 38 (2):
119–124.

Georgiou C. 2009. Balloon tamponade in the management of postpartum haemorrhage: A review. *BJOG* 116: 748–757.

Ghulmiyyah, L., and B. Sibai. 2012. Maternal mortality from preeclampsia/ec
lampsia. *Semin Perinatol* 36 (1): 56–59.

Guttmacher Institute. 2012. "In Brief: Fact Sheet—Facts on Induced Abortion
Worldwide." Accessed November 16, 2015. http://www.guttmacher.org/pubs/fb
_IAW.html.

Hofmeyr, G. J. 2004. Obstructed labor: Using better technologies to reduce mortality. *Int J Gynaecol Obstet* 85:S62–S72.

Hogan, M. C., K. J. Foreman, M. Naghavi, S. Y. Ahn, M. Wang, S. M. Makela, A. D.
Lopez, R. Lozano, and C. J. Murray. 2010. Maternal mortality for 181 countries,
1980–2008: A systematic analysis of progress towards Millennium Development
Goal 5. *Lancet* 375:1609–1623.

Hussein, J., D. V. Mavalankar, S. Sharma, and L. D'Ambruoso. 2011. A review of
health system infection control measures in developing countries: What can be
learned to reduce maternal mortality. *Global Health* 7 (14). doi:10.1186/1744
-8603-7-14.

Kapungu, C. T., A. Koch, S. Miller, and S. E. Geller. 2012. "A community-based continuum of care model for the prevention and treatment of postpartum hemorrhage in low resource settings." In *A Comprehensive Textbook of Postpartum Hemorrhage: An Essential Clinical Reference for Effective Management,* edited by S. Arulkumaran, M. Karoshi, L. Keith, A. B. Lalonde, and C. B-Lynch, 555–561. London: Sapiens Publishing Ltd.

Khan, K. S., D. Wojdyla, L. Say, A. M. Gulmezoglu, and P. F. Van Look. 2006. WHO analysis of causes of maternal death: A systematic review. *Lancet* 367:1066–1074.

Lalonde, André B. 2012. Prevention and treatment of postpartum hemorrhage in low-resource settings. *IJGO* 117 (2): 108–118.

Langer, A., J. Villar, K. Tell, T. Kim, and S. Kennedy. 2008. Reducing eclampsia-related deaths: A call to action. *Lancet* 371:705–706.

Lavender, T., A. Hart, and R. M. Smyth. 2008. Effect of partogram use on outcomes for women in spontaneous labor at term. *Cochrane Database Syst Rev* CD005461.

Lozano, R., H. Wang, K. J. Foreman, J. K. Rajaratnam, M. Naghavi, J. R. Marcus, L. Dwyer-Lindgren, et al. 2011. Progress towards Millennium Development Goals 4 and 5 on maternal and child mortality: An updated systematic analysis. *Lancet* 378:1139–1165.

Magee, L. A., M. Helewa, J. M. Moutquin, and P. von Dadelszen. 2008. Diagnosis, evaluation, and management of the hypertensive disorders of pregnancy. *J Obstet Gynaecol Can* 33:S1–S48.

Miller, S., J. L. Morris, M. M. F. Fathalla, O. Ojengbede, M. Mourad-Youssif, and P. Hensleigh. 2012. "Non-pneumatic anti-shock garments: Clinical trials and results." In *A Comprehensive Textbook of Postpartum Hemorrhage*, edited by Arulkumaran et al., 318–330.

Mobeen, N., J. Durocher, N. Zuberi, N. Jahan, J. Blum, S. Wasim, G. Walraven, and J. Hatcher. 2010. Administration of misoprostol by trained traditional birth attendants to prevent postpartum haemorrhage in home deliveries in Pakistan: A randomised placebo-controlled trial. *BJOG* 118:353–361.

Moran, N. F., and J. Moodley. 2012. The effect of HIV infection on maternal health and mortality. *Int J Gynaecol Obstet* 119 (S1) (Oct.): S26–S29.

Neilson, J. P., T. Lavender, S. Quenby, and S. Wray. 2003. Obstructed labor. *Br Med Bull* 67:191–204.

Nour, N. M. 2008. An introduction to maternal mortality. *Rev Obstet Gynecol* 1 (2): 77–81.

Odon device. n.d. "A New Simple, Low Cost Instrument for Assisted Vaginal Delivery. Accessed June 5, 2016. http://www.odondevice.org/index.php.

Oyelese, Y., and C. V. Ananth. 2010. Postpartum hemorrhage: Epidemiology, risk factors, and causes. *Clin Obstet Gynecol* 53 (1): 147–156.

Prata, N., G. Mbaruku, and M. Campbell. 2005. Using the kanga to measure post partum blood loss. *IJGO* 89 (1): 49–50.

Prata, N., M. A. Quaiyum, P. Passano, S. Bell, D. D. Bohl, S. Hossain, A. J. Azmi, and M. Begum. 2012. Training traditional birth attendants to use misoprostol and an absorbent delivery mat in home births. *Soc Sci Med* 75 (11): 2021–2027.

Ransom, E. I., and N. V. Yinger. 2002. "Making motherhood safer: Overcoming obstacles on the pathway to care. Population Reference Bureau." Accessed March 2014. http://www.eldis.org/go/home&id=16099&type=Document# .U5W1E9gU_cc.

Sibai, B. M. 2002. "The MAGPIE trial." *Lancet* 360:1329.

Singh, S., and J. E. Darroch. 2012. *Adding It Up: Costs and Benefits of Contraceptive Services; Estimates for 2012.* Washington, DC, and New York: Guttmacher Institute. Accessed June 5, 2016. https://www.guttmacher.org/sites/default/files/report _pdf/aiu-2012-estimates_0.pdf.

Sosa, C. G., F. Althabe, J. M. Belizán, and P. Buekens. 2009. Risk factors for postpartum hemorrhage in vaginal deliveries in a Latin-American population. *Obstetrics & Gynecology* 113 (6): 1313–1319. doi:10.097/AOG.0b013e3181a66b05.

Stenson, A. L., S. Miller, and F. Lester. 2012. "The Mechanisms of Action of the Non-Pneumatic Anti-Shock Garment." In *A Comprehensive Textbook of Postpartum Hemorrhage,* edited by Arulkumaran et al., 331–340.

United Nations, "The Millennium Development Goals Report 2015." 2015. Accessed December 2015. http://www.un.org/millenniumgoals/reports.shtml.

van Dillen, J., J. Zwart, J. Schutte, and J. van Roosmalen. 2010. "Maternal sepsis: Epidemiology, etiology, and outcome." *Curr Opin Infect Dis* 23 (3): 249–254.

van Lonkhuijzen, L., J. Stekelenburg, J. van Roosmalen. 2012. "Maternity waiting facilities for improving maternal and neonatal outcome in low-resource countries." *Cochrane Database Syst Rev* 10:CD006759.

von Dadelszen, P., B. Payne, J. Li, J. M. Ansermino, F. Broughton Pipkin, A. M. Côté, M. J. Douglas, et al. 2011. "Prediction of adverse maternal outcomes in pre-eclampsia: Development and validation of the full PIERS model." *Lancet* 377:219–227.

WHO (World Health Organization). 2006a. "Obstetric Fistula: Guiding Principles for Clinical Management and Programme Development." WHO Guidelines. Geneva: WHO.

———. 2006b. "WHO Guidelines on Hand Hygiene in Health Care." World Alliance for Patient Safety. Geneva: WHO.

———. 2007. "WHO Recommendations for the Prevention of Postpartum Haemorrhage." Geneva: WHO. Accessed June 5, 2016. http://whqlibdoc.who.int/hq /2007/WHO_MPS_07.06_eng.pdf.

———. 2008. "Managing Puerperal Sepsis." Education material for teachers of midwifery: Midwifery education modules. 2nd ed. Geneva: WHO.

———. 2009. "Your 5 Moments for Hand Hygiene." Geneva. Accessed February 2014. https://www.google.ca/search?q=WHO,+%E2%80%9CYour+5+moments+for +hand+hygiene,%E2%80%9D&tbm=isch&tbo=u&source=univ&sa=X&ei =XhOjU8byIYqEqga3uICgAQ&ved=0CC4QsAQ&biw=1360&bih=641.

———. 2011a. "The Partnership for Maternal, Newborn, and Child Health." PMNCH Fact Sheet, RMNCH Continuum of Care. Geneva.: WHO. Accessed November 2015. http://www.who.int/pmnch/knowledge/topics/continuum_of_care/en/.

———. 2011b. "Unsafe Abortion: Global and Regional Estimates of the Incidence of Unsafe Abortion and Associated Mortality in 2008." Geneva: WHO. Accessed

February 2014. http://www.who.int/reproductivehealth/publications/unsafe
_abortion/9789241501118/en/.

——. 2012a. "Accountability for Maternal, Newborn, and Child Survival: An Update on Progress in Priority Countries." Geneva: WHO.

——. 2012b. "WHO Recommendations for the Prevention and Treatment of Post partum Haemorrhage." Geneva: WHO. Accessed October 2013. http://apps.who .int/rhl/guidelines/appraisal_pph/en/index.html.

3

Strategies to Reduce Stillbirths in Low-Resource Settings

ZULFIQAR AHMED BHUTTA AND JAI K. DAS

The World Health Organization (WHO) defines stillbirth as the death of a fetus with birth weight of 1,000 grams or more, gestation of twenty-eight weeks or more, or a body length of thirty-five centimeters or more. However, the definition varies by country, and some high-income countries even report stillbirths beyond twenty weeks of gestation (WHO 2014). Figure 3.1 defines stillbirth and neonatal death as it occurs at each stage of pregnancy.

Reducing child mortality has long been on the agenda of many national and international forums. However, despite a significant decline in mortality for children under the age of five—from over 12 million in 1990 to 6.6 million in the year 2012 (UNICEF 2013)—neonatal mortality has been much more resistant to reduction than maternal and child mortality, and the reduction in stillbirth rates has been even slower. There are an estimated 2.6 million annual stillbirths worldwide (Lawn et al. 2014); 1.2 million are intrapartum (occurring after the onset of labor, or as "fresh stillbirth," with skin still intact, implying death within twelve hours of delivery), and 1.4 million were antepartum, or "macerated stillbirth." There are also wide disparities between countries' reported stillbirth rates: from 2 per 1,000 births in Finland to more than 40 per 1,000 in Nigeria and Pakistan (Lawn et al. 2014). Only ten countries account for two-thirds of global intrapartum deaths, most of which could be prevented by adequate care. Table 3.1 gives estimations of stillbirth and intrapartum stillbirth by region.

It has also been observed that the rate of intrapartum stillbirth increases in proportion to overall stillbirth rates. The burden of stillbirth is high in low-resource settings: 67% of all stillbirths occur in rural families, and 55% of those are found in rural sub-Saharan Africa and south Asia

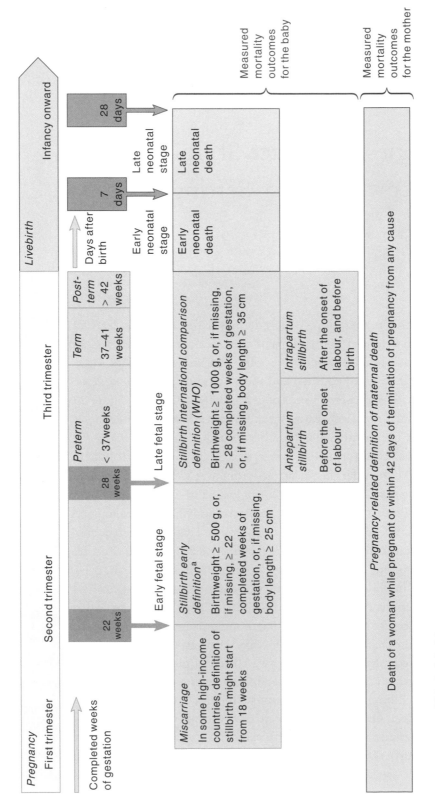

FIGURE 3.1. Stillbirth definition.

a. International Classification of Diseases definition.

Table 3.1   Estimated stillbirth rates and percentage of intrapartum stillbirth by world region, 2008

	Estimated stillbirths per 1,000 total births	Number of stillbirths	Uncertainty range		Estimated intrapartum stillbirths (%)
			Low	High	
High-income countries	3.1	36,300	35,500	38,200	13.7
East Asia	9.0	171,400	116,200	278,600	20.0
Latin America and the Caribbean	9.4	101,800	83,300	125,400	23.1
Eurasia	9.0	33,500	31,300	42,700	20.0
Southeast Asia and Oceania	14.2	164,300	130,400	235,700	30.9
North Africa and West Asia (Middle East)	12.9	112,300	88,900	165,100	16.4
Sub-Saharan Africa	29.0	943,900	701,800	1,388,800	46.5
South Asia	26.7	1,083,000	835,900	1,671,000	56.6
Worldwide	19.1	2,646,800	2,077,010	3,790,420	45.0

Source: Reprinted from Lawn et al. (2011), Table 1. © World Health Organization 2011, with permission from Elsevier.

(Lawn et al. 2014). These areas also face high rates of maternal malnutrition, poor health-care facilities, and limited access to care, including skilled birth attendants and cesarean section (Darmstadt et al. 2014).

One major gap is the scarcity of actual data from high-burden countries, as only 2% of all stillbirths are believed to be reported. In many settings, stillbirths are rarely issued a death certificate, and minimal postmortem investigation protocols and classifications leave most stillbirths unexplained. Because women who deliver stillbirths may not be shown the infant, many cannot adequately respond to household survey questions about the infant's appearance; and the only estimates of the number of stillbirths globally are based on household surveys or modeling.

Inconsistency in terminology and definitions in both high-income and low-income countries also contributes to uncertainty. In high-income countries, there is variability in defining the age of gestation for stillbirth, while in low- and middle-income countries, even where data are available, there is variation not only in the survey definition of stillbirth but in the accuracy of estimation of gestational age. In settings with major delays in access to health care, intrapartum stillbirths may not be delivered for days and thus could be misclassified as macerated. All of these factors can contribute to misclassification and hence hamper accurate estimation of the actual number of stillbirths.

This burden of stillbirth has broad consequences for the wellbeing of society, and women bear the brunt: in addition to the obvious psychological trauma, women who experience a stillbirth may face social taboos, blame, and marginalization. Most stillborn babies are disposed of without any acknowledgment or funeral rituals, as some societies believe that stillbirths are caused by evil spirits or the mother's sins. In other areas, stillbirths may be thought of as a type of natural selection, that is, babies who were never meant to survive (Darmstadt et al. 2014). In addition to societal stigma, the slower progress in reduction in stillbirths is partly attributable to the fact that reporting stillbirths is widely neglected across the globe; they are not mentioned in national or global surveys, including the Global Burden of Disease, and were omitted from the United Nations Millennium Development Goals. Additionally, the pathophysiology underlying stillbirths is not well understood. Multiple causes and pathways contribute to stillbirths, including infectious, genetic, and environmental factors as well as abnormalities in placental vascular development and adverse events in early gestation and intrapartum. The literature on stillbirths is also scarce when compared with that on child or maternal health: for every fifty-four published articles on PubMed that address sudden and unexplained infant death, there is only one on unexplained stillbirths, despite stillbirths being tenfold more common (Froen et al. 2011).

Tackling the existing burden of stillbirth will first require a comprehensive body of interdisciplinary research to fill the current gaps in our knowledge of the epidemiology and pathophysiology of this phenomenon. Only then will we begin to fill the critical need for high-quality evidence to inform promising interventions across the spectrum of maternal and fetal care.

PATHOPHYSIOLOGY

Identifying the causes of stillbirth is imperative to making progress in its prevention. The causes are poorly understood and depend on gestational age, genetics, and environmental factors. As noted above, coming up with global estimates of stillbirth as a cause of death is impeded by multiple, complex classification systems (Lawn et al. 2010); more than thirty-five stillbirth classification systems have been published over the past fifty years, with more than fifteen of these in the past twenty years (Lawn et al.

2011). Because most of these classifications are designed for high-income countries and involve laboratory and pathological examination of the baby and the placenta, they are not applicable in low- and middle-income countries, where the only information available on most stillbirths is verbal autopsy, which can occur a year or even longer after the loss. There are currently no systematic global estimates regarding the causes of stillbirth, because new analyses are required to better define the risk of death at varying gestational ages and also to separate direct from indirect risks and variations between regions.

The most common cause of intrapartum stillbirth in low- and middle-income countries is asphyxia, or a lack of oxygen during birth (Barros et al. 2010). Other known causes of intrapartum stillbirth include labor obstruction, breech presentation, and preterm labor. Overuse of oxytocin or prostaglandins for induction of labor can also cause fetal hypoxia, as can umbilical cord accidents such as a prolapse, a true knot, or fetal entanglement that reduces the flow of blood to the fetus. Breech and multiple pregnancies increase the chances of hypoxia, as they are more often associated with umbilical cord complications. Causes of antepartum stillbirth include a poorly functioning placenta, which may hamper the blood supply to the fetus; this may be the direct cause or may contribute to the baby's death by restricting fetal growth and development. Common adverse conditions include pregnancy-induced hypertension, preeclampsia (causing placental damage and decreased placental blood flow), eclampsia (causing fetal hypoxia, because the mother becomes hypoxic during the seizure), diabetes, antepartum hemorrhage, placental abruption (decreases placental blood flow), syphilis and other maternal and fetal infections, and congenital abnormalities. Obesity or drug abuse during pregnancy can also be underlying factors. Regional stillbirth rates can be increased by country-level variables, such as low per-capita gross domestic product, a low human development index, low prevalence of the use of contraceptives, and a low percentage of girls in secondary education (Froen et al. 2011).

Fetal well-being can be monitored through auscultation or electronically by monitoring fetal heart rate, making it possible to detect fetal hypoxia preceding irreversible organ damage. Interventions such as assisted delivery (forceps or vacuum extraction) or cesarean section at any time during the labor (or even during the antenatal period) can have favorable outcomes once fetal distress is detected. However, these modalities are more common in high-income countries or select areas of low- and middle-income countries.

There is a need to improve collection, analysis, interpretation, and application of epidemiological data as a basis for interventions to reduce stillbirths. The causes of stillbirths and newborn and maternal deaths are closely related, and possible solutions should be based on the continuum of care rather than isolated measures. The five major areas identified to reduce stillbirth are delivery complications, maternal infections, maternal conditions (especially hypertension), fetal growth restriction, and congenital abnormalities (Lawn et al. 2011). Hence intensive efforts should be made to identify these conditions as early as possible, especially in low- and middle-income countries, and identify effective and practical ways to alleviate them.

GLOBAL IMPACT OF DISEASE

We have already discussed the numbers associated with stillbirths, but stillbirth has huge global implications beyond mortality or even health outcomes. When comparing the leading global causes of death in all age categories, all-cause stillbirths would rank fifth, higher than diarrhea, HIV/AIDS, tuberculosis, traffic accidents, or any form of cancer (Froen et al. 2011). This alone highlights the dire need for a focused global strategy not only to curtail stillbirths but to prevent the massive spillover effects, including loss of workdays for both mothers and fathers grieving for their stillborn child, leading to psychological conditions including anxiety, post-traumatic stress disorder, and depression. Many of these psychological conditions go unnoticed and untreated, particularly in low- and middle-income countries, where resources for and attention to mental health are scarce. They can even lead to long-term and chronic conditions with deleterious effects on the parents and the whole family.

Mental and emotional suffering are further aggravated by cultural rituals in many low-resource areas, where mothers are not usually allowed to see, name, or dress the stillborn child, and there are no formal funerals, which could have an impact on mental health, especially that of the mother. In certain parts of the world, society also blames the woman and holds her responsible for the stillbirth, blaming curses or evil spirits. These factors exacerbate the already massive stress on women, who are already underrepresented and lack empowerment. Even in high-resource settings, where psychological support might be available, one in five mothers has appreciable long-term depression, anxiety, or post-traumatic stress disorder after a stillbirth. Additionally and contrary to popular belief, fathers are also affected by negative psychosocial consequences (Froen et al. 2011). The negative environment that surrounds a family affected by stillbirth can even affect the normal growth and development of the surviving children and siblings born later. Stillbirth brings a huge economic burden that is shared by the family and the government, not to mention the additional cost of closer scrutiny for future pregnancies. It is well established that both maternal and child health would benefit substantially from stillbirth-prevention initiatives; studies of the possible costs of such projects would be a useful tool for advocates approaching policy makers (Sather et al. 2010).

TREATMENT AND GUIDELINES FOR CARE

There are effective interventions to prevent and manage the conditions that lead to stillbirth, both antenatal and intrapartum. Many high-income countries have used such interventions to markedly reduce their stillbirth burden. Facilities in these countries provide core packages of maternal and child health care at primary-care and referral levels, and timely facility-based quality care (especially at the time of delivery) is accessible to all. Common interventions to prevent stillbirth include balanced protein-energy supplementation, screening and treatment of syphilis, intermittent presumptive treatment for malaria during pregnancy, insecticide-treated mosquito nets, birth preparedness, emergency obstetric care, cesarean section for breech presentation, and elective induction for postterm delivery (Barros et al. 2010). Community-based approaches within the continuum of maternal and newborn care can help make up for gaps or low coverage of the identified interventions in low- and middle-income countries. (See figure 3.2.)

Nutritional Interventions

Malnutrition, especially in women of reproductive age, is a major problem in low- and middle-income countries, as it can lead to adverse pregnancy and birth outcomes including stillbirth. The current recommendation is to supplement iron and folic acid during pregnancy, but there is evidence of the impact of other nutritional interventions, including general nutrition and dietary advice to pregnant women, balanced protein-energy

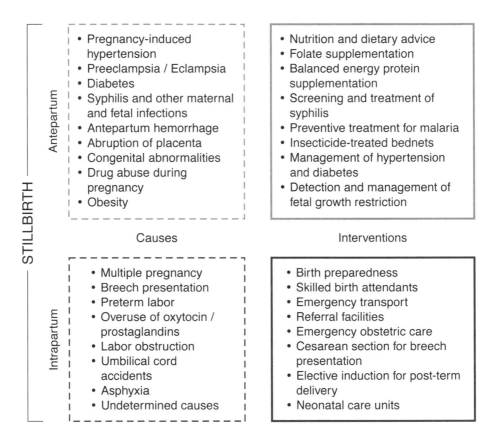

FIGURE 3.2. Framework for the causes of and approach to stillbirth.

supplementation to malnourished women, and lower-calorie diets for overweight pregnant women (Bhutta et al. 2014).

Folic acid supplementation during periconception (before and during pregnancy) can reduce the risk of primary neural tube deficits by as much as 62% (95% CI 49, 71); however, these are one of the less common causes of stillbirth (Blencowe et al. 2010). In women with a previous history of a birth with neural-tube defect, folic-acid supplementation reduces the risk of recurrence by 70% (95% CI 35, 86). A meta-analysis of eight population-based observational studies examining folic-acid food fortification suggests a 46% (95% CI 37, 54) reduction in the incidence of neural tube defect (Blencowe et al. 2010), while a more recent review on fortification suggests a 43% (95% CI 27, 55) reduction (Das et al. 2013). Balanced energy-protein supplementation—defined as nutritional supplementation during pregnancy in which proteins provide less than 25% of the total energy content—reduces stillbirth among undernourished pregnant women by 38% (95% CI 2–60) (Imdad and Bhutta 2012). While there are concerns related to feasibility, delivery strategies, and cost-effectiveness of balanced energy-protein supplementation or any other alternative strategies to promote food intake, these should be considered as an effective intervention in malnourished pregnant women, especially in low-resource areas, to reduce intrauterine growth restriction and hence fetal loss.

Malaria Prevention

Malaria during pregnancy has negative effects on maternal health, birth, and neonatal outcomes. Every year about 50 million pregnant women are exposed to malaria in endemic areas such as sub-Saharan Africa, parts of Latin America, and Asia. Routine antimalarial treatment is often recommended in these areas, including insecticide-treated bed nets or intermittent preventive treatment. The use of insecticide-treated bed nets during pregnancy can reduce blood and placental parasitemia by 24%, low birth weight by 20%, and stillbirths by 32% in the first or second pregnancy. However, intermittent preventive treatment has no significant effect on stillbirth in women in their first or second pregnancy. The combination of intermittent preventive treatment and insecticide-treated bed nets can reduce the risk of low birth weight in the first or second pregnancy by 35% in areas of stable *Plasmodium falciparum* transmission, while data for impact on rates of prematurity and stillbirth (though scarce) is suggestive of possible positive impact (Ishaque et al. 2011) (see Chapter 7).

Syphilis Detection and Treatment

Syphilis in pregnancy can lead to serious adverse events including spontaneous abortion, intrauterine growth restriction, stillbirth, and perinatal death as well as serious consequences in live-born infants. The WHO estimates that between 730,000 and 1,500,000 adverse pregnancy outcomes are caused by untreated maternal syphilis each year, of which about 650,000 are fetal and newborn deaths (Blencowe et al. 2011). Appropriate and timely treatment of pregnant women who have syphilis can prevent these complications, but the major limitation has been the inability to identify such cases, especially in low- and middle-income countries. Syphilis can be easily identified through rapid plasma reagin or venereal disease research laboratory test during the first trimester and then confirmed with fluorescent treponemal antibody absorption assay. Women with positive tests can be treated with penicillin (at least 2.4 million units benzathine penicillin or equivalent). These all are cost-effective strategies and could greatly reduce the existing burden of syphilis and its consequences. Evidence from observational studies suggests that in syphilis-endemic countries, antenatal syphilis screening combined with penicillin treatment can reduce syphilis-specific stillbirths by 82% (95% CI: 67, 90), so it is strongly recommended that maternal syphilis be identified and treated to reduce congenital syphilis and stillbirth (Blencowe et al. 2011) (see Chapter 5).

Detection and Management of Hypertensive Disease of Pregnancy

Hypertensive disorders complicate 5 to 8% of pregnancies and are associated with increased risks of perinatal morbidity and mortality. They include pregnancy-induced hypertension (new arterial hypertension over 140/90 in a pregnant woman after twenty weeks' gestation without the presence of proteinuria of 300 milligrams or more in a twenty-four-hour urine collection), preeclampsia (gestational hypertension plus proteinuria), and eclampsia (gestational hypertension plus proteinuria and seizures). Hypertension could be a primary condition of pregnancy or could be secondary to other causes, such as kidney disease, systemic lupus erythematosus, or diabetes. Maternal risk factors include nulliparity, past history of pregnancy-induced hypertension, long interpregnancy interval (greater than sixty months), and multiple pregnancy (Jabeen et al. 2011). One instance of pregnancy-induced hypertension is a strong predictor of recurrence in the next pregnancy, and these recurrent hypertensive disorders are associated with substantially higher risks of adverse perinatal outcomes including stillbirth. Strategies are needed to improve prevention, detection, and management (especially in low-resource settings) to reduce the burden of adverse pregnancy outcomes and maternal morbidity and mortality.

While identification of patients with preeclampsia continues to be a challenge, improved patient education and counseling strategies are also needed for greater awareness regarding the dangers of preeclampsia and hypertension and earlier diagnosis. There are no current recommendations for intervention in cases of mild hypertension, while treatment is advised for moderate to high hypertension. Evidence suggests that treatment of mild to moderate hypertension during pregnancy does not substantially affect maternal and birth outcomes, although magnesium sulfate can reduce the risk of eclampsia by 59% (Jabeen et al. 2011). Antiplatelet drugs reduce risk of preeclampsia by 17%, preterm birth by 8%, and small size for gestational age in infants by 10%. Calcium supplementation (0.5 to 2.0 grams daily before twenty to thirty weeks of gestation and continued until delivery) reduces the risk of progression to preeclampsia and eclampsia and also improves maternal and birth outcomes, but it is most useful in populations with low calcium intake. Comparing different antihypertensive drugs for very high blood pressure during pregnancy ($MgSO_4$, beta blockers, methyldopa, isradipine, verapamil, nifedipine, glyceryl trinitrate) does not show a benefit of one drug over another. The recommended package of interventions includes screening for hypertension, treatment with antihypertensive drugs, use of magnesium sulfate as needed, and induction of labor or cesarean section. A Delphi exercise of experts (quantitative method aimed at generating consensus amongst experts) has suggested a 20% median reduction in both antepartum stillbirth (IQR 10 to 30) and intrapartum stillbirth (10 to 40) from introduction of these interventions (Jabeen et al. 2011). Optimal management requires close observation for signs and predictive findings as well as serial assessment of maternal symptoms and fetal movement. There is a need for best-practice recommendations to guide clinicians with all forms of preeclampsia and hypertension. (See Chapter 2.)

Detection and Management of Diabetes of Pregnancy

An estimated 60 million women of reproductive age have type 2 diabetes, and gestational diabetes affects up to 15% of pregnant women worldwide. Women with any kind of diabetes have an increased risk of adverse birth outcomes. Preconception dietary advice and counseling can reduce the mean concentration of glycated hemoglobin (HbA1c) during the first trimester of pregnancy and reduce congenital malformations (by 70%) and perinatal mortality (69%); intensified management including dietary advice, monitoring, or pharmacotherapy for women with gestational diabetes also reduces the risk of stillbirths, suggesting that optimal control of serum glucose is a must and is associated with reduced perinatal mortality and other maternal, fetal, and newborn morbidity. Another Delphi exercise of experts suggests that optimum identification and management of diabetes in pregnancy can reduce both antepartum and intrapartum stillbirth owing to gestational diabetes by a median of 10% (Syed et al. 2011).

Detection and Management of
Fetal Growth Restriction

Intrauterine growth restriction describes a fetus that has not achieved its growth potential owing to some pathologic process. Effective screening for intrauterine growth restriction also requires accurate dating of conception and the mother's accurate menstrual history. Potential growth restriction can be diagnosed through clinical examination, including fundal height measurement or ultrasound screening and formal assessment of fetal movement by the mother. Fetal-movement counting is one of the oldest methods of monitoring fetal well-being, but there is no conclusive evidence regarding its effectiveness. Abnormal blood-flow patterns in fetal circulation can be detected by Doppler ultrasound and may suggest poor fetal growth and outcome. Current evidence suggests that Doppler velocimetry of umbilical and fetal arteries in high-risk pregnancies reduces the risk of perinatal mortality by 29% (95% CI: 2,48) through early delivery, while false-positive results might increase cesarean section rates (Alfirevic, Stampalija, and Gyte 2010). Confirmation of fetal growth restriction by Doppler velocimetry alone does not determine the appropriate course of action; other factors should be considered, like gestation and the availability of additional monitoring methods (including computerized cardiotocography, biophysical profile, and color Doppler), delivery facilities, and neonatal intensive-care units (Alfirevic Stampalija, and Gyte et al. 2010). Amniotic-fluid volume assessment can aid in the differential diagnosis of intrauterine growth restriction and increase the accuracy of the diagnosis of placental insufficiency (SOGC Clinical Practice Guide 2013). Serial ultrasound estimation of fetal weight along with umbilical-artery Doppler studies should be initiated and, if available, a placental assessment and Doppler studies of other vessels such as the middle cerebral artery, the umbilical vein, and ductus venosus can be considered (SOGC Clinical Practice Guide 2013).

The outcomes in cases of fetal growth restriction depend largely upon gestational age and the sophistication of the setting (including the presence of obstetricians, pediatricians, or neonatologists and access to cesarean section). It is important that every woman be screened for clinical risk factors for intrauterine growth restriction through a complete history and followed up accordingly. Although stillbirth rates are higher when fetal growth restriction is not detected antenatally, there is only low-quality evidence that antenatal identification of fetal growth restriction improves outcome. Unfortunately, significant problems remain in terms of defining growth-restricted fetuses at high risk of adverse outcome, accurately identifying these fetuses in utero, and determining interventions to improve outcomes. These issues need to be addressed by large multicenter studies employing consistent definitions, randomly assigned interventions, and long-term follow-up.

Birth Preparedness

Birth preparedness includes counseling the mother and family during pregnancy (or ideally before a planned pregnancy) and preparing them for the ideal course during pregnancy and possible complications. This would include seeking proper and timely antenatal care including nutrition and vaccination, identifying the skilled birth attendant and place of delivery, procurement of proper and sterile delivery materials, and a plan for a referral, including transport and facility, in case of complications to the mother or newborn.

Basic and Comprehensive
Emergency Obstetric Care

Tackling high-risk pregnancies and complications during childbirth, with interventions to improve skilled care at birth and delivery within facilities, are key to reducing intrapartum stillbirths. Basic emergency obstetric care includes six signal functions that should be available at first-level facilities that provide childbirth care: parenteral antibiotics, parenteral oxytocics, parenteral anticonvulsants for preeclampsia or eclampsia, assisted vaginal delivery (including vacuum or forceps assistance for delivery, episiotomy, advanced skills for manual delivery of shoulder dystocia, skilled vaginal delivery of the breech infant), manual removal of the placenta, and removal of retained products. Comprehensive emergency obstetric care includes basic obstetric care, cesarean section, and blood transfusion. Safe cesarean section is a crucial component of any systematic attempt to reduce stillbirth rates. Deciding who will benefit from the procedure and when to perform it are central to a successful outcome.

Evidence suggests that as the proportion of cesarean section births increases from 0% to 8%, each 1% increase decreases the risk of intrapartum stillbirth by 1.61 per 1,000 births (Goldenberg, McClure, and Bann 2007). However, all too often, especially in low-income countries, cesarean sections are performed on the wrong women, are provided too late to change the outcome, or are of poor quality. The percentage of deliveries by cesarean section may be useful for population monitoring, but much more important is confirming that the operations are performed on the right women and in a timely manner. In an attempt to reduce stillbirths, physicians in many high- and middle-income countries perform cesarean sections in 30% or more of deliveries. Though avoiding most stillbirths does not require such high rates of cesarean section, several studies do suggest that cesarean section rates of 5 to 10% substantially reduce stillbirth. Cesarean section rates in sub-Saharan Africa and parts of south Asia can be 1% or less. The poorest women and women from rural areas often have little or no access to this lifesaving intervention. A review to estimate the effect of basic and comprehensive emergency obstetric care during labor and birth suggests (through the Delphi process) that intrapartum-related deaths are reduced 85% by comprehensive emergency obstetric care, 40% by basic emergency obstetric care, and 25% by skilled birth care (Lee et al. 2011; Yakoob et al. 2011) (see Chapter 2).

Induction to Prevent Postterm Pregnancies

If pregnancy continues beyond term, it increases the risk of complications and mortality. Inducing labor at term or postterm (forty-one weeks or more) when compared with spontaneous labor or later induction of labor, results in 69% fewer perinatal deaths, 50% fewer cases of babies with meconium aspiration syndrome, and an 11% reduction in the rates of cesarean section (Gulmezoglu, Crowther, and Middleton 2006). Labor induction beyond forty-one weeks of gestation should be recommended to improve birth and neonatal outcomes. While planned cesarean section for singleton breech presentation at term reduces mortality perinatally and within three months of delivery by 67%, women allocated to planned cesarean section reported less urinary incontinence, more abdominal pain, and less perineal pain (Hofmeyr, Hannah, and Lawrie 2003). Thus planned cesarean section should be considered for breech singleton pregnancies and pregnancies beyond forty-one weeks.

Skilled Care at Birth

Substantial reduction of stillbirths requires skilled birth attendants, screening, and prophylactic and therapeutic interventions. Unfortunately, many birth attendants in low- and middle-income countries (this includes midwives, nurses, and sometimes even doctors) are not equipped with the basic skills to prevent stillbirth or manage complicated labor. Strong and well-structured training programs are needed to help bring about a real change.

Other Promising Interventions

A range of other interventions have the potential to reduce stillbirth but the evidence is scarce and would require more research. These include birth spacing and family planning, reduction of female genital mutilation, reduction in indoor air pollution, reduction in tobacco use during pregnancy, multiple micronutrient supplementation, prevention of mother-to-child transmission of HIV, periodontal care, antibiotics and antisepsis for high-risk pregnancies, anthelmintic drugs, antibiotics for premature rupture of membranes or preterm premature rupture of membranes, management of intrahepatic cholestasis, cervical cerclage, amniotic-fluid volume assessment, maternal hyperoxygenation for suspected impaired fetal growth, maternal plasma exchange, and a range of other environmental and genetic factors. However, new interventions should also be evaluated for their ethical and social-justice implications before being recommended (Rubens et al. 2010).

CONCLUSION

The WHO recently launched Every Newborn action plan and the *Lancet*'s newborn series call for reduction of national stillbirth rates to fewer than 10 per 1,000 live births by 2035, but reaching these targets will require much more concerted effort from many quarters, including researchers, academicians, pediatricians, general physicians, paramedics, community activists, policy makers, and donors.

- There is a need for global standard definitions of gestational age and stillbirth. Data collection systems need to be standardized and strengthened; areas of highest risk currently have the least information available. Data collection systems should take into account feasible modalities in low- and middle-income countries, both for vital registration and facility data. This should include standard death certificates for stillbirths and linkages to a standardized verbal autopsy tool.

- It is imperative to create a revised standardized classification system for cause-of-death coding that is feasible in low- and middle-income countries. This would catalyze, facilitate, and provide targeted support and also leverage support from international and national governments to inform evidence-based policies and to scale up effective interventions.
- There is a need to better understand the mechanisms and pathways underlying intrauterine deaths and stillbirth. The genetic risks for stillbirth should be assessed, and potentially modifiable environmental and other influences should be identified. Targeted population-based studies could identify these factors in special contextual settings.
- Screening for intrauterine growth restriction can identify fetuses at risk for stillbirth in underdeveloped regions; this could be carried out through fundal height measurement or ultrasound and later monitoring of the fetal heart rate or biophysical profile or uterine Doppler flow where feasible. Early delivery of infants correctly identified as being at high risk of intrauterine death must be ensured.
- There is a need to improve the coverage of existing low-cost and proven interventions, and a special focus should be to improve access to quality care at the time of birth. Attention and resources should be directed toward preventing or better managing some of the maternal conditions that increase the risk of stillbirth, including nutrition status, screening and treatment for syphilis, prevention of malaria, maternal antibiotic treatment when there are ruptured membranes, antenatal antiretroviral treatment of women with HIV, better screening and management of diabetes and hypertension, and prevention of preeclampsia and eclampsia through the use of calcium or aspirin prophylaxis.
- To prevent intrapartum stillbirths, skilled birth delivery with essential emergency obstetric care and timely referral through efficient transport mechanisms must be prioritized in low-resource settings. Quality of care at referral facilities also needs special attention and focus.
- Improving access to essential interventions in low- and middle-income countries will require not only deployment of community health workers but increasing their capacity and sustaining their work over time. Efforts should also be focused on improving

community awareness of stillbirth and the empowerment of women, as their voices should be central on this issue. Employing more physicians and improving women's access to trained medical professionals will yield dramatic positive results in high-burden countries.

- A strong multidisciplinary momentum is required to generate the desired attention and allocate sufficient resources to support policies, programs, and actions at the global, regional, national, and community levels. Stillbirth interventions must be considered part of the broader continuum of maternal, newborn, and child health and be integrated into national policies and guidelines to ensure safe full-term pregnancies and healthy newborns.

REFERENCES

Alfirevic, Z., T. Stampalija, and G. M. Gyte. 2010. Fetal and umbilical Doppler ultrasound in high-risk pregnancies. *Cochrane Database Syst Rev,* no. 1: CD007529.

Barros, F. C., Z. A. Bhutta, M. Batra, T. N. Hansen, C. G. Victora, and C. E. Rubens. 2010. Global report on preterm birth and stillbirth (3 of 7): Evidence for effectiveness of interventions. *BMC Pregnancy Childbirth* 10 (S1): S3. doi:10.1186/1471-2393-10-S1-S3

Bhutta, Z. A., J. K. Das, R. Bahl, J. E. Lawn, R. A. Salam, V. K. Paul, M. J. Sankar, et al. 2014. Can available interventions end preventable deaths in mothers, newborn babies, and stillbirths, and at what cost? *Lancet* 384:347–370.

Blencowe H., S. Cousens, M. Kamb, S. Berman, and J. E. Lawn. 2011. Lives Saved Tool supplement detection and treatment of syphilis in pregnancy to reduce syphilis related stillbirths and neonatal mortality. *BMC Public Health* 11 (S3): S9.

Blencowe, H., S. Cousens, B. Modell, and J. Lawn. 2010. Folic acid to reduce neonatal mortality from neural tube disorders. *Int J Epidemiol* 39 (S1): i110–i121.

Darmstadt, G. L., M. V. Kinney, M. Chopra, S. Cousens, I. Kak, V. K. Paul, J. Martines, Z. A. Bhutta, and J. E. Lawn. 2014. Who has been caring for the baby? *Lancet* 384: 174–188. doi:10.1016/S0140-6736(14)60458-X. Epub 2014 May 19.

Das, J. K., R. A. Salam, R. Kumar, and Z. A. Bhutta. 2013. Micronutrient fortification of food and its impact on woman and child health: A systematic review. *Syst Rev* 2 (1): 67. doi:10.1186/2046-4053-2-67

Froen, J. F., J. Cacciatore, E. M. Mcclure, O. Kuti, A. H. Jokhio, M. Islam, and J. Shiffman. 2011. Stillbirths: Why they matter. *Lancet* 377:1353–1366.

Goldenberg, R. L., E. M. McClure, and C. M. Bann. 2007. The relationship of intrapartum and antepartum stillbirth rates to measures of obstetric care in developed and developing countries. *Acta obstet gynecol Scand* 86:1303–1309.

Gulmezoglu, A. M., C. A. Crowther, and P. Middleton. 2006. Induction of labour for improving birth outcomes for women at or beyond term. *Cochrane Database Syst Rev,* no. 6: CD004945. doi:10.1002/14651858.CD004945.pub3.

Hofmeyr, G. J., M. E. Hannah, and T. A. Lawrie. 2003. Planned caesarean section for term breech delivery. *Cochrane Database Syst Rev,* no. 3: CD000166. doi:10.1002/14651858.CD000166.pub2

Imdad, A., and Z. A. Bhutta. 2012. Maternal nutrition and birth outcomes: Effect of balanced protein-energy supplementation. *Paediatr Perinat Epidemiol* 26 (S1): 178–190. doi:10.1111/j.1365–3016.2012.01308.x.

Ishaque S., M. Y. Yaqoob, A. Imdad, R. L. Goldenberg, T. P. Eisele, and Z. A. Bhutta. 2011. Effectiveness of interventions to screen and manage infections during pregnancy on reducing stillbirths: A review. *BMC Public Health* 11 (S3): S3. doi:10.1186/1471-2458-11-S3-S3.

Jabeen, M., M. Y. Yakoob, A. Imdad, and Z. A. Bhutta. 2011. Impact of interventions to prevent and manage preeclampsia and eclampsia on stillbirths. *BMC Public Health* 11 (S3): S6. doi:10.1186/1471-2458-11-S3-S6.

Lausman, A., and J. Kingdom. 2013. Intrauterine growth restriction: Screening, diagnosis, and management. *SOGC Clinical Practice Guideline,* no. 295 (August). Accessed May 26, 2016. http://sogc.org/wp-content/uploads/2013/08/gui295CPG1308E.pdf.

Lawn, J. E., H. Blencowe, S. Oza, D. You, A. C. C. Lee, P. Waiswa, M. Lalli, Z. Bhutta, A. J. D. Barros, and P. Christian. 2014. Every newborn: Progress, priorities, and potential beyond survival. *Lancet* 384:189–205. doi:10.1016/S0140-6736(14)60496-7. Epub 2014.

Lawn, J. E., H. Blencowe, R. Pattinson, S. Cousens, R. Kumar, I. Ibiebele, J. Gardosi, I. T. Day, and C. Stanton. 2011. Stillbirths: Where? When? Why? How to make the data count? *Lancet* 377:1448–1463. doi:10.1016/S0140-6736(10)62187-3. Epub 2011.

Lawn, J. E., M. G. Gravett, T. M. Nunes, C. E. Rubens, and C. Stanton. 2010. Global report on preterm birth and stillbirth (1 of 7): Definitions, description of the burden and opportunities to improve data. *BMC Pregnancy Childbirth* 10 (S1): S1. doi:10.1186/1471-2393-10-S1-S1.

Lee, A. C. C., S. Cousens, G. L. Darmstadt, H. Blencowe, R. Pattinson, N. F. Moran, G. J. Hofmeyr, R. A. Haws, S. Z. Bhutta, and J. E Lawn. 2011. Care during labor and birth for the prevention of intrapartum-related neonatal deaths: A systematic review and Delphi estimation of mortality effect. *BMC Public Health* 11 (S3): S10. doi:10.1186/1471-2458-11-S3-S10.

Rubens, C., M. Gravett, C. Victora, T. Nunes; GAPPS Review Group. 2010. Global report on preterm birth and stillbirth (7 of 7): Mobilizing resources to accelerate innovative solutions (Global Action Agenda). *BMC Pregnancy Childbirth* 10 (S1): S7. doi:10.1186/1471-2393-10-S1-S7.

Sather, M., A-V. R. Fajon, R. Zaentz, and C. E. Rubens. 2010. Global report on preterm birth and stillbirth (5 of 7): Advocacy barriers and opportunities. *BMC Pregnancy Childbirth* 10 (S1): S5. doi:10.1186/1471-2393-10-S-S5.

Syed, M., H. Javed, M. Y. Yakoob, and Z. A. Bhutta. 2011. Effect of screening and management of diabetes during pregnancy on stillbirths. *BMC Public Health* 11 (S3): S2. doi:10.1186/1471-2458-11-S3-S2.

UNICEF. 2013. *Levels & Trends in Child Mortality: Estimates Developed by the UN Inter-agency Group for Child Mortality Estimation.* New York: UNICEF.

WHO (World Health Organization). 2014. "Maternal, Newborn, Child and Adolescent Health: Stillbirths." Accessed May 26, 2016. http://www.who.int/maternal _child_adolescent/epidemiology/stillbirth/en/.

Yakoob, M. Y., M. A. Ali, M. U. Ali, A. Imdad, J. Lawn, N. Van Den Broek, and Z. A. Bhutta. 2011. The effect of providing skilled birth attendance and emergency obstetric care in preventing stillbirths. *BMC Public Health* 11 (S3): S7. doi:10.1186/ 1471-2458-11-S3-S7.

4

Obstetric Fistula

L. LEWIS WALL

A *fistula* is an abnormal communication between two body cavities lined with epithelium that are not normally connected. An *obstetric fistula* is one that develops as the result of obstetrical trauma, usually between the vagina and the bladder *(vesicovaginal fistula)* or between the vagina and the rectum *(rectovaginal fistula)* (see Figure 4.1). Genitourinary fistulas are rare in higher-resource countries with well-developed health-care systems, where they are often the result of surgical misadventure (a complication of hysterectomy or other pelvic surgery), radiation therapy, or invasive cancer itself (Brown et al. 2012; Hilton and Cromwell 2012). Rectovaginal fistulas in industrialized countries are most commonly caused by inflammatory bowel disease, surgical misadventure, or complications of episiotomies or lacerations during vaginal delivery (Champagne and McGee 2010). In lower-resource countries where the health-care infrastructure is poorly developed or does not function well, the major cause of genitourinary fistula is pressure necrosis of the vesicovaginal septum from prolonged obstructed labor (Wall 2006; Wall et al. 2004; Muleta, Rasmussen, and Kiserud 2010; Onsrud, Sjoveian, and Mukwege 2011). In some cases a fistula may also develop as the direct result of tearing or cutting of tissues, such as during an instrumental delivery in which the perineum and anorectum are lacerated or as the result of traditional genital cutting procedures such as *gishiri* among the Hausa of West Africa (Tukur, Jido, and Uzoho 2006). A significant number of fistula cases also result from sexual trauma owing to the exploitation of young girls who are not yet physically ready for intercourse or as acts of terrorism in politically unstable regions (Longombe, Claude, and Ruminjo 2008).

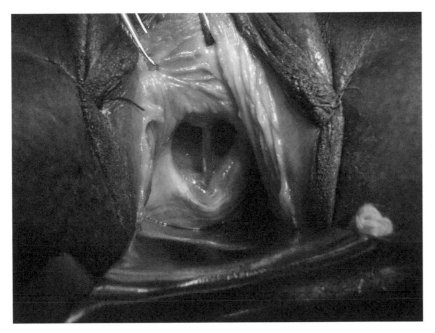

FIGURE 4.1.
Obstetric vesicovaginal fistula. A metal probe has been passed through the urethra and is clearly visible within the bladder.

PATHOPHYSIOLOGY OF OBSTETRIC FISTULA

The pathophysiology of fistula formation differs completely between obstetric fistula and postsurgical vesicovaginal fistula. The latter develops as the result of a discrete injury to otherwise normal tissue; the former (after prolonged obstructed labor) is the result of a field injury in which the surrounding tissues themselves have also been seriously injured (Wall 2006).

A posthysterectomy fistula usually develops as the result of a specific injury to the bladder that allows urine to escape into the pelvis. The escaping urine pools at the vaginal cuff, where it interferes with normal wound healing. Eventually the urine drains out between the nonhealing edges of the vaginal incision, and a fistula tract forms between the bladder and the vagina. In most cases these fistulas are discrete, relatively small (only a few millimeters in size), and easily identifiable near the vaginal apex. The surrounding tissue is usually normal.

The pathophysiology is radically different in an obstetric fistula, which forms not as the result of a discrete injury to normal tissue but rather as the result of pressure necrosis of the vesicovaginal septum (Arrowsmith, Hamlin, and Wall 1996). When labor is obstructed, the fetus cannot pass through the birth canal in spite of adequate contractions. Obstructed labor usually develops from cephalopelvic disproportion or sometimes from fetal malpresentation. In these cases, the space in the birth canal is too tight to allow normal obstetrical mechanics, and labor comes to a halt. The fetal head (or other presenting part) becomes trapped in the pelvis. However, because labor is involuntary once it begins, the uterus continues to contract in a futile effort to force the fetus past the point of obstruction (Figure 4.2). The soft tissues of the mother's pelvis (bladder, rectum, urethra, cervix, and so on) become trapped between the fetal head and her pelvic bones. Because the pressure of the fetal head often compresses the bladder neck and urethra tightly against the pubic symphysis during obstructed labor, many women in this condition are unable to urinate.

Not only does this problem greatly increase the pain such women experience, but as the bladder becomes more and more overdistended, its walls become thinner and thinner, making them progressively more vulnerable to ischemic injury the longer labor continues. Over time, the uterine contractions apply enough pressure to interrupt the blood flow to the entrapped tissues. If labor is not terminated promptly, the compressed tissues will become asphyxiated and die. When necrosis of the vesicovaginal septum occurs, a fistula forms, but the tissues surrounding the fistula are often severely injured even though they are still living. The result may be the formation of wide, thick bands of scar tissue that dramatically change the contours of the vagina and make surgical repair much more difficult.

Figure 4.3 illustrates the five major components that contribute to the ultimate location and nature of an obstetric fistula: the degree of fetopelvic disproportion, the level of the obstruction in the birth canal, the force applied to the entrapped tissues, the duration of the compression, and the inherent resiliency of the tissues affected (largely influenced by maternal health and nutritional status). The complex interplay of these five factors means that there is no absolute time limit at which a fistula will form during obstructed labor. When the obstruction is tangential and the uterine contractile forces are relatively weak, labor may be prolonged for several days with relatively little tissue damage; on the other hand, if the obstruction is severe and the uterine contractions are strong and unyielding, substantial damage may occur in a relatively short period of time. The only reliable way to prevent the formation of a fistula during obstructed labor is early diagnosis and intervention.

The degree of damage that obstructed labor produces in the female pelvis is also quite variable. Some fistulas are only a millimeter or two in size, yet in other cases nearly all of the soft tissues of the pelvis are obliter-

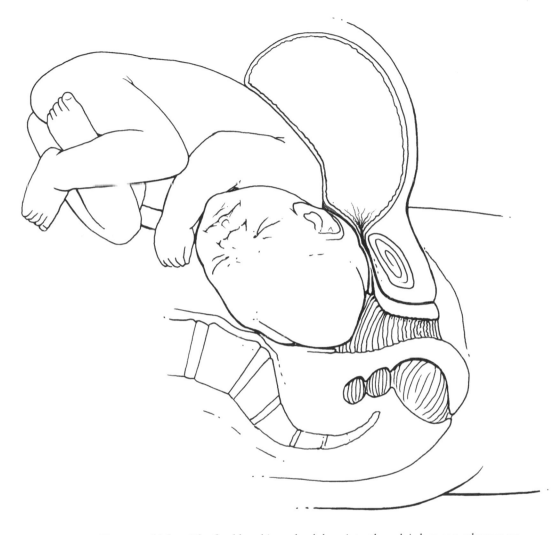

FIGURE 4.2. Obstructed labor. The fetal head is wedged deep into the pelvis but can advance no further. The parietal bones are overlapping. Pressure from the fetal head has compressed the soft tissues of the vagina, urethra, and bladder neck, preventing the laboring woman from urinating. The bladder is becoming progressively more distended and vulnerable to pressure necrosis.

ated, creating injuries that are truly breathtaking. John St. George once described a fistula patient whom he had examined shortly after her delivery: "The patient, who was aged 18, was brought to the hospital three days after delivery, following labour which lasted seven days. She was incontinent of urine and faeces . . . very pale . . . dehydrated, toxic, and unable to walk. Vaginal examination revealed a gaping opening with offensive

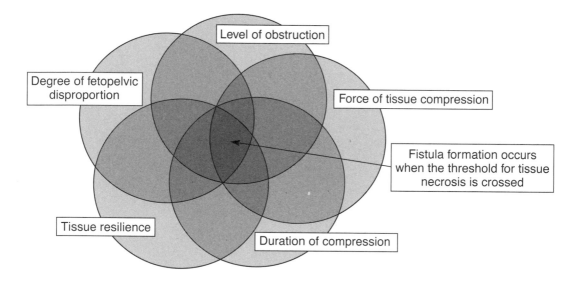

FIGURE 4.3. Interplay of pathophysiological factors in obstetric fistula formation.

purulent lochia and discharge. The lateral walls of the vagina had sloughed, revealing both pubic rami and the right ischial tuberosity. The perineum was torn, leaving an indefinite anal sphincter. A large vesico-vaginal fistula and a small recto-vaginal fistula, both with infected edges, were seen" (St. George 1969, 742).

Owing to the variability of factors depicted in Figure 4.3, almost any area of the pelvis may be injured as the result of obstructed labor. Although attention generally focuses on genitourinary and rectovaginal fistulas, a wide spectrum of other injuries known collectively as the obstructed-labor injury complex is often seen in women who have suffered from prolonged obstructed labor (Table 4.1) (Arrowsmith et al. 1996). The presence of these comorbidities complicates the long-term treatment and recovery of women with obstetric fistulas.

In developing countries some vesicovaginal fistulas may be classified as diseases of medical progress, that is, they are side effects or complications of otherwise generally beneficial developments in medical care that would not arise otherwise (Moser 1956). For example, before surgical operations such as hysterectomy were available, women did not develop fistulas as a complication of such surgery. As these surgical procedures became more accessible, the number of associated complications also rose, even though the total number of fistulas fell owing to the greater

Table 4.1 Spectrum of injuries in the obstructed labor injury complex

Acute obstetric injury
- Hemorrhage, especially post-partum hemorrhage resulting from uterine atony
- Intrauterine infection and/or systemic sepsis
- Deep venous thrombosis
- Massive vulvar edema
- Pathological uterine contraction ring (Bandl's ring)
- Uterine rupture

Gynecologic injury
- Amenorrhea
- Vaginal scarring and stenosis, often with loss of coital function
- Cervical damage, including complete loss of the cervix
- Secondary pelvic inflammatory disease
- Secondary infertility

Musculoskeletal injury
- Osteitis pubis and related injuries to the pelvic bones
- Diffuse trauma to the pelvic floor

Dermatological injury
- Chronic excoriation of the skin from maceration by urine and feces

Psychosocial injury
- Social isolation
- Separation and divorce
- Worsening poverty
- Malnutrition
- Depression, sometimes leading to suicide

Urologic injury
- Vesicovaginal fistula and complex combinations of other fistulas (urethrovaginal, ureterovaginal, vesicocervical, vesicouterine, and so on)
- Urethral damage, including complete urethral loss
- Bladder stone formation
- Urinary stress incontinence
- Secondary hydroureteronephrosis and chronic pyelonephritis
- Renal failure

Gastrointestinal injury
- Rectovaginal fistula
- Acquired rectal atresia
- Anal sphincter injury with resulting anal incontinence

Neurological injury
- Foot-drop
- Neuropathic bladder dysfunction

Fetal or neonatal injury
- Approximately 95% perinatal-case fatality rate
- Neonatal sepsis
- Neonatal birth asphyxia
- Neonatal birth injury, including scalp necrosis, nerve palsies, intracranial hemorrhage

Source: Reprinted from Arrowsmith, Hamlin, and Wall (1996), Table 1. © 1996 Williams & Wilkins.

availability of surgical operations such as cesarean section. In developed countries the number of obstetric and genitourinary fistulas has decreased dramatically, but the percentage of fistulas that result from surgical misadventure and radiation therapy has increased. The spread of bioscientific medical and surgical technology to low-resource countries will most likely replicate this pattern.

In a review of 164 genitourinary fistulas at Komfo Anokye Teaching Hospital in Kumasi, Ghana, between 1977 and 1982, nearly 92% of cases were associated with obstetric complications, but twelve women (7.2% of cases) developed fistulas during complicated hysterectomies for large uterine tumors (Danso et al. 1996). Similar observations have been made in other parts of the world as better obstetric care reduces the prevalence of prolonged labor and access to other medical and surgical interventions increases (Onsrud, Sjoveian, and Mukwege 2011; Kochakarn and Pummagnura 2000). For example, in 230 cases of vesicovaginal fistula treated at Ramathibodi Hospital in Bangkok, Thailand, between 1969 and 1997, only ten fistulas were the result of prolonged or difficult childbirth; the rest occurred as complications of radiation therapy, hysterectomy, invasive cervical cancer, pelvic fracture, or other causes (Kochakarn and Pummagnura 2000). When a follow-up study was later done at the same institution covering the years 1998 to 2005, during which an additional forty-five fistula cases were reported, none was the result of obstetric trauma; the majority of new cases were complications of laparoscopic hysterectomies (Kochakarn and Pummagnura 2007).

CLASSIFICATION OF OBSTETRIC FISTULAS

Although many different variations have been proposed, there is as yet no generally accepted classification system for obstetric fistulas. The simplest classification systems describe the location of the fistula and the structures involved, for example, urethrovaginal fistula, midvaginal vesicovaginal fistula, juxtacervical fistula, uterovaginal fistula, ureterovaginal fistula, rectovaginal fistula, "circumferential" fistula (in which the urethra is detached from the rest of the bladder), and so on. There is a growing consensus that the most important variables with respect to the surgical cure of obstetric fistulas are location, size, and the amount of scarring in the surrounding tissues (Goh et al. 2008; Nardos, Browning, and Chen 2009; Frajzyngier et al. 2013). The most important functions of a classification system are to allow the communication of standardized clinical information among medical centers, researchers, and surgeons caring for fistula patients, and, as with various cancer-staging systems, to collect information that supports accurate prognosis, that is, How will this patient fare after surgery? When all is said and done, is this a fistula that can be closed with satisfactory clinical results?

The simplest classification system that attempts to answer such questions is one proposed by the World Health Organization, which divides fistulas into "simple" and "complicated" (Lewis and de Bernis 2006). Classification elements are shown in Table 4.2.

This is certainly a useful protocol for screening cases that should be sent to an experienced fistula surgeon. However, more useful for research purposes is the classification system described by Judith Goh (2004) (Table 4.3), which is similar to the staging systems used in cancer treatment and research. The Goh system has been validated and appears to correlate reasonably well with surgical outcomes (Goh et al. 2008; Goh et al. 2009).

Table 4.2   WHO classifications of simple versus complicated fistulas

Criterion	Simple case with good prognosis	Complicated case with uncertain prognosis
Number of fistulas	Single fistula	Multiple fistulas
Site	Isolated vesicovaginal or rectovaginal fistula	Combined vesicovaginal and rectovaginal fistula, involvement of the cervix
Size (diameter)	Less than or equal to four centimeters	Greater than four centimeters
Involvement of the urethra and continence mechanism	No	Yes
Vaginal scarring	No	Yes
Circumferential defect (complete separation of the urethra from the bladder)	No	Yes
Degree of tissue loss	Minimal	Extensive
Ureteral and bladder involvement	Ureters are inside the bladder, not draining into the vagina	Ureters drain directly into the vagina; bladder stones may be present
Previous attempts at repair	None	Previous attempts at repair have failed

Source: Modified from Lewis and de Bernis (2006), Annex A. © World Health Organization 2006.

Table 4.3   Goh classification and characteristics of genitourinary fistulas

Location: Distance from the external urethral meatus
  1. Distal edge of the fistula greater than 3.5 centimeters from external meatus
  2. Distal edge 2.5 to 3.5 centimeters from external meatus
  3. Distal edge 1.5 to 2.5 centimeters from external meatus
  4. Distal edge less than 1.5 cm from external meatus

Size: Largest dimension of the fistula in centimeters
  A. less than 1.5 centimeters
  B. 1.5 to 3 centimeters
  C. Greater than 3 centimeters

Special considerations
  i. None or mild fibrosis and vaginal length greater than or equal to six centimeters, normal capacity
  ii. Moderate or severe fibrosis and/or marked reduction in vaginal length and/or capacity
  iii. Special circumstances, for example, postirradiation, ureteric involvement, circumferential defect (urethra completely separated from the bladder), previous repair, and so on.

Source: Reprinted from Goh (2004). © Royal Australian and New Zealand College of Obstetricians and Gynaecologists 2004.

EPIDEMIOLOGY OF OBSTETRIC FISTULA

Who gets an obstetric fistula, and why? Obstetric fistulas are caused by prolonged obstructed labor when the diagnosis is delayed and competent obstetric care is not available. As Figure 4.3 demonstrates, a combination of factors must coincide before tissue necrosis occurs and a fistula develops. As stated above, there is no clearly delimited length of time that a woman must be in obstructed labor before a fistula occurs, so appropriate intervention should follow diagnosis of obstructed labor as quickly as possible. The woman afflicted with a fistula typically gives a history of having labored for several days, but fistulas may occur in labors lasting less than twenty-four hours if the conditions for injury are right (Emmet 1879). AbouZahr (2003) has estimated that obstructed labor occurs in roughly 4.6% of human births, giving a worldwide incidence of around 6 million cases per year. Case series document that up to 7% of women in obstructed labor develop an obstetric fistula, depending on whether they receive timely access to competent emergency obstetric care (Wall 2012a).

Because obstetric fistula is a highly stigmatizing condition, women suffering from this condition are often part of a hidden population, living on the margins of society and not easily accessible to researchers or to public view. For example, the government of Kenya estimates that 3,000 new cases of fistula occur in that country every year, but only 7.5% are reported and receive treatment (Roka et al. 2013). Estimates based on relatively soft data suggest that between 30,000 and 130,000 new fistula cases occur in sub-Saharan Africa each year (Wall 2006; Vangeenderhuysen, Prual, and Ould el Joud 2001), and because fistula patients often live for decades after their initial injuries, this means that there are hundreds of thousands (if not several millions) of women worldwide living in the miserable circumstances associated with an obstetric fistula. Who are they?

Several studies comparing women with fistulas with normal parous controls have delineated risk factors linked to obstetric fistula formation (Roka et al. 2013; Ojanuga and Ekwmpu 1999): young age at marriage (with consequent childbearing before pelvic growth is complete), earlier age at first pregnancy, short stature (linked to smaller pelvic capacity), illiteracy or low levels of education, poverty, residence in rural areas (linked to greater distances to health-care facilities), lack of antenatal care, and most important, a greater history of prolonged labor compared with parous controls. The pathway to obstetric fistula offered in Figure 4.4 suggests how these risk factors are linked.

THE EXISTENTIAL SITUATION OF THE FISTULA PATIENT

In a very real sense, the development of an obstetric fistula is a body blow to the unfortunate woman who is afflicted with this condition. Obstructed labor is a traumatic and physically exhausting event that may last for days. To have one's child stillborn at the end of a week of obstructed labor is heartbreaking. This by itself is enough to cause profound psychological trauma in many women (Furuta, Sandall, and Bick 2012), but to combine the pain of obstructed labor and the loss of her child with constant leakage of urine or stool is overwhelming. To add foot-drop, chronic dermatitis, or any of the multiple other injuries that can occur as part of the obstructed-labor injury complex makes these circumstances nearly unendurable.

In one fell swoop, the fistula victim regresses from being an autonomous adult in full control of her bodily functions to an infantile being who is no longer able to contain her bodily wastes. Women who develop a fistula at the end of their first pregnancy go from being poised on the threshold of motherhood, with all of the cultural status and social

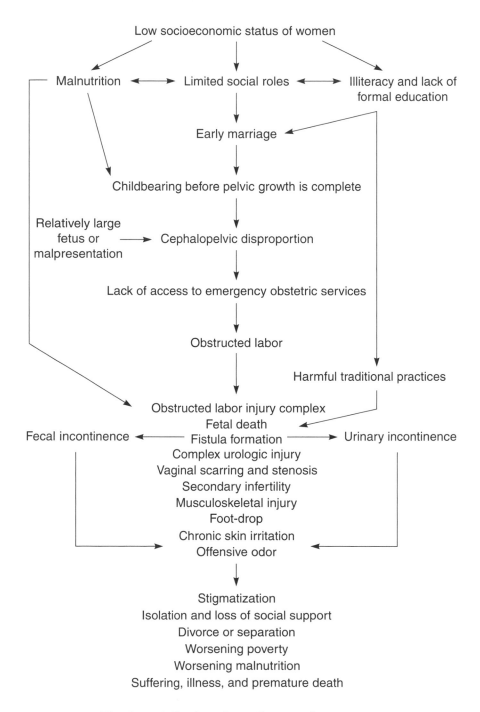

FIGURE 4.4. The obstetric fistula pathway: Causes and consequences.

expectations this entails, to childless, damaged goods with limited future prospects. If a woman has other young children to look after, her injuries may make the tasks she is expected to perform difficult, if not impossible, with damaging consequences for the dependent children. Containing the leakage of urine and stool and minimizing the smell that inevitably results from incontinence may be physically exhausting, if not impossible. The increasing strain on friendships, family, and social relationships produced by the unending trickle of urine often results in physical isolation, social ostracism, and ruptured family ties. In many cultures the constant presence of liquid or solid excrement renders fistula sufferers ritually—as well as physically—unclean. This prevents them from participating in social or religious rituals that would normally be a source of comfort and meaning in their lives. It is no surprise that psychological surveys of women with obstetric fistulas reveal widespread depression, deep dissatisfaction with their lives, constant worries about social and economic relationships, and profound levels of insecurity (Wall 2002; Yeakey et al. 2009).

How such women are treated and how they respond varies widely depending on individual circumstances. In some cases their husbands remain loyal and supportive in spite of their injuries, even fathering other children despite the fistula. In some cases the strain on family relationships is too great for the marriage to bear, and the women are sent away to live with their parents or to survive on their own as best they can. In other cases these women are abused and treated cruelly as the stigma associated with a fistula boils over into overt physical violence. Some women endure their condition with a profound dignity in spite of the terrible circumstances in which they find themselves, while others succumb to despair and commit suicide. Each case is different but involves similar challenges: how to mend a broken body while supporting and sustaining the spirit of the woman who lives within it.

ETHICAL PREREQUISITES FOR FISTULA REPAIR

The fundamental prerequisite for ethical fistula surgery is straightforward: The operation should not be performed unless the patient will receive care that meets or exceeds the minimal requirements for safe, effective, competent, and compassionate surgery. The best interests of the patient should be the first priority of the operating team. Surgeons should have adequate experience in fistula-repair surgery under equivalent circumstances (which are sometimes less than ideal). There should be adequate anesthesia (usually spinal), lighting, intravenous fluids, medications (antibiotics, analgesics), suture material, and surgical equipment. There should be competent postoperative nursing care, including the ability to monitor vital signs and ensure adequate catheter drainage. Patients should receive adequate pain relief, both during and after surgery. To operate on a fistula patient without anesthesia because the operating surgeon finds it more convenient is flatly unethical (Waaldijk 1994). Patients should be provided with adequate food, clothing, and shelter while recovering from their operations. If the surgeon does not speak the local language, an interpreter should be readily available. There must be a backup plan for emergency situations when the operating surgeon is unavailable and problems arise. An old surgical adage says that "patients don't die from complications; they die from the complications of complications." The obstetric-fistula surgeon must understand that what might be a minor complication in a European or North American hospital could end catastrophically in an impoverished setting where resources may be scarce. Fistula repair is elective, scheduled surgery; the logistics of surgical planning must reflect this, and high standards of care must be upheld (Wall et al. 2008).

TREATMENT AND GUIDELINES FOR CARE

Initial Evaluation of the Patient with a Suspected Fistula

The initial evaluation of a patient suspected of having an obstetric fistula should begin by confirming the presence of the injury. A fistula should be suspected when a woman complains of continuous urine loss starting after a prolonged labor, but the diagnosis must be confirmed. This is usually fairly straightforward. On speculum examination there is usually a pool of urine in the posterior vagina, and a defect through which the urine escapes can usually be seen (or palpated). However, smaller fistulas (particularly those that persist after previous attempts at repair) may not be readily discernible. Sometimes the fistula cannot be identified until an examination under anesthesia is carried out in the operating room using a speculum, lateral retraction of the vagina, and high-quality lighting.

The diagnosis of a fistula can usually be confirmed with a simple dye test. Sterile water is mixed with five milliliters of methylene blue or indigo carmine dye. A size 14 Foley catheter is inserted into the urethra and attached to a sixty-milliliter irrigating syringe. The urethra should be compressed with a gauze sponge to prevent leakage of dye around the catheter. The bladder is then filled incrementally with colored water while the vagina is inspected. Leakage of dye documents the location of the fistula (though it should be kept in mind that patients may have more than one fistula). The size and location of the fistula should be recorded, along with appropriate measurements and any complicating factors according to the preferred fistula-classification system.

Small fistulas, especially if they are fresh (less than three months old), may heal spontaneously if the bladder is catheterized and allowed to drain continuously for several weeks. Such a strategy may alleviate the need for surgery, particularly in patients who are markedly debilitated and need time to recuperate from their travail or who have other major comorbidities that preclude immediate operative intervention.

Basic Principles of Obstetric Fistula Repair

Although the conditions under which operations are performed and the tools that are available to aid the surgeon have been enormously refined over the last 150 years, the basic principles necessary to achieve successful closure of an obstetric fistula have not changed since Sims and others enumerated them in the nineteenth century (Sims 1852; Emmet 1868):

- excellent exposure of the fistula achieved through broad mobilization of the surrounding tissues so that the hole can be closed without tension
- watertight closure
- adequate emptying of the bladder postoperatively so that repair does not become overdistended and break down

However, application of these straightforward principles to any individual case may be quite challenging, especially when the fistula is complex. Successful fistula closure often requires dexterity, ingenuity, and improvisation. No single drawing or series of drawings can describe the steps necessary to achieve successful closure of fistulas in all their possible variation. The basic principles of fistula repair (using a simple midvaginal fistula as an example) are illustrated in Figures 4.5 and 4.6.

Successful fistula repair starts by exposing the entire fistula as completely as possible so that it may be closed without tension. Many fistula

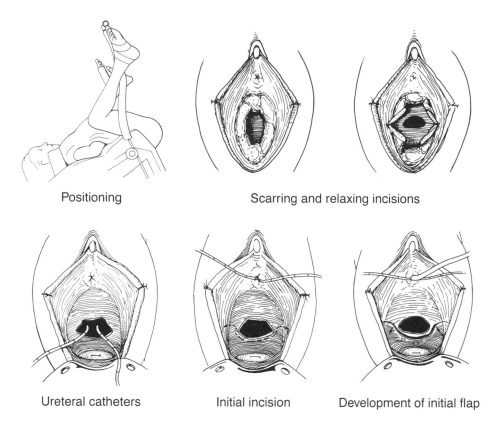

Positioning   Scarring and relaxing incisions

Ureteral catheters   Initial incision   Development of initial flap

FIGURE 4.5. *Positioning the patient.* For transvaginal repair of an obstetrical fistula, the patient must be positioned to gain maximum exposure of the operative site. This is best achieved by putting the woman in a high lithotomy position with the buttocks extending well over the edge of the operating table and the table tilted into steep, head-down Trendelenberg position. Good lighting (including the use of a surgical headlamp) is mandatory.

Exposure of the fistula. The illustration on the left-hand side depicts a vagina that has been narrowed by heavy scarring, making the fistula difficult to see. Relaxing incisions have been made in several places to gain exposure in the illustration on the right-hand side.

Catheterization of the ureters. Knowledge of the location of the ureters is extremely important in fistula repair since closure of the fistula may lead to inadvertent ureteral damage. The use of small caliber (5 Fr) whistle-tip or olive-tip ureteral catheters is very helpful. The ureters can usually be visualized through the fistula, particularly if it is large. After ureteral catheterization, a small clamp should be introduced into the bladder through the urethra and used to pull the free ends of the ureteral catheters out through the urethra so that they will not be directly in the operative field. After the fistula is closed, the ureteral catheters may generally be removed.

Initial incision. The initial incision is made along the posterior border of the fistula at the vesicovaginal junction. The incision should be extended as far laterally as possible, even out along the lateral vaginal sidewalls. The purpose of the large incision is to allow wide mobilization of the tissues around the fistula so that it can be closed without any tension on the suture line. This is particularly important when there is heavy scarring around the fistula.

Posterior extension of the initial incision. Once the initial incision has been made, a flap of tissue should be developed posteriorly, freeing the vagina from the bladder. Much of this dissection can be carried out bluntly, using a finger, once the incision has been made.

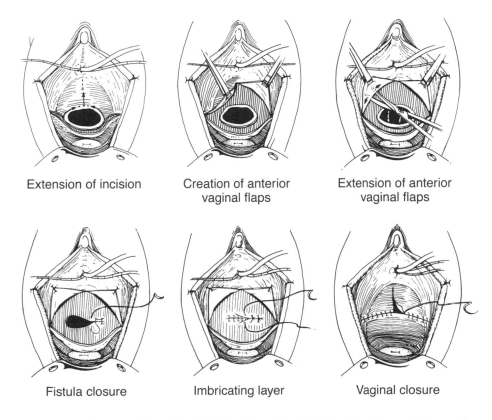

Extension of incision	Creation of anterior vaginal flaps	Extension of anterior vaginal flaps
Fistula closure	Imbricating layer	Vaginal closure

FIGURE 4.6. Anterior extension of the initial incision. The initial incision is carried circumferentially around the entire fistula and then up the anterior vaginal wall toward the urethra. Once again, the purpose is to mobilize all tissues away from the fistula as extensively as possible so that the defect can be closed without tension.

Creation of anterior vaginal flaps. After the circumferential incision has been completed, the dissection is carried laterally to create broad vaginal flaps.

Penetrating the retropubic space of Retzius. In many cases it is necessary to dissect up under the pubic rami to free the fistula completely, particularly if extensive scarring is present. This further increases lateral mobility of the bladder and the vagina.

Initial closure of the fistula. The defect in the bladder is closed using absorbable suture and a continuous stitch. If possible, a second layer should be added for reinforcement. After the fistula is closed, a dye test should be performed instilling roughly 250 milliliters of sterile water colored with indigo carmine or methylene blue dye, to check the integrity of the repair.

Second layer closure of the fistula. A second layer of imbricating stitches (either interrupted or continuous) may be placed to reinforce the initial repair.

Vaginal closure. Once the fistula has been closed and the integrity of the repair has been assured by a dye test, the vaginal mucosa may be closed using continuous or interrupted absorbable sutures. The ureteral catheters may be removed at the end of the case, unless special considerations are present. An indwelling Foley catheter should be placed to insure continuous drainage of the bladder until it has healed.

operations fail because the fistula was never completely mobilized. Sometimes this may require opening almost all of the anterior vagina, as well as dissecting into the retropubic space of Retzius. When extensive vaginal scarring is present, relaxing incisions or episiotomies may be needed to obtain full exposure.

Once the fistula has been fully exposed and mobilized, it may be closed with a continuous running suture of delayed-absorbable material such as 3–0 polyglactin 910 (Vicryl, Ethicon, Somerville, NJ). Interrupted sutures may also be used. There is some debate as to whether a second layer of imbricating sutures is required in routine fistula repair. Where possible, such a closure seems prudent, but extensive scarring or substantial loss of bladder tissue may sometimes make a two-layer closure impossible. The use of absorbable sutures is preferred. If permanent sutures are used in fistula repair, they may become the nidus around which a bladder or vaginal stone forms. This can lead to the breakdown of the closure and always creates pain and discomfort for the patient. If permanent sutures are used, they should be removed seven to ten days after surgery to prevent such problems.

After fistula closure, the integrity of the repair should be confirmed with a dye test. Approximately 150 to 250 milliliters of a solution of sterile water and indigo carmine or methylene blue dye should be instilled into the bladder through a transurethral catheter. As the bladder is filled, the site of the repair should be carefully inspected for any leakage of dye. If a leak is discovered, the repair must be revised until it is watertight; otherwise failure is almost guaranteed.

Once the fistula has been repaired, the overlying vagina is closed using either interrupted or running absorbable sutures. Most surgeons place a tight gauze pack in the vagina for one or two days after surgery to improve hemostasis and support the healing tissues.

Following surgery, the bladder must be drained to prevent overdistension of the suture line while the wound heals. The conventional wisdom of postoperative fistula care is to drain the bladder for two weeks or more, but there are few hard data to support the fourteen-day rule. Nardos, Member, and Browning (2012) have shown that catheter drainage can be decreased to ten days without compromising the results of surgery. It may well be that catheters can be removed as early as three or four days after surgery if the patient is able to void normally and empties her bladder completely. It may also be that clean intermittent self-catheterization rather than continuous catheterization works well in patients with uncomplicated fistulas. Decreasing the duration of postoperative catheterization is important, because a shorter duration could shorten the time patients must spend on the ward, thus increasing the surgical capacity of busy fistula units. Nevertheless, such changes in clinical care should be evaluated through well-designed clinical trials before they are implemented (Barone et al. 2012).

A further controversy in fistula repair involves the use of tissue flaps. Because obstetric fistula results from a crush injury in the pelvis that produces tissue necrosis, the idea that wound healing could be improved by interposing a flap of healthy tissue with a robust blood supply into the surgical repair is attractive. The most accessible location for developing such a flap is the vulva. There is always a suitable fat pad overlying the bulbo-cavernosus muscle within one of the labia majora. Originally described by Martius (Elkins, Delancey, and McGruie 1990), the bulbocavernosus flap is created by opening the labium, freeing up the underlying fat pad, transecting its superior attachments while maintaining the vascular pedicle inferiorly, and then rotating the flap into the vagina through a tunnel created at the base of the labium and tacking it into place over the fistula repair using absorbable sutures (Elkins, Delancey, and McGruie 1990). The bed from which the graft was harvested is then closed in layers, the labial incision is closed with a running suture, and a pressure dressing is applied to prevent formation of a hematoma. The vaginal epithelium is then closed over the fistula repair.

However, few clinical studies have evaluated the efficacy of the Martius bulbocavernosus flap in fistula repair. In a retrospective review of forty-six obstetric fistula repairs in India, done with and without the use of a Martius flap (Rangnekar et al. 2000), the authors reported that patients whose repair used a flap had better postoperative results. On the other hand, Browning (2004) analyzed 440 fistula repairs in Ethiopia with and without the use of a Martius flap and found no significant difference in outcomes between the two groups. He attributed the high rates of success attained in both groups to the experience of the surgeon rather than the use of a flap.

PERSISTENT INCONTINENCE AFTER FISTULA REPAIR

No one is as disheartened as a patient who has had an obstetric fistula repair but remains wet after surgery. For this reason, patients should have realistic expectations about fistula surgery. Preoperative counseling concerning the process of surgery and its possible outcomes should be part of every surgical operation. One of the best ways to do this is by training obstetric-fistula patients who have undergone surgery themselves to be peer counselors, who can then explain the process to other women in their own terms. Even with expert care, there is still a risk that the patient may be incontinent after surgery. The risk of persistent incontinence goes up with the number of previous attempts at fistula repair. Even when the fistula has been closed successfully, the patient may still experience transurethral incontinence, a discrepancy that has been called the "continence gap" (Wall and Arrowsmith 2007). Postoperative incontinence after fistula repair is a result of either a persistent fistula ("failed closure") or transurethral incontinence in the presence of successful closure of the fistula ("closed but wet.")

In such cases it is important to determine whether a fistula is still present using the dye test described above. A dye test may reveal a small fistula relatively far from the operative site that was previously overlooked or defects at the site of fistula repair. If the repair was unsuccessful, it is probably prudent to wait at least six weeks before attempting another repair. If the residual defect is small, prolonged catheterization for several weeks may allow the fistula to heal. Each case must be evaluated individually.

If there is urine in the vagina but the dye test reveals no leakage of dye, a previously undetected ureterovaginal fistula should be suspected. Careful inspection of the vagina may reveal clear urine spurting from the injured ureter, but this is not always obvious. In problematic cases, a ureterovaginal fistula may be confirmed by giving the patient an oral dye (such as phenazopyridine hydrochloride, which is orange). The presence of blue dye in the bladder but orange urine entering the vagina confirms the diagnosis of a ureterovaginal fistula. If intravenous urography is available, a ureterovaginal fistula may be documented radiographically; unfortunately, this technology is usually not available in low-resource settings.

Once extraurethral urine loss has been excluded, the patient will probably be found to have transurethral urinary incontinence from one of the following conditions: urinary stress incontinence owing to an incompetence urethral closure mechanism (often caused by trauma to urethra or bladder neck); detrusor overactivity (uninhibited bladder contractions); incomplete bladder emptying; a bladder stone (more common if some time has elapsed since the fistula repair, particularly if nonabsorbable sutures were used during surgery); or combinations of the above. In the past, it was largely assumed that all of these women had stress incontinence. More recent investigations have disproven this assumption (Goh et al. 2013).

Under ideal circumstances, patients who fall into the continence gap should undergo urodynamic assessment. Unfortunately, most fistula centers lack the capability to perform subtracted cystometry and other technical evaluations of bladder function. Nonetheless, systematic evaluation of such patients will often produce a working diagnosis that can guide further therapy. The patient should be examined with a full bladder and asked to cough. If transurethral loss of urine is observed coincident with the cough, the patient likely has stress incontinence. Such patients may benefit from a course of rigorous, supervised pelvic muscle rehabilitation. Because such interventions carry very low risk, they may be offered to all such patients as the first line of therapy. Individual instruction and supervision by a trained physical therapist will be extremely beneficial. If stress incontinence surgery is performed, the most effective treatment is likely to be some form of sling operation that supports and partially closes the urethra and bladder neck. Such operations are best done using autologous abdominal or rectus fascia (Browning 2006). The synthetic mesh sling operations popular for ordinary stress incontinence in higher-resource countries are associated with high rates of erosion and should be avoided in women who have had an obstetric fistula (Ascher-Walsh et al. 2010).

An attractive alternative to sling surgery in women with severely damaged urethras is the removable urethral plug (Femsoft, Rochester Medical Corporation, Stewartville, MN) (Goh and Browning 2005). The insert closes the urethra, is removed by the patient every three hours to void, and is then reinserted. As is the case with other advanced-technology treatments (such as urinary-diversion procedures that require ongoing supervision or the use of catheters, bags, or appliances), long-term access to supplies may be problematic. Logistical issues of this kind should be considered before embarking upon complicated surgical strategies.

A great deal of information can be obtained by simple retrograde filling of the bladder with sterile water through a catheter at the bedside (Videla and Wall 1998). The diagnosis of stress incontinence has been described. Similarly, if there is a sudden gush of fluid accompanied by a rise in the column of water attached to the filling catheter during filling, the problem is likely to be detrusor overactivity, particularly when this finding is accompanied by a history of frequency and urgency. These patients often benefit from a bladder-retraining program and anticholinergic medications. The anticholinergic drugs most widely prescribed in the high-resource countries are rarely available at an affordable price in the countries where fistulas are prevalent. The most commonly available drug is probably hyoscine butylbromide (Buscopan, Boehringer Ingelheim, Ingelheim, Germany), given in doses of ten to twenty milligrams four times per day. Alternatively, generic oxybutynin chloride may be helpful if available, given in doses of five milligrams three to four times per day. However, particularly in rural areas it may be difficult to gain consistent access to supplies of these medications.

Patients who are still incontinent after fistula closure should have a postvoid residual urine volume measured to make sure the bladder is emptying completely. The innervation of the detrusor muscle runs through the trigone of the bladder, which is often injured during obstructed labor. This may lead to neuropathic bladder-emptying problems. This area is also dissected extensively during fistula repair, which may further contribute to neuropathic injury. The use of a metal catheter when measuring the postvoid residual also allows the bladder to be probed for the presence of a stone; if suspected, the presence of a stone may be confirmed by cystoscopy.

Incontinence associated with incomplete bladder emptying may resolve with regular, clean, intermittent self-catheterization. A system should be in place to ensure that patients who need therapy of this kind have access to a regular supply of catheters.

The Inoperable Fistula

Just as some injuries cannot be fixed, some fistulas cannot be closed. In some instances so much bladder has been destroyed that the defect simply cannot be repaired. When the entire urethra has sloughed away, continence is unlikely to be restored. Such patients may be offered urinary diversion in an attempt to improve their quality of life. The simplest diversion is an ileal conduit, in which the ureters are transplanted into a loop of small bowel, which drains through a stoma in the abdomen. This is a form of "incontinent" urinary diversion that simply moves the fistula from the pelvis to the abdominal wall, where the urine can be collected in a bag. Although such a procedure may make the urine loss easier to contain, unless the patient has access to good stoma care and adequate ostomy supplies, the patient with an ileal conduit in a very low-resource setting may be even more stigmatized by this operation than she was by the original fistula (Wall 2005).

Operations such as the Mainz II pouch or ureterosigmoidostomy are "continent" urinary diversions in which the ureters are transplanted into the colon, which then serves as a storage reservoir for urine (Morgan et al. 2009). These patients have constant liquid stools, and if the anal-sphincter mechanism is deficient (or if there is an unrecognized rectovaginal fistula), such operations may do more harm than good. Patients undergoing ureterosigmoidostomy also have an increased risk of rectal cancer as well as a propensity to develop electrolyte imbalances, which must be followed and treated. Such operations can be performed successfully in low-resource settings, but doing so requires surgical experience and good postoperative medical and nursing support, as well as a long-term plan to care for the ongoing needs of such patients (Morgan et al. 2009). Not every medical facility in a low-resource country will be prepared to perform such operations skillfully and with acceptable postoperative morbidity and mortality. These operations also require general (as opposed to spinal) anesthesia, which may not be available in all settings.

STRUCTURAL VIOLENCE AND FISTULA PREVENTION

Obstetric fistulas develop when labor is obstructed and the obstruction is not promptly relieved. Since labor can become obstructed by malposition of the fetus as well as cephalopelvic disproportion, any pregnant woman may develop obstructed labor if the "perfect storm" of interlocking obstetric conditions is present. This means that the key to prevention of obstetric fistula lies ultimately in the careful surveillance of every labor so that those that do not progress normally are identified early and appropriate interventions occur in a timely fashion. In affluent countries with well-developed health-care systems, it is expected that diligent care of this kind will be provided to all laboring women as a matter of course. Obstructed labor rarely (if ever) results in an obstetric fistula in the world's wealthy nations. Obstetric fistula persists only where competent, high-quality obstetric care is lacking. Obstetric fistula is rooted in poverty and deprivation. Obstetric fistula is a "neglected tropical disease" like leprosy, filariasis, and the other unusual maladies that cluster among the world's poorest citizens (Wall 2012b). In short, obstetric fistula is an expression of structural violence.

Direct violence is personal violence such as that experienced by the victim of a mugging or an accident (see Chapter 10). Indirect violence is also injurious, but it is mediated by intervening socioeconomic factors ("structural violence") (Galtung 1969). Gilligan (1997) defines structural violence as the higher rates of death and disability among the very poorest, compared with those who have more resources. He goes on to explain that a substantial portion of such harm is the result of that society's choices regarding distribution of wealth. Structural violence is relevant to clinical medicine because it illuminates the interface between human biology and the socioeconomic environment in which health care takes place (Farmer et al. 2006). Obstetric fistula is a particularly vivid example of structural violence, because it is produced directly by the physical violence of obstructed labor and the social, political, and economic circumstances in which obstructed labor occurs.

Obstetric fistula occurs when labor is obstructed, diagnosis is delayed, and prompt competent treatment is absent. In their classic paper on maternal mortality, Thaddeus and Maine (1994) described the three types of delays that lead to maternal death and serious birth injury: delay in deciding to seek care when an obstetric complication arises; delay in arriving at a suitable health-care facility; and delay in receiving proper care after arrival. These delays all represent particular facets of the socioeconomic matrix that must be navigated by the laboring woman if she is to deliver a healthy baby without developing an obstetric fistula or another adverse pregnancy outcome (Wall 2012c). Since most cases of obstructed labor require cesarean delivery, access to cesarean section is a useful proxy for how the reproductive morbidity of obstructed labor is distributed across any society. In West Africa, for example, the overall rate of cesarean section is estimated to be only 1.3%, well below the absolute minimum required to meet basic maternal-health needs (5.4%) and far below the optimal suggested rate of 15% (Dumont et al. 2001). Cross-national statistical analysis of cesarean delivery shows that even among the poorest countries with the lowest rates of cesarean section, access to this potentially lifesaving technology is markedly skewed by geographic location and wealth: the richest quintile of the population has the best access to obstetric services, and those in urban settings have far better access to cesarean section than do the rural poor (Ronsmans, Holtz, and Stanton 2006). Obstetric fistula is a disease of poverty and social injustice.

When labor is obstructed, whether the laboring woman will develop an obstetric fistula is determined by the interplay of remote, intermediate, and acute factors (Wall 2012a). The most critical factors are those that directly affect the immediate clinical situation, but they are influenced by the intermediate and remote factors that determine the nature of the setting in which the acute clinical scenario plays out (see Figures 4.7 and 4.8).

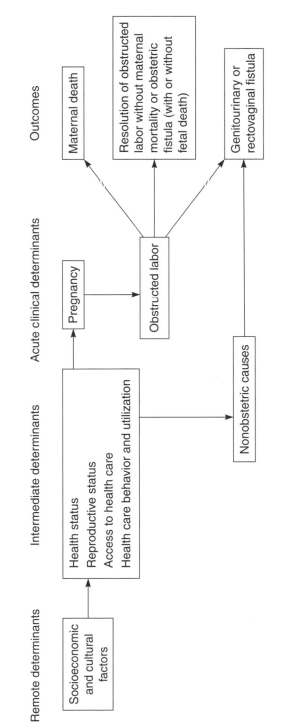

FIGURE 4.7. A framework for analyzing the determinants of obstetric fistula formation.

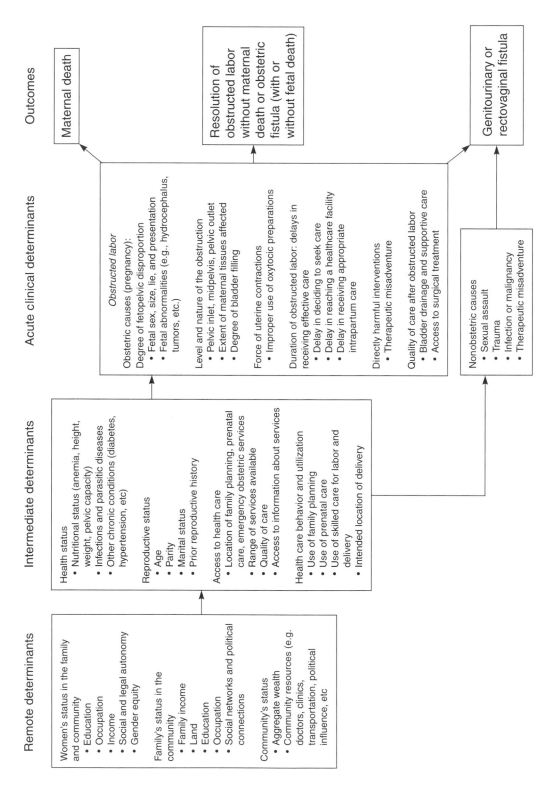

FIGURE 4.8. A detailed framework for analyzing the determinants of obstetric fistula formation.

Review of these factors makes it obvious that the eradication of obstetric fistula is an enormous long-term development project that requires the participation of all levels of society (Shiffman and Smith 2007). Fistula eradication will require a long-term social, political, and economic commitment to the education of girls and women; the development of schools, roads, communication systems, clinics and hospitals; the training of midwives, surgical technicians, community-based physicians, and specialist obstetricians who work within a health-care system that provides obstetric care to all women irrespective of their socioeconomic status.

First and foremost, however, fistula eradication demands a commitment to gender equity: girls and women must be valued equally with boys and men. Because the risks of childbearing are borne exclusively by women (who often have little say in when or whether they become pregnant), the reproductive-health needs of women must be placed at the top of the health-care agenda as a basic matter of social justice. The history of the Western world demonstrates that a condition like obstetric fistula can be eliminated and that maternal morbidity and mortality can be reduced to previously unimaginable levels (Loudon 1992). The worldwide persistence of obstetric fistula is a searing indictment of the social, political, and economic systems that have allowed this ancient scourge of womankind to survive even though the solutions have been known for over a century (Cook, Dickens, and Syed 2004).

REFERENCES

AbouZahr, C. 2003. Global burden of maternal death and disability. *Br Med Bull* 67:1–11.

Arrowsmith, S. D., E. C. Hamlin, and L. L. Wall. 1996. Obstructed labor injury complex: Obstetric fistula formation and the multifaceted morbidity of maternal birth trauma in the developing world. *Obstet Gynecol Surv* 51 (9): 568–574.

Ascher-Walsh, C. J., T. L. Capes, Y. Lo, A. Idrissa, J. Wilkinson, K. Echols, B. Crawford, and R. Genadry. 2010. Sling procedures after repair of obstetric vesicovaginal fistula in Niamey, Niger. *Int Urogynecol J* 21:1385–1390.

Barone, M. A., V. Frajzyngier, S. Arrowsmith, J. Ruminjo, A. Seuc, E. Landry, K. Beattie, et al. 2012. Non-inferiority of short-term urethral catheterization following fistula repair surgery: Study protocol for a randomized controlled trial. *BMC Women's Health* 12:5. doi:10.1186/1472-6874-12-5.

Brown, H. W., L. Wang, C. H. Bunker, and J. L. Lowder. 2012. Lower reproductive tract fistula repairs in inpatient US women, 1979–2006. *Int Urogynecol J* 23:403–410.

Browning, A. 2006. Lack of value of the Martius fibrofatty graft in obstetric fistula
    repair. *Int J Gynecol Obstet* 93 (1): 33–37.

———. 2006. Prevention of residual urinary incontinence following successful repair
    of obstetric vesico-vaginal fistula using a fibro-muscular sling. *BJOG*
    111:357–361.

Champagne, B. J., and M. F. McGee. 2010. Rectovaginal fistula. *Surg Clin North Am*
    90 (1): 69–82.

Cook, R. J., B. M. Dickens, and S. Syed. 2004. Obstetric fistula: The challenge to
    human rights. *Int J Gyn Obstet* 87 (1): 72–77.

Danso, K. A., J. O. Martey, L. L. Wall, and T. E. Elkins. 1996. The epidemiology of
    genitourinary fistulae in Kumasi, Ghana, 1977–1992. *Int Urogynecol J* 7 (3): 117–120.

Dumont, A., L. de Bernis, M. H. Bouvier-Colle, and G. Breart for the MOMA Study
    Group. 2001. Caesarean section rate for maternal indication in sub-Saharan
    Africa: A systematic review. *Lancet* 358 (9290): 1328–1333.

Elkins, T. E., J. O. L. DeLancey, and E. G. McGruie. 1990. The use of modified
    Martius graft as an adjunctive technique in vesicovaginal and rectovaginal
    fistula repair. *Obstet Gynecol* 75 (4): 727–733.

Emmet, T. A. 1868. *Vesicovaginal Fistulas from Parturition and Other Causes, with Cases of
    Recto-Vaginal Fistula*. New York: William Wood.

———. 1879. The necessity for early delivery, as demonstrated by the analysis of one
    hundred and sixty-one cases of vesico-vaginal fistula. *Trans Am Gynecol Soc*
    3:114–134.

Farmer, P. E., B. Nizeye, S. Stulac, and S. Keshavjee. 2006. Structural violence and
    clinical medicine. *PLoS Medicine* 3 (10): 1686–1691.

Frajzyngier, V., G. Li, E. Larson, J. Ruminjo, and M. A. Barone. 2013. Development
    and comparison of prognostic scoring systems for surgical closure of genitouri-
    nary fistula. *Am J Obstet Gynecol* 208:112e1–e11.

Furuta, M., J. Sandall, and D. Bick. 2012. A systematic review of the relationship
    between severe maternal morbidity and post-traumatic stress disorder. *BMC
    Pregnancy Childbirth* 12:125.

Galtung, J. 1969. Violence, peace, and peace research. *J Peace Res* 6 (3): 167–191.

Gilligan, J. 1997. *Violence: Reflections on a National Epidemic*. New York: Vintage Books.

Goh, J. T. 2004. A new classification for female genital tract fistula. *Aust N Z J Obstet
    Gynaecol* 44:502–504.

Goh, J. T. W., and A. Browning. 2005. Use of urethral plugs for urinary incontinence
    following fistula repair. *Aust N Z J Obstet Gynaecol* 45:237–238.

Goh, J. T. W., A. Browning, B. Berhan, and A. Chang. 2008. Predicting the risk of
    failure of closure of obstetric fistula and residual urinary incontinence using a
    classification system. *Int Urogynecol J* 19:1659–1662.

Goh, J. T. W., H. G. Krause, A. Browning, and A. Chang. 2009. Classification of
    female genito-urinary tract fistula: Inter- and intra-observer correlations.
    J Obstet Gynaecol 35:160–163.

Goh, J. T. W., H. Krause, A. B. Tessema, and G. Abraha. 2013. Urinary symptoms and
    urodynamics following obstetric genitourinary fistula repair. *In Urogynecol J*
    24:947–951.

Hilton, P., and D. A. Cromwell. 2012. The risk of vesicovaginal and urethrovaginal fistula after hysterectomy performed in the English National Health Service: A retrospective cohort study examining patterns of care between 2000 and 2008. *BJOG* 119:1447–1454.

Kochakarn, W., and W. Pummagnura. 2000. Vesico-vaginal fistula: Experience of 230 cases. *J Med Assoc Thail* 83 (10): 1129–1132.

———. 2007. A new dimension in vesicovaginal fistula management: An 8-year experience at Ramathibodi Hospital. *Asian J Surg* 30 (4): 267–271.

Lewis, G., and L. de Bernis, eds. 2006. *Obstetric Fistula: Guiding Principles for Clinical Management and Programme Development.* Geneva: World Health Organization.

Longombe, A. O., K. M. Claude, and J. Ruminjo. 2008. Fistula and traumatic genital injury from sexual violence in a conflict setting in Eastern Congo: Case studies. *Repro Health Matters* 16 (31): 132–41.

Loudon, I. 1992. The transformation of maternal mortality. *BMJ* 305:1557–1560.

Morgan, M. A., M. L. Polan, H. H. Melecot, B. Debru, A. Sleemi, and A. Husain. 2009. Experience with a low-pressure colonic pouch (Mainz II) urinary diversion for irreparable vesicovaginal fistula and bladder exstrophy in East Africa. *Int Urogynecol J* 20:1163–1168.

Moser, R. H. 1956. Diseases of medical progress. *N Engl J Med* 255:606–614.

Muleta, M., S. Rasmussen, and T. Kiserud. 2010. Obstetric fistula in 14,928 Ethiopian women. *Acta Obstet Gynecol Scand* 89:945–951.

Nardos, R., A. Browning, and C. C. G. Chen. 2009. Risk factors that predict failure after vaginal repair of obstetric vesicovaginal fistulae. *Am J Obstet Gynecol* 200 (5): 578.e1–e4.

Nardos, R., B. Member, and A. Browning. 2012. Outcome of obstetric fistula repair after 10-day versus 14-day Foley catheterization. *Int J Gynecol Obstet* 118:21–23.

Ojanuga, D., and C. C. Ekwmpu. 1999. An investigation of sociomedical risk factors associated with vaginal fistula in northern Nigeria. *Women Health* 28 (3): 103–116.

Onsrud, M., S. Sjoveian, and D. Mukwege. 2011. Cesarean delivery-related fistulae in the Democratic Republic of Congo. *Int J Gynecol Obstet* 114:10–14.

Rangnekar, N. P., N. I. Ali, S. A. Kaul, and H. R. Pathak. 2000. Role of the Martius procedure in the management of urinary-vaginal fistulas. *J Am Coll Surg* 191:259–263.

Roka, Z. G., M. Akech, P. Wanzala, J. Omolo, S. Gitta, and P. Waiswa. 2013. Factors associated with obstetric fistulae occurrence among patients attending selected hospitals in Kenya, 2010: A case control study. *BMC Pregnancy Childbirth* 13:56. http://www.dbiomedcentral.com. doi:10.1186/1471-2393-13-56.

Ronsmans, C., S. Holtz, and C. Stanton. 2006. Socioeconomic differentials in caesarean rates in developing countries: A retrospective analysis. *Lancet* 368:1516–1523.

Shiffman, J., and S. Smith. 2007. Generation of political priority for global health initiatives: A framework and case study of maternal mortality. *Lancet* 370:1370–1379.

St. George, J. 1969. Factors in the prediction of successful vaginal repair of vesico-vaginal fistulae. *J Obstet Gynaecol Br Commonw* 76:741–745.

Thaddeus, S., and D. Maine. 1994. "Too far to walk": Maternal mortality in context. *Soc Sci Med* 38:1091–1110.

Tukur, J., T. A. Jido, and C. C. Uzoho. 2006. The contribution of gishiri cut to vesicovaginal fistula in Birnin Kudu, northern Nigeria. *Afr J Urol* 12 (3): 121–125.

Vangeenderhuysen, C., A. Prual, and D. Ould el Joud. 2001. Obstetric fistulae: Incidence estimates for sub-Saharan Africa. *Int J Gynecol Obstet* 73:65–66.

Videla, F. L. G., and L. L. Wall. 1998. Stress incontinence diagnosed without multichannel urodynamic studies. *Obstet Gynecol* 91:965–968.

Waaldijk, K. 1994. The immediate surgical management of fresh obstetric fistulas with catheter and/or early closure. *Int J Gynecol Obstet* 45:11–16.

Wall, L. L. 2002. Fitsari 'dan Duniya: An African (Hausa) praise-song about vesico-vaginal fistulas. *Obstet Gynecol* 100:1328–1332.

———. 2005. Hard questions concerning fistula surgery in Third World countries. *J Womens Health* 14 (9): 863–866.

———. 2006. Obstetric vesicovaginal fistula as an international public health problem. *Lancet* 368:1201–1209.

———. 2012a. A framework for analyzing the determinants of obstetric fistula formation. *Stud Fam Plann* 43:255–272.

———. 2012b. Obstetric fistula is a "neglected tropical disease." *PLoS Negl Trop Dis* 6 (8): e1769. doi:10.1371/journal.pntd.0001769.

———. 2012c. Preventing obstetric fistulas in low-resource countries: Insights from a Haddon Matrix. *Obstet Gynecol Sur* 67:111–121.

Wall, L. L., and S. D. Arrowsmith. 2007. The "continence gap": A critical concept in obstetric fistula repair. *Int Urogynecol J* 18 (8): 843–844.

Wall, L. L., J. Karshima, C. Kirschner, and S. D. Arrowsmith. 2004. The obstetric vesicovaginal fistula: Characteristics of 899 patients from Jos, Nigeria. *Am J Obstet Gynecol* 190:1011–1119.

Wall, L. L., J. Wilkinson, S. D. Arrowsmith, D. Ojengbede, and H. Mabeya. 2008. A code of ethics for the fistula surgeon. *Int J Gynecol Obstet* 101:84–87.

Yeakey, M. P., E. Chipeta, F. Taulo, and A. O. Tsui. 2009. The lived experience of Malawian women with obstetric fistula. *Cult Health Sex* 11:499–513.

PART TWO

Infectious Diseases
and Pregnancy

5

Sexually Transmitted Infections

KHADY DIOUF

Worldwide, an estimated 499 million curable sexually transmitted infections (STIs) occur every year (WHO 2012). These include gonorrhea, chlamydia, syphilis, and trichomoniasis. When left untreated, they can lead to ectopic pregnancy, infertility, chronic pelvic pain (gonorrhea and chlamydia), preterm birth (trichomoniasis), stillbirth (syphilis) and devastating sequelae in the fetus and the newborn infant (syphilis, herpes simplex).

In addition to these curable STIs, chronic viral infections resulting from herpes simplex virus (HSV), human papillomavirus (HPV), and hepatitis B also afflict populations worldwide. Herpes simplex virus is the most common cause of genital ulcer disease and can lead to neonatal HSV, with its devastating consequences (WHO 2007). Cancers associated with HPV include cervical cancer, the second most common cancer in women, other anogenital cancers; and there is mounting evidence of an association with oropharyngeal cancers (de Sanjose et al. 2012). Hepatitis B, which can be sexually transmitted, can lead to hepatocellular carcinoma, one of the leading causes of mortality in developing countries in Asia and Africa. Human immunodeficiency virus (HIV) has claimed millions of lives since the onset of the epidemic in the 1980s, and there are around 34 million people currently living with the virus, over 90% of whom reside in developing countries. Perinatal transmission of HIV and syphilis continue to present huge challenges and still lead to thousands of perinatal infections every year. The presence of an STI such as herpes or syphilis also greatly increases the risk of HIV acquisition and transmission (WHO 2007). In addition to these health consequences, STIs can also have a huge social and economic impact (WHO 2007). Given this large burden on global health, focusing on STI prevention and control can help achieve Millennium Development Goals 4, 5, and 6: to reduce child mortality (goal 4), improve maternal health (goal 5), and combat major diseases such as HIV (goal 6).

However, challenges in STI control are numerous. Surveillance data from the World Health Organization indicate no decline in STI infections between 2005 and 2008 (WHO 2013). The challenges of diagnosing STIs in resource-limited settings include lack of trained personnel, lack of adequate laboratory facilities, and limited availability of point-of-care testing for common STIs. In 2001, the World Health Organization (WHO) published a treatment algorithm for common symptoms of STIs including genital ulcers, lower abdominal pain, and vaginal discharge, the keystone of syndromic management. The recommendation for practitioners in resource-limited settings emphasized this approach over etiologic management of STIs, which focuses on diagnosing and treating a specific STI (WHO 2001). Though syndromic management is still advocated by WHO, it has become clear that without adequate surveillance data, including mapping of antimicrobial resistance (in the case of gonorrhea) and widely available point-of-care testing for common STIs, the goal of STI control will certainly be difficult to reach.

This chapter reviews the diagnosis and management of selected sexually transmitted infections prevalent in developing countries. Reproductive tract infections that are not sexually transmitted are beyond the scope of this discussion. The chapter focuses on the syndromic management of sexually transmitted infections and identifies key points for the global-health practitioner who will encounter these patients. It also discusses challenges in case management and highlights interventions intended to improve STI control globally.

EPIDEMIOLOGY AND GLOBAL BURDEN OF DISEASE

Determinants of STI Epidemic

More than thirty pathogens are transmissible sexually, and some are easily spread within vulnerable populations. Epidemics are usually identified within certain high-risk groups (for example, female sex workers), who are the core group; they come into contact with the bridging population (for example, clients), who provide a point of entry into the main population. Both biological and behavioral factors account for the vulnerability of certain populations to the acquisition and transmission of STIs. Owing to cervical ectopy and behavioral risk factors (early age at sexual intercourse, older male partners, and so on), young women may be at higher risk for STIs (including HIV) than their male counterparts (Donovan 1997).

Factors such as access to health care, socioeconomic status, and political commitment also play an important role in the vulnerability of populations and in controlling epidemics. For example, when the HIV epidemic was slowly spreading in sub-Saharan Africa in the mid-1980s, the government of Senegal created the National AIDS Council, which quickly adopted several measures to stop the spread of HIV: condom use was promoted, high-risk groups such as commercial sex workers were encouraged to be registered and benefited from free and regular quarterly checkups (including STI testing and treatment), and a sentinel surveillance system was put in place (Open Society Institute 2007). More than twenty years into the epidemic, Senegal has managed to keep rates of HIV infection under 2%, lower than most of its sub-Saharan counterparts. Of course, HIV 2, a less virulent strain, was more prevalent in Senegal and also contributed to the timely control of the epidemic. Compared with HIV 1, HIV 2 is less easily transmissible from mother to child and between adult partners and leads to slower disease progression. Despite these successes, Senegal is still struggling to control the epidemic in certain high-risk groups, among whom HIV prevalence is similar to that in high-burden sub-Saharan countries.

SEXUALLY TRANSMITTED INFECTIONS AND HIV

Largely neglected in prior decades, STIs have attracted greater interest because of their role in spreading the HIV epidemic. The presence of both ulcerative and nonulcerative STIs greatly increases the risk of HIV acquisition and transmission and contributes to epidemiological synergy. Studies indicate a three- to tenfold increased risk of HIV acquisition and transmission in subjects with another sexually transmitted infection (Fleming and Wasserheit 1999). It is estimated that 40% of HIV transmissions are

Table 5.1   Global incidence estimates of curable sexually transmitted infections
in adults aged fifteen to forty-nine, 2005 and 2008 (millions of cases)

Infection	2005	2008	% change
Chlamydia trachomatis	101.5	105.7	4.1
Neisseria gonorrhoea	87.7	106.1	21.0
Syphilis	10.6	10.6	0
Trichomonas vaginalis	248.5	276.4	11.2
Total	448.3	498.9	11.3

Source: Reprinted from WHO (2012), Table 1. © World Health Organization 2012.

facilitated by the presence of an STI in one of the partners (WHO 2007; Freeman et al. 2006). (See Chapter 6.)

INCIDENCE OF COMMON CURABLE STIs

According to the latest WHO update on the incidence of the most common curable STIs (WHO 2012), chlamydia, gonorrhea, syphilis, and trichomonas together accounted for 498.9 million new cases in 2008 (Table 5.1). As stated above, compared with surveillance data from 2005, there was no decline in the incidence of new cases of these four curable STIs.

According to the published data, the male-to-female ratio of new common curable STIs is slightly higher than 1:1 (53% in males and 47% in females). Additionally, the regional incidence of these estimates indicates large numbers of cases in resource-limited regions (Figure 5.1).

Though countries with adequate surveillance systems have managed to identify high-risk populations based on incidence numbers, much work needs to be done to expand accurate surveillance systems so that interventions can be targeted to these groups. In addition, there is a great deal of uncertainty regarding the regional and global estimates. The World Health Organization is working on strengthening surveillance data by improving the uniformity of data collection methods (WHO 2007).

Chlamydia and Gonorrhea

Untreated gonococcal and chlamydial infections may result in pelvic-inflammatory disease in up to 40% of infected women. Infertility related to tubal disease may be responsible for up to 85% of infertility cases in

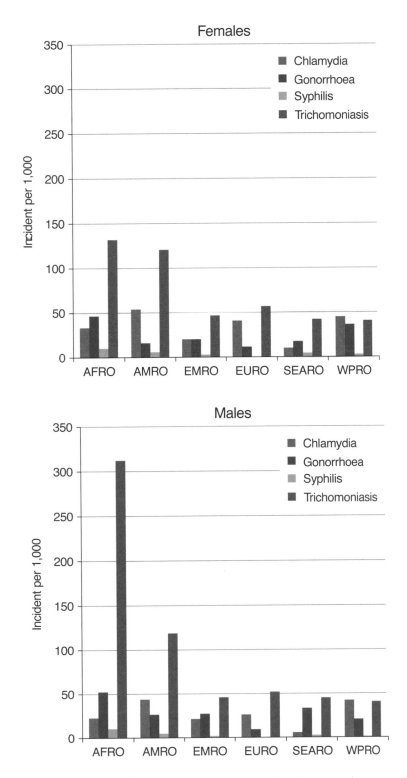

FIGURE 5.1. Incidence of sexually transmitted infections, by sex and region, 2005.
AFRO=African Region; AMRO=Americas Region; EURO=European Region;
EMRO=Eastern Mediterranean Region; SEARO=Southeast Asia Region;
WPRO=Western Pacific Region

sub-Saharan Africa. Additionally, over 4,000 children born each year to women with untreated infections become blind from ophthalmia neonatorum, an ocular gonorrhea infection acquired during passage through the birth canal (WHO 2013).

Syphilis

Over 12 million people, including more than 1 million pregnant women, are infected with syphilis worldwide (Newman et al. 2013). Untreated maternal syphilis can lead to adverse outcomes in over half of affected pregnancies. Among those, 21% will result in stillbirths and about 9% in neonatal deaths, according to a recent meta-analysis (Gomez et al. 2013). Syphilis also increases the risk of HIV transmission more than threefold (Fleming and Wasserheit 1999).

Trichomoniasis

Trichomoniasis, a common cause of vaginitis, is a sexually transmitted infection caused by the protozoan *T. vaginalis*. Though it is often asymptomatic in women, it can manifest as a malodorous vaginal discharge with pruritus and occasional discomfort upon urination. Though limited, the available data on trichomoniasis suggests a high global burden of disease: there is an estimated 8% prevalence and 276 million new cases per year (WHO 2007). Trichomoniasis may lead to adverse pregnancy outcomes, including preterm rupture of membranes and preterm delivery. Like most STIs, it is also a facilitator for HIV acquisition and transmission.

THE BURDEN OF CHRONIC VIRAL STIs

Alongside the curable STIs discussed above, HIV and other viral STIs (HPV, hepatitis B, and HSV) are chronic infections with a large amount of morbidity and mortality. Apart from the discussion of its synergistic relationship with other STIs, HIV is beyond the scope of this chapter, as it is discussed extensively in another section of this book (Chapter 6).

Herpes simplex virus is the most common cause of genital ulcer disease worldwide. Genital HSV may be caused by either HSV 1 or HSV 2. There were an estimated 23.6 million new cases of HSV 2 infection in 2003, and over 536 million adults age fifteen to forty-nine were living with HSV 2, representing about 16% of the global population. Of the total number of infections, 314.8 million were diagnosed in women and 220.7 million were diagnosed in men. It is unclear why the prevalence is so much higher among women, but biological and socioeconomic factors may play some part. Sub-Saharan Africa, Asia, and Central and South America carry the largest burden of disease, with HSV seropositivity rates somewhere between 10 and 80%. The virus may still be transmitted to sex partners many years after initial infection. In addition to being a chronic infection that may lead to recurrence of painful genital ulcers, HSV has been shown to facilitate HIV transmission (Fleming and Wasserheit 1999; Freeman et al. 2006; Looker, Garnett, and Schmid 2008). Additionally, an acute primary infection with HSV around the time of delivery is associated with a 60% risk of transmission to the fetus (Straface et al. 2012).

Human papillomavirus is the most common viral infection of the female reproductive tract, with a worldwide prevalence of 11%. However, there are large regional disparities, for example, the prevalence is about 16% in Latin America but roughly 24% in sub-Saharan Africa (Knaul et al. 2012). The virus causes cervical cancer, the fourth most common cause of cancer worldwide and the second most common cause of cancer in women. In 2012, there were an estimated 266,000 deaths from cervical cancer and 528,000 new cases worldwide. Over 85% of these cases occur in developing countries, where there is limited capability for screening and treatment (GLOBOCAN). Human papillomavirus has also been implicated in other cancers of the anogenital tract as well as in head and neck cancers (de Sanjose et al. 2012) and in genital warts. Human-papillomavirus subtypes 16 and 18 are implicated in most cases of cervical cancer, whereas HPV 6 and 11 are responsible for genital warts.

Hepatitis B is another common cause of chronic infection and death worldwide. The virus can be acquired through sexual contact, via mother-to-child transmission, or through contact with blood and other body fluids of an infected person, making it an occupational hazard for health workers. More than 240 million people are living with chronic infection, which can lead to liver cirrhosis, liver cancer (hepatocellular carcinoma), and death. Hepatitis B is implicated in an estimated 600,000 deaths yearly from liver cirrhosis and cancer. Hepatitis B prevalence is highest in sub-Saharan Africa and East Asia, where most infections occur at birth or during childhood, and where 5 to 10% of the adult population is chronically infected. Hepatitis B is preventable with the use of a safe vaccine. Many countries have integrated the hepatitis B vaccine into the routine childhood immunization series (Te and Jensen 2010), which has lowered prevalence.

In addition to the health consequences mentioned, STIs have devastating social and economic consequences. Alongside lost wages from inability to work, stigmatization and domestic violence are some of the consequences that affect women who have been diagnosed with an STI (Neal, Lichtenstein, and Brodsky 2010).

PATHOPHYSIOLOGY

Sexually transmitted diseases are passed on via the mucous membranes of the vagina, penis, urethra, and rectum during sexual contact with an infected person. However, many STIs are also transmissible via other routes. Mother-to-child transmission of pathogens can occur during pregnancy through the placenta (HIV, syphilis, hepatitis B), during childbirth, by means of through contact of the infant with infected blood or vaginal fluid (HIV, gonorrhea, chlamydia), or through breast milk (HIV). Contact with infected blood products or other body fluids (saliva) may also pose an infectious risk, such as in hepatitis B transmission. Pathogens that are responsible for STIs can be bacterial *(Neisseria gonorrheae, Chlamydia trachomatis),* viral (HIV, HSV, HBV), or parasitic *(Phthirius pubis).* Diseases caused by these pathogens can often be asymptomatic but are usually grouped into the syndrome they cause, such as genital ulcers, vaginal discharge, and lower abdominal pain.

TREATMENT AND GUIDELINES FOR CARE

There are three approaches to the management of patients presenting with STI-related symptoms: etiologic management, clinical diagnosis, and syndromic management. Etiologic diagnosis is challenging in many resource-limited settings: laboratory resources may be lacking, and diagnostic tests may not be reliable. Clinical diagnosis may be inaccurate, owing to the nonspecific nature of STI-related symptoms, and may miss mixed infections. The World Health Organization updated its guidelines in 2001 to recommend a syndrome-based approach to the management of sexually transmitted infections in areas with logistical challenges to etiologic diagnosis (WHO 2003).

Syndromic management of STIs is based on the identification of a group of symptoms (syndrome) reported by patients, such as vaginal discharge, genital ulcer, or lower abdominal pain. Based on the syndrome as well as local epidemiologic surveillance data, patients are treated for the most common and likely etiologic agents. The World Health Organization has developed syndromic management algorithms for genital ulcer, lower abdominal pain, and vaginal discharge (WHO 2001).

As a global-health practitioner, it is important for you to be familiar with the syndromic management of STIs. You should also get to know the local prevalence of STIs; that information may be available from the country's ministry of health. Though general algorithms have been developed by WHO for some of the syndromes, most countries have adapted WHO flow charts to reflect disease prevalence and available drugs in their own communities.

GENITAL ULCER SYNDROME

The most common cause of genital ulcers worldwide is herpes simplex virus. Lesions can present as single or multiple painful vesicles, which may develop to become painful ulcers over the course of days. In a patient presenting with this complaint, not only should appropriate counseling be provided regarding condom use, but syphilis and HIV counseling and testing should also be provided if possible. Antiviral treatment for HSV can be offered if available, and the patient should be counseled regarding the goals for antiviral therapy, not to effect a cure but to reduce the number of symptomatic days and the risk of transmission to an uninfected partner. If the exam is concerning for other causes of genital ulcer disease (GUS), or there is no clinical improvement within seven days, the patient should be treated for syphilis (if that has not already occurred).

The primary stage of syphilis is characterized by a chancre, which in women usually presents as a painless, isolated ulcer either on the labia or cervix. It usually begins at the site of inoculation as a small raised lesion and develops into a red, usually painless lesion with a scooped-out appearance. Chancres are highly contagious. In the secondary stage, a rash can appear on any part of the body but usually involves the palms of the hands and soles of the feet. Condyloma lata (flat, wart-like lesions) can be present. Most people then enter the latent phase of syphilis, during which they can be asymptomatic for several years. Tertiary syphilis can develop years later and lead to neurologic and cardiovascular manifestations.

Other Sexually Transmitted Causes of GUS

In patients presenting with GUS, the decision to treat for chancroid, *granuloma inguinale,* or *lymphogranuloma venereum* should be based on local epidemiologic surveillance data. Because these conditions are relatively rare in the United States, diagnosis can present challenge for providers unfamiliar with the pathogens; however if the disease is relatively common in the area where you practice, treatment should be instituted. *Knowing local epidemiologic surveillance data is key.* Figure 5.2 presents symptoms and treatment of genital ulcers.

Lymphogranuloma venereum (LGV)

Lymphogranuloma venereum is a sexually transmitted infection that is endemic to many parts of the developing world and is caused by specific serovars of *Chlamydia trachomatis* (L1, L2, L3). It often presents as a single nontender lesion at the site of contact (primary stage), followed by unilateral or bilateral lymphadenopathy that evolves several weeks after the primary lesion (secondary or lymphatic stage). These lesions may coalesce as a bubo and eventually drain spontaneously. The tertiary stage is characterized by rectal narrowing or elephantiasis with possible destruction of genitalia. Additionally, LGV can be transmitted to the newborn through the birth canal at the time of delivery. Treatment is a twenty-one-day course of doxycycline; erythromycin can be used as an alternative when doxycycline is contraindicated, such as during pregnancy.

Chancroid

Chancroid is a sexually transmitted infection caused by *Haemophilus ducreyi* and is characterized by painful necrotizing genital ulcers with inguinal lymphadenopathy in up to 50% of cases. It is a rare disease in the United States, where outbreaks have been documented in certain high-risk groups (sex workers) (Hammond et al. 1980; Schmid et al. 1987), but it still occurs among the population at large in regions of Africa, Asia, and the Caribbean. Erythromycin is the mainstay of therapy; single-dose azithromycin or ciprofloxacin and intramuscular ceftriaxone regimens may improve patient compliance. There is data to suggest that longer-course therapy may be indicated in patients who are also HIV infected.

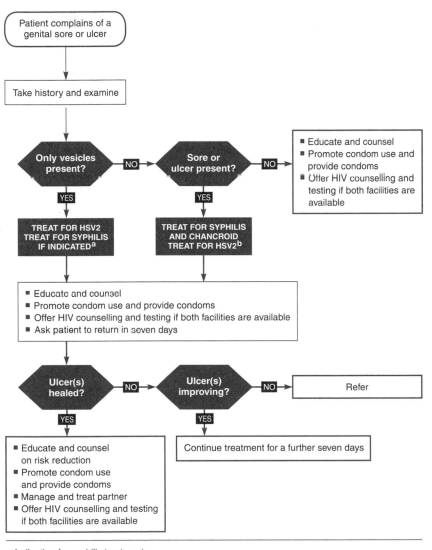

a. Indication for syphilis treatment:
   • RPR positive; and
   • Patient has not been treated for syphilis recently.
b. Treat for HSV2 where prevalence is 30% or higher, or adapt to local conditions.

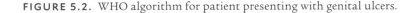

FIGURE 5.2. WHO algorithm for patient presenting with genital ulcers.

Granuloma inguinale

Granuloma inguinale is a sexually transmitted infection caused by *Klebsiella granulomatis* endemic to certain regions of the world such as Brazil, New Guinea, Southern Africa, and areas of Asia (Bezerra, Jardim, and Silva

2011). It usually begins with a painless nodule at the site of inoculation, which then bursts and leads to an ulcer that is slow growing and bleeds easily. Unlike chancroid and LGV, *Granuloma inguinale* is not associated with lymphadenopathy.

One key point regarding genital ulcers is that mixed infections are not uncommon in low-resource areas. Therefore, if a patient is not improving at the follow-up visit, other etiologies should be considered and treated if necessary.

Another salient fact is that genital ulcers may also be caused by diseases that are prevalent in tropical regions but are not sexually transmitted. For example, amoebiasis and leishmaniasis can present with genital ulcerations.

Schistosomiasis (owing to *Schistosoma haematobium* and to a lesser extent *S. mansoni*) is a well-described entity in the developing world that can lead to genital ulcers (vulvar and cervical), ectopic pregnancy, and infertility (Kjetland et al. 2012). It is also a reported risk factor for HIV transmission in endemic areas (Holen 2012). More than 200 million cases are reported worldwide, over 90% of which occur in Africa. Schistosomiasis is increasingly reported in developed countries among immigrant populations, as well as in returning travelers from the tropics who have had exposure to the parasites in fresh water (Chen et al. 2012; Catteau et al. 2011). It may present with wartlike growths on the vulva or cervical lesions mimicking cervical cancer. These entities should be included in the differential diagnosis, especially if standard treatment using syndromic management fails to resolve symptoms.

LOWER ABDOMINAL PAIN

Lower abdominal pain can be a presenting symptom in women with pelvic inflammatory disease (PID); sexually active women presenting with this complaint should be evaluated for PID. Untreated pelvic inflammatory disease may lead to many reproductive sequelae, including chronic pelvic pain, infertility, and ectopic pregnancy. Pelvic inflammatory disease is the leading cause of infertility in many resource-limited settings, though other infectious causes of infertility such as pelvic tuberculosis (which may account for 15 to 20% of tubal infertility in such areas) have been reported. Pelvic inflammatory disease is most com-

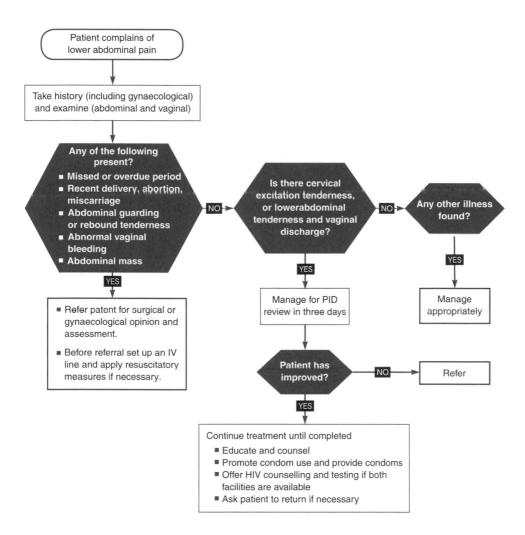

FIGURE 5.3. WHO algorithm for patient presenting with lower abdominal pain.

monly the result of sexually transmitted infections such as gonorrhea and chlamydia. Figure 5.3 illustrates the history and treatment of pelvic inflammatory disease.

Though treatment for PID is important in the scenario presented, a larger differential diagnosis should be considered for patients presenting with lower abdominal pain. In addition to pregnancy complications such as ectopic pregnancy, gastrointestinal and urinary etiologies should be investigated if necessary. As discussed for the GUS algorithm, one must also consider potential genital manifestations of other tropical diseases.

GENITAL TUBERCULOSIS AS A CAUSE OF INFERTILITY

As a practitioner in a resource-limited setting, one must consider other causes of PID leading to infertility. Primary and secondary infertility are common presentations of female genital tuberculosis; in fact, tuberculosis may account for up to 20% of tubal infertility in endemic countries. Pelvic pain or abnormal bleeding can also be presenting symptoms in both premenopausal and postmenopausal patients. Genital tuberculosis can also appear similar to ovarian carcinomatosis with peritoneal seeding.

ABNORMAL VAGINAL DISCHARGE

Worldwide, the most common causes of infectious vaginitis are *Candida albicans, Trichomonas vaginalis,* and bacterial vaginosis. Women presenting with abnormal vaginal discharge should be treated for the most common causes of vaginitis (*T. vaginalis* and bacterial vaginosis and, where appropriate, *C. albicans*). However, abnormal vaginal discharge per se is poorly predictive of cervical infection. If risk assessment is of concern for cervical infection, the patient should also be treated for gonorrhea and chlamydia.

Other common causes of abnormal vaginal discharge may be diseases such as genital amoebiasis, which may present as foul-smelling, bloody vaginal discharge (Richens 2004). There have been reports of neglected cases of genital amoebiasis leading to necrotizing vulvitis, which then require radical vulvectomy. The infection can be sexually transmitted, and partners should be treated. Figure 5.4 presents diagnosis and treatments for vaginal infection.

SELECTION OF TREATMENT DRUGS

Because treatment of STIs should be easily implementable and accessible for most populations, drugs should be highly effective, inexpensive, and

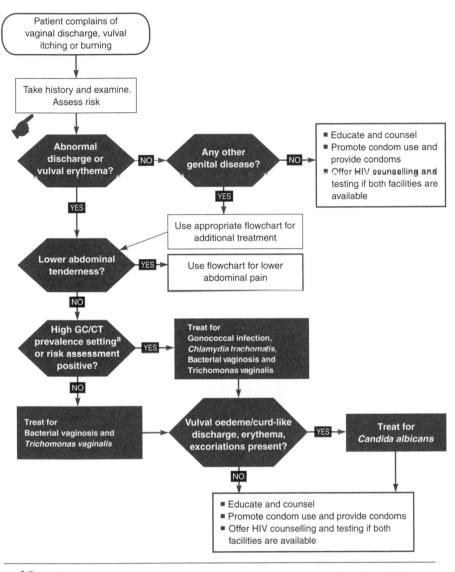

FIGURE 5.4. WHO algorithm for patient presenting with abnormal vaginal discharge.

low in toxicity. They should also require one-dose oral administration and be safe in most populations, including pregnant women. They should also be available in WHO's Essential Drugs List for countries. Tables 5.2, 5.3, and 5.4 show the WHO-recommended list of drugs for the treatment of

STIs. Note that this list is not all-inclusive and refers mostly to illnesses identified within the syndromic management of STIs. Where appropriate, the management of other common causes of genital disease such as donovanosis and schistosomiasis is mentioned in the text.

The tables below are extracted from the WHO list of drugs for STI-associated syndromes.

Table 5.2   Available treatments for genital ulcer disease

Disease	Drug options	Alternatives	Penicillin allergy and non-pregnant
Syphilis	Benzathine benzylpenicillin	Procaine benzylpenicillin	Doxycycline Tetracycline
Chancroid	Ciprofloxacin Erythromycin Azithromycin	Ceftriaxone	
Granuloma inguinale	Azithromycin Doxycyclinel	Erythromycin Tetracycline Trimethoprim/ sulfamethoxazole	
LGV	Doxycycline Erythromycin	Tetracycline	
Genital herpes	Acyclovir Valaciclovir Famciclovir		

Source: Reprinted from WHO (2003), At a Glance: Genital Ulcer Disease. © World Health Organization 2003.

Table 5.3   Available treatments for cervical infection

Infection	Drug options	Alternatives
Gonorrhoea	Ciprofloxacin Ceftriaxone Spectinomycin Cefixime	
Chlamydia	Doxycycline Azithromycin	Amoxicillin Ofloxacin Erythromycin (if Tetracycline is contraindicated) Tetracycline

Source: Reprinted from WHO (2003), At a Glance: Cervical Infection. © World Health Organization 2003.

Table 5.4   Available treatments for vaginal infection

Infection	Drug options	Alternatives
Bacterial Vaginosis	Metronidazole	Clindamycin Metronidazole gel Clindamycin vaginal cream
T. vaginalis	Metronidazole Tinidazole	None
Candida	Miconazole Clotrimazole Fluconazole	Nystatin

Source: Reprinted from WHO (2003), At a Glance: Vaginal Infection. © World Health Organization 2003.

MANAGEMENT OF HPV-RELATED DISEASE

Two prophylactic HPV vaccines are currently available and could substantially reduce the prevalence of cervical cancer worldwide. Cervarix, manufactured by Glaxo-Smith-Kline, is a bivalent vaccine targeting high-risk HPV 16 and 18. Gardasil, a quadrivalent vaccine targeting HPV 6, 11, 16, and 18, is manufactured by Merck and is currently approved in over 120 countries. The World Health Organization currently recommends that countries include HPV in their routine immunization series. The Global Alliance for Vaccines and Immunisation (GAVI) started supporting HPV immunization in over twenty countries in 2013 for as low as $4.50 per injection. More countries are expected to roll out HPV immunization in the coming years. The targeted group for immunization comprises girls aged nine to thirteen, before sexual debut. The vaccination is thought to be safe and immunogenic in HIV-infected individuals.

Human papillomavirus vaccination is not a replacement for cervical cancer screening. In resource-limited settings, screen-and-treat approaches are preferred alternatives to cytology-based screening. The more recent WHO recommendations suggest approaches such as HPV testing alone or HPV followed by visual inspection with acetic acid (VIA) as a primary screening modality. Human papillomavirus testing alone for screening has been shown to reduce morbidity and mortality despite a potential risk of overtreatment (Sankaranarayanan and Ferlay 2006). Treatment for dysplasia is usually cryotherapy or a loop electrosurgical excision procedure (LEEP) if the patient is not eligible for cryotherapy. Treatment for cervical cancer is often based on the resources available but may include radiation therapy alone or combined with surgery. Palliative care resources are scarce or nonexistent in much of Africa, Asia, and Latin America.

In patients presenting with lesions of concern for genital warts, other entities must also be considered. As mentioned above, genital schistoso-miasis may mimic HPV-related lesions such as warts and cervical cancer (Richens 2004). In a resource-limited setting, vaginal warts can be managed with triacetic acid (TCA 80 to 90%), podophyllin (10 to 25%), or cryo-therapy. A suspicion of cervical warts should trigger screening for cervical cancer; TCA and podophyllin should not be used on cervical warts.

LIMITATIONS OF THE SYNDROMIC APPROACH TO THE MANAGEMENT OF STIs

There are obvious advantages to the syndromic management of STIs for resource-limited settings, including limited need for testing facilities, minimal training required for personnel to follow management algorithms, and the capability to treat mixed infections (WHO 2001). However, there are also many shortcomings. The syndromic approach aims to identify patients via a set of standardized clinical symptoms; however, a majority of people with STIs (including gonorrhea, chlamydia, and syphilis) may be asymptomatic or may not recognize short-lived symptoms and will not seek care when they are most symptomatic and often most infectious. Missing this subclinical pool of the population not only affects proper case management but also limits the efficacy of national STI-surveillance systems. It may also lead to overtreatment of patients, increased drug resistance, and undertraining of medical personnel who rely on management algorithms.

The availability of cheap, rapid point-of-care (POC) tests would allow quick, targeted, on-site diagnosis and treatment. Currently, POC testing is available for syphilis and HIV in resource-limited settings. These antibody tests are easily performed with whole blood from a finger prick or a noninvasive specimen such as saliva. Studies that integrated POC testing for syphilis in prevention of mother-to-child transmission programs for HIV have shown its feasibility and increase in uptake of testing for syphilis and HIV (Tucker, Bien, and Peeling 2013). It is hoped that POC tests for gonorrhea, chlamydia, and other STIs will become increasingly available in resource-limited settings to circumvent limitations associated with the syndromic management of STIs.

CONCLUSION

Physicians practicing in resource-poor countries are often faced with challenging diagnostic dilemmas. To circumvent diagnostic issues, WHO has advocated for over a decade the syndromic management of sexually transmitted infections. Any physician wishing to practice in resource-limited settings should become familiar with these algorithms and should understand the epidemiology of the region so they can appropriately offer therapy. In addition, differential diagnoses should be broadened in tropical regions to include common causes of genital-tract diseases, which are not always sexually transmitted.

REFERENCES

Bezerra, S. M., M. M. Jardim, and V. B. Silva. 2011. Granuloma inguinale (Donovanosis). *An Bras Dermatol* 86 (3): 585–586.

Catteau, X., A. Fakhri, V. Albert, B. Doukoure, and J. C. Noel. 2011. Genital schistosomiasis in European women. *ISRN Obste Gynecol* 242140. doi:10.5402 /2011/242140. Epub 2011 Jun 9.

Chen, W., E. A. Flynn, M. J. Shreefter, and N. A. Blagg. 2012. Schistosomiasis: An unusual finding of the cervix. *Obstet Gynecol* 119 (2, pt. 2): 472–475.

de Sanjose, S., B. Serrano, X. Castellsague, M. Brotons, J. Munoz, L. Bruni, and F. X. Bosch. 2012. Human papillomavirus (HPV) and related cancers in the global alliance for vaccines and immunization (GAVI) countries. *Vaccine* 30 (4): D1–83, vi.

Donovan, P. 1997. Confronting a hidden epidemic: The Institute of Medicine's report on sexually transmitted diseases. *Family Plann Perspect* 29 (2): 87–89.

Fleming, D. T., and J. N. Wasserheit. 1999. From epidemiological synergy to public health policy and practice: The contribution of other sexually transmitted diseases to sexual transmission of HIV infection. *Sex Transm Infect* 75 (1): 3–17.

Freeman, E. E., H. A. Weiss, J. R. Glynn, P. L. Cross, J. A. Whitworth, and R. J. Hayes. 2006. Herpes simplex virus 2 infection increases HIV acquisition in men and women: Systematic review and meta-analysis of longitudinal studies. *AIDS* (London) 20 (1): 73–83.

GLOBOCAN. Estimated cancer incidence, mortality, and prevalence worldwide in 2012. Geneva: World Health Organization. Accessed May 22, 2014. http:// globocan.iarc.fr/Pages/fact_sheets_cancer.aspx.

Gomez, G. B., M. L. Kamb, L. M. Newman, J. Mark, N. Broutet, and S. J. Hawkes. 2013. Untreated maternal syphilis and adverse outcomes of pregnancy: A systematic review and meta-analysis. *Bull World Health Organ* 91 (3): 217–226.

Hammond, G. W., M. Slutchuk, J. Scatliff, E. Sherman, J. C. Wilt, and A. R. Ronald. 1980. Epidemiologic, clinical, laboratory, and therapeutic features of an urban outbreak of chancroid in North America. *Rev Infect Dis* 2 (6): 867–879.

Holen, O. 2012. Schistosomiasis: A probable risk of HIV transmission. *Tidsskrift Norske Laegeforen* 132 (6): 646.

Kjetland, E. F., P. D. Leutscher, and P. D. Ndhlovu. 2012. A review of female genital schistosomiasis. *Trends in Parasitology* 28 (2): 58–65.

Knaul, F. M., A. Bhadelia, J. Gralow, H. Arreola-Ornelas, A. Langer, and J. Frenk. 2012. Meeting the emerging challenge of breast and cervical cancer in low- and middle-income countries. *Int J Gynaecol Obstet* 119 (S1): S85–S88.

Looker, K. J., G. P. Garnett, and G. P. Schmid. 2008. An estimate of the global prevalence and incidence of herpes simplex virus type 2 infection. *Bull World Health Organ* 86 (10): 805–812. doi:10.2471/BLT.07.046128. PMCID: PMC2649511.

Neal, T. M., B. Lichtenstein, and S. L. Brodsky. 2010. Clinical implications of stigma in HIV/AIDS and other sexually transmitted infections. *Int J STD AIDS* 21 (3): 158–160.

Newman, L., M. Kamb, S. Hawkes, G. Gomez, L. Say, A. Seuc, and N. Broutet. 2013. Global estimates of syphilis in pregnancy and associated adverse outcomes: Analysis of multinational antenatal surveillance data. *PLoS Medicine* 10 (2): e1001396.

Open Society Institute. 2007. HIV/AIDS policy in Senegal: A civil society perspective. http://www.opensocietyfoundations.org/reports/hivaids-policy-senegal-civil-society-perspective.

Richens, J. 2004. Genital manifestations of tropical diseases. *Sex Transm Infect* 80 (1): 12–17.

Sankaranarayanan, R., and J. Ferlay. 2006. Worldwide burden of gynaecological cancer: The size of the problem. *Best Pract Res Clin Obstet Gynaecol* 20 (2): 207–225.

Schmid, G. P., L. L. Sanders Jr., J. H. Blount, and E. R. Alexander. 1987. Chancroid in the United States: Reestablishment of an old disease. *JAMA* 258:3265–3268.

Straface, G., A. Selmin, V. Zanardo, M. De Santis, A. Ercoli, and G. Scambia. 2012. Herpes simplex virus infection in pregnancy. *Infect Dis Obstet Gynecol,* no. 385697. doi:10.1155/2012/385697. Epub 2012 Apr 11.

Te, H. S., and D. M. Jensen. 2010. Epidemiology of hepatitis B and C viruses: A global overview. *Clin Liver Dis* 14 (1): 1–21, vii. doi:10.1016/j.cld.2009.11.009.

Tucker, J. D., C. H. Bien, and R. W. Peeling. 2013. Point-of-care testing for sexually transmitted infections: Recent advances and implications for disease control. *Curr Opin Infect Dis* 26 (1): 73–79.

WHO (World Health Organization, Department of Reproductive Health and Research). 2001. *Guidelines for the Management of Sexually Transmitted Infections.* Geneva: World Health Organization .

———. 2007. *Global Strategy for the Prevention and Control of Sexually Transmitted Infections- Breaking the Chain of Transmission, 2006–2015.* Geneva: World Health Organization.

———. 2011. *Sexually Transmitted Infections Epidemiology: Training Course in Sexual and Reproductive Health Research.* Geneva: World Health Organization.

———. 2012. *Global Incidence and Prevalence of Selected Curable Sexually Transmitted Infections, 2008.* Geneva: World Health Organization.

———. 2013. *Baseline Report on Global Sexually Transmitted Infection Surveillance.* Geneva: World Health Organization.

6

HIV and Pregnancy

CHRISTIN PRICE AND SIGAL YAWETZ

The world's medical community first became aware of what is now known as acquired immunodeficiency syndrome (AIDS) more than three decades ago, when an epidemic of obscure opportunistic infections and Kaposi sarcoma was observed in several major U.S. urban centers among men who had sex with men. Soon thereafter, a similar epidemic was described in U.S. hemophiliacs. Within a short few years, an epidemic of AIDS among heterosexuals, predominantly women, was reported in Africa (Quinn et al. 1986). Since then, the epidemic has spread to nearly every country of the world, with the greatest impact in sub-Saharan Africa and Southeast Asia, followed by Latin America, the Caribbean, and Eastern Europe. In the areas most strongly affected, the AIDS epidemic affected not only morbidity, mortality, and survival but every aspect of the human condition. It is now estimated that during the first three decades of one of the worst epidemics of modern times, nearly 70 million individuals have contracted the human immunodeficiency virus (HIV) worldwide, and 35 million of them have died.

EPIDEMIOLOGY: THE GLOBAL IMPACT OF HIV

The World Health Organization (WHO) reported that at the end of 2011, 34 million people were living with HIV worldwide, with the majority in sub-Saharan Africa (24 million), followed by South, Southeast, and East Asia (5 million), and the Caribbean, Eastern Europe, and Central Asia (3.5 million). Women account for about 54% of adults living with HIV/AIDS.

Compared with men, women acquire HIV infection at a younger age, with peak prevalence between twenty and twenty-four years of age. Hence, the majority of women living with HIV are of childbearing age. Infection in infants and young children occurs most often through vertical or mother-to-child transmission (MTCT), which may occur in utero, at delivery, or during breast-feeding. As a result of interventions to reduce MTCT of HIV, new infections among children have declined dramatically. In 2012, the number of newly infected children was roughly 260,000 (230,000 to 320,000) in low- and middle-income countries, a 35% reduction compared with 2009.

EPIDEMIOLOGY OF MOTHER-TO-CHILD TRANSMISSION OF HIV

One of the greatest achievements in HIV prevention has been to improve the prevention of mother-to child transmission (PMTCT). Without any intervention, HIV transmission rates from an infected mother to her child may be as high as 35 to 40%. This can be reduced to less than 2% by prevention strategies that include HIV testing of women, laboratory monitoring of pregnant women, provision of antiretrovirals to HIV-infected mothers during the period of fetal and infant exposure, scheduled cesarean delivery (before rupture of membranes) in selected settings, administering postpartum antiretrovirals to infants born to HIV-infected mothers, and either formula feeding or provision of antiretroviral drugs to breast-feeding mothers or their infants (or both). The major impediment to success has been limited access to these interventions, predominantly in low-resource settings. Yet even in high-resource settings, there are many missed opportunities for prevention of MTCT of HIV. Among these are late or absent prenatal-HIV testing, unrecognized primary HIV acquisition during pregnancy and lactation, delayed or lack of prenatal care, limited access to antiretrovirals and laboratory monitoring, incomplete medication adherence, and inability to access or safely use formula feeding.

HIV Testing in Pregnancy

The World Health Organization recommends provider-initiated HIV testing for all pregnant women as a routine component of their first antenatal visit. In most areas of the world, where the HIV epidemic is generalized and HIV incidence rates during pregnancy are higher, retesting is recommended in the third trimester (or during labor or shortly after delivery) to diagnose infections acquired during pregnancy. In the United States, where the HIV epidemic in women is at a low level, a first prenatal-HIV test is universally recommended, and a second test during the third trimester is recommended only for women at high risk of HIV acquisition. The screening test of choice for all patients, including pregnant women, is an HIV-antibody test performed by enzyme-linked immunosorbent assay on a blood sample or an approved rapid point-of-care test of blood or oral mucosa.

Timing of Mother-to-Child Transmission of HIV

In non-breast-feeding populations, most HIV MTCT occurs during delivery (intrapartum), most likely through direct contact of maternal HIV from blood and genital secretions with the infant's mucous membranes. A smaller proportion of transmissions occur before the time of delivery, or in utero, with the majority of those during the third trimester. In breast-feeding populations it is estimated that up to 40% of HIV transmissions occur postnatally. Although transmission risk from breast milk may be highest earlier in the nursing infant's life, risk persists throughout breast-feeding (Miotti et al. 1999; Coutsoudis et al. 2004).

Risk Factors for HIV Mother-to-Child Transmission

The strongest predictor for MTCT of HIV is the last antenatal maternal-viral-load value (Garcia et al. 1999). Although lower maternal viral loads are associated with lower risk, residual MTCT has been reported at very low, and even undetectable, viral loads. More recent studies have demonstrated that in addition to the last antenatal viral-load value, the duration of virologic suppression during pregnancy is also a predictor of transmission risk (Tubiana et al. 2010; Read et al. 2012; Townsend et al. 2008). For breast-feeding mothers, maternal-plasma and breast-milk viral load are important risk factors (Rousseau et al. 2004). Antiretrovirals reduce the viral load but also have a protective effect against MTCT that is independent of their effect on viral-load reduction. This may be a direct effect on the virus in genital secretions and might also provide preexposure prophylaxis for the infant through transplacental passage of some antiviral drugs. Short or absent antiviral therapy during pregnancy is associated with elevated HIV 1 transmission risk (Read et al. 2012). Other maternal risk factors for MTCT of HIV include low CD4 (cluster of differentiation 4) cell count in the mother, anemia, more advanced WHO clinical disease stage, and the presence of concomitant sexually transmitted infections (STIs). Preterm delivery is also associated with a higher MTCT risk. In the absence of antiviral therapy, membrane rupture for longer than four hours has been associated with increased HIV transmission rates as well. Earlier studies have also shown a direct positive association between HIV 1 transmission and illicit drug use or cigarette smoking.

ANTENATAL CARE: INITIAL EVALUATION OF HIV-INFECTED PREGNANT WOMEN

All HIV-infected women presenting to care or diagnosed during pregnancy should have an initial evaluation as per local HIV-management guidelines as well as routine antenatal HIV evaluation. A complete history should include any history of HIV-associated complications and opportunistic infections including tuberculosis, substance use, immunizations, antiviral therapy and adherence history, and prior laboratory evaluation, including resistance assays, if available. A complete examination should assess for signs of immunodeficiency such as hepatosplenomegaly, lymphadenopathy, skin lesions, oral thrush, STIs, and signs of any other opportunistic process or complication. A laboratory evaluation, when feasible, should include CD4 cell count, quantitative plasma HIV RNA polymerase chain reaction (PCR) (also known as the HIV viral load), a complete blood count, liver function tests, and serum creatinine. Serologic screening for coinfections should include tests for syphilis and viral hepatitis. Evaluation for current or past sexually transmitted diseases such as herpes simplex, gonorrhea, or chlamydia should also be obtained. All HIV-infected adults (including pregnant women) should be routinely screened for active and latent tuberculosis. As discussed below, the most important predictor for MTCT is the maternal viral load. Since control of viremia (virus in the bloodstream) is achieved through effective combination antiretroviral therapy (cART), and since such therapy also has a preventive effect that is independent of the viral load, a plan for initiation and continued adherence to combination antiviral therapy should be made as early as possible during prenatal care.

ANTENATAL CARE:
ANTIRETROVIRAL THERAPY FOR PMTCT

Antiretroviral Therapy in Nonpregnant Adults

Without antiviral therapy, most HIV-infected individuals develop progressive immunosuppression (as measured by a decline in CD4 cell count) leading to illnesses (including AIDS-defining complications) and eventually death. Effective antiviral therapy inhibits HIV replication, ideally to viral-load levels below the limit of detection, and improves immune function; results include decreased complication rates, longer survival, and improved quality of life. It is now evident that ART reduces morbidity and mortality in all HIV-infected individuals regardless of their clinical or immunological status (Kitahata et al. 2009). The benefits of therapy are stronger for those initiating therapy at CD4 cell counts of less than or equal to 500 cells/mm^3 and even more so for those at less than or equal to 350 cells/mm^3. It is also known that antiretroviral therapy reduces the risk of sexual transmission of HIV and thus has an additional benefit in HIV prevention; this is often referred to as "treatment as prevention" (Cohen et al. 2011). In high-resource settings, ART is thus recommended for all HIV-infected individuals regardless of their clinical or immunological status to reduce the risk of disease progression and prevent transmission, as long as patients are willing to commit to long-term therapy. However, given limited resources, guidelines for when to initiate ART in HIV-infected adults in most settings differ by locale, and eligibility for ART is often determined by clinical and immunological parameters. The latest guidelines from WHO recommend that HIV-infected adults be started on ART for their own health if they have CD4 cell counts less than or equal to 500 cells/mm^3, with a priority given to individuals who have CD4 cell counts less than or equal to 350 cells/mm^3 (WHO 2013). However, the guidelines now also recommend treatment for the following individuals regardless of CD4 cell count: those with active tuberculosis disease, coinfection with hepatitis B and resultant severe liver disease, HIV-positive individuals in a serodiscordant partnership (to reduce risk of transmission to the uninfected partner), and pregnant and breast-feeding HIV-positive women (WHO 2013). Hence all pregnant and breast-feeding women with HIV should receive highly active antiretroviral therapy (HAART) for the purpose of PMTCT for the duration of fetal and infant exposure, regardless of their treatment eligibility for their own health.

Antiretroviral Therapy for Prevention of HIV Transmission from Mother to Child

For women who do not meet their local treatment eligibility criteria for their own health, pregnancy represents an additional indication for antiretroviral therapy, as highlighted by the WHO recommendations noted above—the prevention of mother-to-child transmission. The pivotal study showing that antiretroviral therapy administered to pregnant mothers reduces transmission of HIV to their infants was the Pediatric AIDS Clinical Trials Group's trial 076 (PACTG 076), which was conducted in the United States. Mothers randomized to receive zidovudine (AZT) alone during pregnancy had a 70% reduction in transmission, from 25.0 to 6.7% (Connor et al. 1994). It is important to note that formula feeding replaced breast-feeding in this trial. Since then numerous studies in diverse settings have demonstrated that administration of ART antepartum and intrapartum to pregnant women as well as postpartum to infants or to breast-feeding mothers (or to both) significantly reduces transmission. Review of these studies is beyond the scope of this chapter; however, findings from the major studies are summarized in the U.S. Department Health guidelines for the management of HIV in pregnant women (AIDSinfo 2014). However, several important conclusions may be drawn from the results of these studies. In general, combination antiretroviral regimens with three active agents are more effective than single- or dual-agent regimens in reducing perinatal transmission and should be used whenever possible. When cART with three active agents is not feasible, single-agent (AZT, single-dose nevirapine) or dual-agent (AZT/3TC) regimens have still been shown to reduce perinatal transmission when administered to pregnant women.

In addition to the number of antiretroviral drugs administered, studies have also shown that for prevention of perinatal transmission, administration of ART throughout the antepartum, intrapartum, and postpartum periods is superior to administration only during the antepartum and intrapartum periods or intrapartum and postpartum periods (Tubiana et al. 2010; Townsend et al. 2008; AIDSinfo 2014). The majority of the trials in resource-constrained countries have included intrapartum ART administration. When antepartum ART was administered to pregnant women in addition to intrapartum treatment, the rate of perinatal HIV transmission was further reduced. This was demonstrated even when antepartum therapy was initiated as late as thirty-six weeks gestation;

however, the earlier ART was started in pregnancy, the more effectively it reduced perinatal transmission. The European National Study of HIV in Pregnancy and Childhood demonstrated that with each additional week of a triple-drug regimen during the antepartum period, there was a 10% incremental reduction in risk of transmission regardless of maternal viral load, mode of delivery, or sex of the infant (Townsend et al. 2008). In a trial comparing ART started early (at twenty weeks) versus late (at thirty-five weeks) during pregnancy and comparing the length of infant treatment after delivery (three days versus six weeks), the rate of in utero HIV transmission was higher in the late arm of the study and remained so regardless of the length of infant treatment (Lallemant et al. 2000).

The current WHO guidelines recommend that all pregnant women who do not meet criteria for starting ART for their own health should begin cART and continue this throughout the entire duration of mother-to-child transmission risk (at a minimum), or throughout pregnancy and breast-feeding (Table 6.1). Ideally, all women with HIV who become pregnant should begin ART as early as possible and continue lifelong ART (Option B+, Table 6.1). There are many advantages to this, including simplified delivery of ART (no CD4 testing is required), maternal benefits of avoiding stopping and restarting ART with each pregnancy, and decreased risk of transmission to uninfected partners. For WHO clinical staging system, please refer to http://www.who.int/hiv/pub/guidelines/HIVstaging 150307.pdf.

When a pregnant woman has not received antepartum ART, intrapartum ART should be initiated as soon as possible, then postpartum ART should be given to the infant and to the mother if breast-feeding (to reduce risk of transmission). Similarly, if neither antepartum nor intrapartum ART is available, postpartum ART for the infant and for the breast-feeding mother will still provide protection from HIV transmission. In such cases combination therapy with at least two active agents is superior to a single agent when ART is given to the infant postpartum (Nielson-Saines 2012).

Choice of Antiretroviral Agents in Pregnancy

In general, the same regimens used for treating nonpregnant adults should be used in pregnant women unless there are known adverse effects for the woman, fetus, or infant that outweigh the benefits of a drug. Pregnancy should not preclude a woman from receiving a regimen that is optimal for her own health. However, international treatment guidelines for the man-

Table 6.1 Program options for ART for PMTCT

National PMTCT program option	Pregnant and breast-feeding women with HIV		HIV-exposed infant	
Use of lifelong ART for all pregnant and breast-feeding women (Option B+)	Regardless of WHO clinical stage or CD4 cell count		Breast-feeding	Replacement feeding
	Initiate ART and maintain after delivery and cessation of breast-feeding			
Use of lifelong ART only for pregnant and breast-feeding women eligible for treatment (Option B)	Eligible for treatment	Not eligible for treatment	Six weeks of infant prophylaxis with once-daily NVP	Four to six weeks of infant prophy-laxis with once-daily NVP (or twice-daily AZT)
	Initiate ART and maintain after delivery and cessation of breast-feeding	Initiate ART and stop after delivery and cessation of breast-feeding		

Source: Adapted from WHO (2013), © World Health Organization 2013.

agement of pregnant women consider additional factors when making recommendations for specific agents. Those include prior experience with the use of a drug in pregnancy, the pharmacokinetics of drugs during pregnancy, and what is known about potential adverse effects to pregnant mothers, fetuses, and infants. Recommendations for antiviral therapy in pregnant women are updated frequently based on clinical trials and collective experience. The most recent version of the U.S. Public Health Service task force guidelines can be found online at http://www.aidsinfo.nih.gov/. The most recent version of the World Health Organization guidelines may be found at http://www.who.int/hiv/pub/guidelines/en/. Both sets of guidelines endorse cART for all HIV-infected pregnant women. All guidelines now recommend cART with three active agents.

The WHO guidelines recommend triple therapy (three antiretrovirals) for the duration of mother-to-child transmission risk. Whenever feasible, therapy should be continued for life (option B+, Table 6.1). However, in some countries, for women who are not eligible for ART for their own health, stopping ART after the period of mother-to-child transmission risk could be considered (option B, Table 6.1).

According to the WHO guidelines, first-line ART should consist of two nucleoside reverse-transcriptase inhibitors (NRTIs) and one nonnucleoside reverse-transcriptase inhibitor (NNRTI). A fixed-dose combination of

Table 6.2 Summary of first-line ARV regimens for adults

First-line ART	Preferred first-line regimen	Alternative first-line regimens
Adults (including pregnant and breast-feeding women)	TDF + 3TC (or FTC) + EFV	AZT + 3TC + EFV AZT + 3TC + NVP TDF + 3TC (or FTC) + NVP

Source: Adapted from WHO (2013), © World Health Organization 2013.

tenofovir (TDF) plus lamividine (3TC) or emtricitabine (FTC) plus efavirenz (EFV) is the preferred option for first-line ART (Table 6.2). This is based on evidence that this particular once-daily combination is less frequently associated with severe adverse events, has fewer drug interactions, and has a better virologic and treatment response compared with other once- or twice-daily regimens (WHO 2013).

If the preferred first-line regimen (or a particular component of it) is contraindicated or unavailable, alternative regimens include AZT plus 3TC plus either EFV or nevirapine (NVP) or TDF plus 3TC or FTC plus NVP. World Health Organization now recommends discontinuing any stavudine (d4T)-containing regimens because of its well-recognized metabolic toxicity (WHO 2013). Please note that updated guidelines are posted regularly; the WHO website may provide more up-to-date guidelines than those included in this chapter.

The U.S. guidelines recommend combination ART (cART) with at least three agents. For ART-naïve women, two NRTIs and either a protease inhibitor with low-dose ritonavir or an NNRTI are preferred. The preferred two-NRTI backbone includes TDF plus 3TC or FTC, abacavir plus 3TC, or AZT plus 3TC. Ritonavir-boosted lopinavir (LPV) and ritonavir-boosted atazanavir (ATV) are the preferred protease inhibitors for use in antiretroviral-naïve pregnant women. Efavirenz is the preferred NNRTI, if therapy is initiated after the first eight weeks of pregnancy. To avoid a severe hypersensitivity reaction, testing for the HLA-B5701 allele is recommended before initiating regimens containing abacavir, which should not be used in women testing positive for this allele.

Risks of Antiretrovirals in Pregnancy

Though the benefits to maternal health and reduction of HIV transmission to infants appear to greatly outweigh the risks of adverse outcomes related to ART use, there are a few possible outcomes in mothers and in infants exposed to ART in utero that are worth noting in this chapter. For a complete list of potential adverse and potential teratogenic effects of antiviral agents, please consult Appendix B to the U.S. Public Health Service task force perinatal treatment guidelines (AIDSinfo 2014) and the antiretroviral pregnancy registry at http://www.apregistry.com.

Mitochondrial Toxicity and Nucleoside Reverse-Transcriptase Inhibitors

Nucleoside reverse-transcriptase inhibitors (NRTIs) may cause mitochondrial toxicity, including hepatosteatosis, lactic acidosis, pancreatitis, neuropathy, and cardiomyopathy, through their effect on mitochondrial gamma DNA polymerase. There is likely to be a maternal genetic predisposition to this adverse effect. The risk for mitochondrial toxicity is highest for zalcitabine, followed (in decreasing order) by didanosine, stavudine, AZT, lamivudine, and TDF. Such toxicity has been reported in pregnant women and may have some similarities to other pregnancy-related syndromes such as hemolysis, elevated liver enzymes, and low-platelets (HELLP) syndrome, and acute fatty liver of pregnancy. As a result it is recommended to avoid the combination of didanosine and stavudine in pregnancy. Additionally, data from a French cohort raised concerns for elevated risk of mitochondrial syndromes in infants exposed in utero to NRTIs (mostly AZT and lamivudine) (Barret et al. 2003). However, such risk was not identified in other cohort studies from the United States and Europe (Perinatal Safety Review Working Group 2000). As a general precaution, long-term clinical follow-up is recommended for any child exposed in utero to antiretrovirals. Despite those concerns, two NRTIs remain the recommended backbone of cART for pregnant women in all areas of the world.

Efavirenz and Teratogenicity

Based on early animal studies raising the possibility of neural-tube birth defects (including anencephaly, microphthalmia, and cleft palate) among primates exposed in utero to EFV as well as a few case reports of neural-tube defects in humans, there has been concern about the use of EFV during the first few weeks of pregnancy or in nonpregnant HIV-infected women of childbearing age. As a result, the U.S. Food and Drug Administration and European Medicines Agency still advise against EFV use in this population unless the potential benefit outweighs potential risks. However, the British HIV Association (Taylor et al. 2012) recently changed its recommendation to allow EFV use in the first trimester. More recent data have shown no increase in overall birth defects related to EFV compared with other antiretrovirals in pregnancy and showed an incidence of neural-tube defects comparable to that in the general population in the United States (Ford, Calmy, and Mofenson 2012). As a result, and as previously discussed, the WHO guidelines recommend EFV as a first-line antiviral agent for all adults, including pregnant women, and for women of child-bearing age, while the U.S. guidelines recommend EFV when antiviral therapy is initiated after the first eight weeks of pregnancy.

Nevirapine Hypersensitivity

Severe hypersensitivity reactions including hepatitis, rash, and fever may occur during the first eighteen weeks of NVP therapy, especially in women with CD4 cell counts greater than 250 cells/mm^3. Recent studies in the general population have shown that, compared with those taking EFV, adults treated with NVP were more likely to discontinue treatment owing to adverse events (with the most common events being severe hepatotoxicity, skin reactions, and hypersensitivity reactions) (Shubber et al. 2013). The rates of NVP-associated adverse events in pregnant women, however, were comparable to frequencies in nonpregnant women within the same cohort, though there was a nonsignificant trend toward increased likelihood of severe skin and hepatotoxic adverse events in pregnant women with CD4 cell counts greater than 250 cells/mm^3 (Ford 2013). It is recommended that an NVP-containing regimen be initiated in women with CD4 cell count greater than 250 cells/mm^3, but only if the benefit clearly outweighs the risk. These reactions were not observed in women receiving single-dose NVP for PMTCT.

Antiretroviral Therapy and Preterm Birth

Data remain conflicting on whether certain antiviral regimens are associated with an increased rate of prematurity. Such an effect was reported initially by the European Collaborative and Swiss Cohort Study, demonstrating higher preterm delivery rates among women using combination antiviral therapy, as compared with single- and dual-NRTI therapy. Although several studies from the United States found no such effect, a recent meta-analysis did demonstrate elevated prematurity rates in pregnant women treated with protease-inhibitor (PI)-based therapy, compared with all other regimens (Kourtis et al. 2007). Two studies from Botswana addressed this issue. One study showed higher preterm delivery rates in women using ritnoavir-LPV-based therapy when prospectively compared with those taking triple-NRTI-combination therapy. However, another study using NNRTI-based therapy as the combination-therapy comparator found no association between the regimen and prematurity (Powis et al. 2011; Parekh et al. 2011). Protease inhibitors remain an important component of antiviral therapy for both maternal health and PMTCT, and two PI-based regimens are among the preferred antiretroviral regimens in pregnancy by U.S. treatment guidelines. Protease inhibitors should therefore not be withheld in pregnancy. However, clinicians should be aware that there may be a small increased risk of prematurity in pregnant women using these agents.

Pharmacokinetics and Dosing of Antiretroviral Agents during Pregnancy

Changes in the pharmacokinetics of antiviral drugs may necessitate dose adjustments during the second trimester of pregnancy. For most antiviral agents, standard adult doses and body weight adjustments are recommended. For the preferred regimens, no change in dosing is recommended when using NRTIs and NNRTIs in pregnancy. However, some PIs may require dose adjustments. Atazanavir concentrations are lower during the second and third trimesters of pregnancy and when given concomitantly with TDF or with an H2-receptor antagonist. Therefore the use of ATV without ritonavir boosting is not recommended during pregnancy. When used with low-dose ritonavir (100 milligrams) and TDF, it is recommended that the ATV dose be increased during the second trimester, from 300 to 400 milligrams daily. Similarly, LPV levels are lower in late pregnancy, and therefore the once-daily dosing that is acceptable in nonpregnant adults is not recommended for pregnant women. For PI-experienced patients, an increase in the dose of LPV to 600 milligrams with RTV 150 milligrams twice daily is recommended in the second and third trimesters. For PI-naïve patients it may not be necessary, but if standard dosing of RTV 100 milligrams with LPV 400 milligrams twice daily is used, monitoring virologic response is prudent.

Monitoring of HIV Parameters during Treatment in Pregnancy

Monitoring during ART therapy is essential to evaluate treatment response, adherence, and toxicity. Historically, clinical outcomes and CD4 T-cell counts were used to monitor individuals on ART. However, it has become increasingly apparent that HIV viral load is a more sensitive and time-dependent marker of treatment success or failure. Thus the 2013 WHO guidelines now recommend viral-load monitoring every six to twelve months while a person is on ART. After six months of ART, a viral load of more than 1,000 copies/mL on two consecutive tests can be considered a marker of treatment failure or nonadherence (WHO 2013). When feasible, more frequent virologic monitoring during pregnancy may be beneficial to confirm response to therapy and ongoing virologic control. When possible, checking a viral load two to four weeks after initiating therapy, monthly until the viral load is undetectable, and at least every three months thereafter, is recommended (AIDSinfo 2014). A viral-load value obtained at thirty-four to thirty-six weeks of gestation may be useful in determining the optimal mode of delivery (see below). When virologic testing is not available, CD4 count and clinical monitoring (for signs of AIDS-related complications and opportunistic infections) are still recommended. Use of CD4 cell count becomes less significant if lifelong treatment of pregnant and breast-feeding women is continued, following the updated 2013 WHO guidelines, since they are already on treatment. Laboratory evaluation for safety (liver enzymes, glucose, creatinine, and a complete blood count) should be pursued according to the antiviral agents used and local guidelines for HIV therapy.

ANTENATAL CARE: PREVENTING AND TREATING SELECTED COINFECTIONS AND COMPLICATIONS

Pneumocystis and Toxoplasmosis

Co-trimoxazole therapy is used in HIV-infected patients as prophylaxis for pneumocystis pneumonia and toxoplasmosis and has some benefit in malaria and other bacterial infection prevention as well. In general, it is recommended that all adults be provided with co-trimoxazole prophylaxis if their CD4 cell count is less than 350 cells/mm^3 (though some countries may adopt a threshold of less than 200 cells/mm^3) or WHO stage 3 or 4 regardless of CD4 cell count. This should be continued until CD4 cell count reaches greater than 200 cells/mm^3 (for pneumocystis and toxoplasmosis prophylaxis) or greater than 350 cells/mm^3 (in areas of high prevalence of malaria) after six months of ART (WHO 2013). For infants born to HIV-infected mothers, co-trimoxazole prophylaxis should be initiated four to six weeks after birth and continued until the period of exposure risk is over and the infant has tested negative for HIV infection.

Tuberculosis

All HIV-infected adults (including pregnant women) and children should be routinely screened for active and latent tuberculosis (TB), bearing in mind that extrapulmonary and atypical presentations of tuberculosis are more common in HIV patients, especially those with advanced immune suppression. In TB-endemic areas, a clinical algorithm should be used to assess for symptoms of active TB, including cough, fever, weight loss, or night sweats. Those with symptoms should undergo diagnostic evaluation in accordance with national guidelines to identify active TB or an alternative diagnosis. In areas of high HIV prevalence, WHO-approved molecular tests such as Xpert MTB/RIF (a nucleic acid amplification test that detects both MTB DNA as well as Rifampicin resistance within two hours) should be the primary diagnostic test for TB in individuals with HIV (WHO 2010b). Newly identified TB-HIV coinfected patients with no evidence of drug resistance to typical TB drugs should be initiated on a TB regimen including six months of rifampicin (initial two months with isoniazid, rifampicin, pyrazinamide, and ethambutol followed by an additional four months of rifampicin and isoniazid). In addition, these individuals should be started on ART as soon as possible within the first two months of TB treatment regardless of CD4 count (WHO 2010b; WHO 2011a). For those with baseline drug resistance, guidelines recommend a regimen that includes pyrazinamide, a later-generation fluoroquinolone, a parenteral agent, ethionamide (or prothionamide), and cycloserine, or p-aminosalicylic acid if cycloserine cannot be used). For full guidelines regarding multi-drug-resistant TB, see WHO Guidelines at http://www.who.int/tb/challenges/mdr/programmatic_guidelines_for_mdrtb/en/.

Women without symptoms are less likely to have active TB and should be screened or treated for latent infection. Screening tests for latent TB include either a tuberculin skin test (TST) or interferon γ release assays (IGRA). Those with a positive test and those living in TB-endemic areas with an unknown screening-test result should be offered isoniazid preventive therapy (IPT) after active infection is excluded (Aberg et al. 2014; WHO 2011b, 2013). Similarly, all HIV-infected close contacts of persons with infectious TB should be assessed for active infection and, if excluded, treated for latent TB regardless of their screening results (Aberg et al. 2014).

For HIV-infected patients with active tuberculosis, directly observed therapy is highly recommended.

Cryptococcal Infection

Early initiation of ART is the most effective strategy for reducing the incidence and mortality from cryptococcal disease in all HIV-infected adults (including pregnant women). All HIV-infected individuals should be screened with a serum Cryptococcal antigen (CrAg). There is no evidence to support the use of antifungal prophylaxis in HIV-infected patients with a negative or unknown CrAg. However, HIV-infected patients who have a positive serum CrAg and show signs or symptoms of cryptococcal meningitis should undergo a lumbar puncture with cerebrospinal fluid examination using India ink stain or CSF CrAg to assess for cryptococcal meningitis.

Hepatitis B and C

Coinfection with HIV and hepatitis B or C is a significant cause of morbidity and mortality in HIV-infected individuals, with the highest burden of coinfection in Southeast Asia and sub-Saharan Africa. All HIV-infected individuals should be screened for hepatitis B and C before initiation or change in antiviral therapy (WHO 2013). Screening for hepatitis B consists of a hepatitis B surface antigen (HBsAg), hepatitis B surface antibody (HBsAb), and hepatitis B total-core antibody (HBcAb). Women infected with HIV who have chronic hepatitis B (HBsAg+, HBsAb–) should be assessed for evidence of liver damage, and if detected, prescribed antiviral therapy effective for both HIV and hepatitis B, regardless of CD4 cell count. Effective therapy should include either TDF+FTC or TDF+3TC. In low-resource settings, those without liver damage should initiate therapy when they become eligible for HIV treatment for their own health (WHO 2013). Individuals who are neither infected with nor immune to hepatitis B (HBsAg–, HBsAb–, HBcAb–) should be vaccinated against hepatitis B (Aberg et al. 2014). Newborns of chronically infected (HBsAG+) mothers should receive hepatitis B immune globulin in combination with the hepatitis-B vaccine series.

A hepatitis C antibody test is used to screen for hepatitis C infection. If the antibody is positive, a nucleic acid test (NAT) for hepatitis C ribonucleic acid (RNA) should be obtained to assess for chronic hepatitis C infection. Those with chronic infection should have a minimum of aminotransferase/platelet ratio index (APRI) or fibrosis (FIB4) tests to assess the degree of liver fibrosis. At present drugs used to treat hepatitis C are not used during pregnancy, and there are no proven interventions to reduce the risk of mother-to-child transmission of hepatitis C. For their own health, all HIV-infected patients with chronic hepatitis C infection should initiate antiviral therapy for HIV when they are eligible and should be referred for hepatitis C treatment postpartum (WHO 2011b).

Cervical Cancer Screening

Women with HIV have a higher rate of HPV-associated precancerous cervical and vaginal lesions and invasive cervical cancer. In addition, in HIV-infected women, the risk of persistent human papillomavirus (HPV) infection increases with decreasing CD4 count and increasing HIV viral load. Ideally, all HIV-infected women should undergo cervical cancer screening upon initiation of care. This should be repeated at six months and, if normal, annually thereafter. If the screening test shows any abnormalities, further evaluation is indicated (Aberg et al. 2014).

Sexually Transmitted Infections

All HIV-infected individuals should be screened for the following sexually transmitted diseases (STDs): syphilis, trichomonas, gonorrhea, and chlamydia infections. Treatment is indicated for any pregnant woman who tests positive (see Chapter 5).

Immunizations for HIV-Infected Adults

Immunization recommendations in HIV differ widely according to locale. A list of recommended immunizations for HIV-infected adults in the United States may be found at http://aidsinfo.nih.gov/contentfiles/recommended_immunizations_fs_en.pdf. It is important to note that live-attenuated vaccines (for example, measles, mumps, and rubella, *Varicella*, oral polio, oral typhoid, and yellow fever) should be avoided in pregnancy.

INTRAPARTUM CARE

Intrapartum HIV Testing and Antiviral Therapy

Women receiving antiviral therapy should continue their regimen without interruption during labor. Women who are not on therapy should initiate cART as soon as possible. If available, intravenous AZT during labor should be administered to women whose HIV RNA near term was greater than 1,000 copies/mL or who were not on antiviral therapy. Women whose HIV status is not known should undergo HIV-antibody testing and, if results are positive, should be started on maternal and infant prophylaxis while confirmatory testing is carried out.

Mode of Delivery

In resource-abundant settings, before the wide availability of effective cART and viral-load monitoring in pregnancy, a large meta-analysis demonstrated that scheduled cesarean delivery (performed before the onset of labor and rupture of membranes) reduced the risk of vertical HIV transmission by 50% compared with vaginal delivery or urgent cesarean section (International Perinatal HIV Group 1999). However, since rates of transmission of approximately 1% can now be achieved with cART during pregnancy, the benefit of scheduled cesarean deliveries in preventing transmission is much harder to evaluate. For pregnant women receiving cART whose last antenatal viral load was less than 1,000 copies/mL, there is no evidence to suggest a MTCT-prevention benefit to scheduled cesarean deliveries. Therefore, in the United States, a planned cesarean section for prevention of vertical transmission is not recommended for pregnant women on antiviral therapy whose viral load is less than 1,000 copies/mL. A scheduled cesarean delivery at thirty-eight weeks' gestation is still recommended for women with an unknown HIV viral load or HIV RNA levels greater than 1,000 copies/mL near the time of delivery. Women with HIV RNA levels lower than 1,000 copies/mL who need a cesarean delivery for standard obstetrical indications may schedule the delivery at thirty-nine weeks' gestation (AIDSinfo 2014). In Britain, the recommendations are more stringent, and vaginal delivery is recommended for HIV-infected pregnant women who have a viral load of less than 50 copies/mL (Taylor et al. 2012). A planned cesarean delivery is considered for women with a viral load at thirty-six weeks of 50 to 399 copies/mL, taking into account the actual viral load and its trajectory, length of antepartum ART, adherence issues, obstetric considerations, and the woman's preferences (Taylor et al. 2012). Where viral-load testing is not available, elective cesarean section before the rupture of membranes may be considered for untreated women.

Other Intrapartum Interventions

The risk and benefits of obstetric procedures that could increase fetal exposure to maternal blood should be weighed, and when not clearly indicated, certain procedures should generally be avoided, including artificial rupture of membranes, routine use of fetal scalp electrodes for monitoring, and liberal use of forceps, a vacuum extractor, or episiotomy. Because there are few data on the actual HIV-transmission risk of these practices, especially in the cART era, decisions should be made on a case-by-case basis.

POSTNATAL CARE

Infant Feeding and Risk of Transmission

In breast-feeding populations it is estimated that up to 40% of MTCT of HIV occurs during breast-feeding. However, in many settings infant morbidity and mortality are significantly higher among infants who are fed formula. Therefore, in areas of the world where infant formula is readily available and safe, strict formula feeding is recommended for infants whose mothers are HIV infected; however, such infant-feeding recommendations cannot be universal. Since the availability, risks, and benefits of infant formula greatly vary by locale, national or subnational health authorities must decide whether to counsel HIV-infected mothers in their jurisdiction to breast-feed while receiving antiviral therapy or avoid breast-feeding. In locales where authorities support breast-feeding for HIV-exposed infants, mothers should remain on triple antiviral therapy for the duration of breast-feeding and exclusively breast-feed their infants for the first six months of life. Age-appropriate complementary foods should be introduced thereafter, with breast-feeding continued for the first twelve months of life. Breast-feeding should then stop once a nutritionally adequate and safe diet without breast milk can be provided (WHO 2013). These recommendations are based on evidence that the maximum benefit of breast-feeding in preventing mortality from diarrhea, pneumonia, and malnutrition is in the first twelve months of life, and that the risk of transmitting HIV to infants continues throughout the breast-feeding period but is significant lower when the mother is on ART (WHO 2013).

Postpartum Testing and Management of HIV-Exposed Infants

All infants born to HIV-infected mothers should receive postnatal antiviral therapy for prevention beginning at birth. Infants of mothers who receive antiretrovirals and are breast-feeding should receive six weeks of infant prophylaxis with daily NVP (WHO 2013). Infants receiving exclusive formula feeding should be given four to six weeks of twice daily AZT or daily NVP (WHO 2013). Co-trimoxazole prophylaxis should be initiated four to six weeks after birth and continued until the infant tests negative for HIV infection and the period of exposure risk is over. An HIV testing algorithm for exposed infants may be found at http://www.who.int/hiv /pub/paediatric/diagnosis/en/. Testing schedules depend on test availability and the period of exposure. In general, for HIV-exposed infants, virologic tests for HIV DNA, RNA, or P24 Ag are recommended beginning at four to six weeks of age and until eighteen months of age, and serologic tests are recommended thereafter. Infants diagnosed with HIV should be immediately referred for care.

Other Postpartum-Care Considerations

As indicated above, HIV-infected women continue to benefit from ART for their own health, regardless of their pretreatment HIV viral load and CD4 cell count. They should therefore remain on antiviral therapy postpartum whenever feasible. However, if women do not meet criteria for therapy for their own health in their locale, they should, at a minimum, continue therapy for the duration of infant risk, including the entire duration of breast-feeding. If a woman's sex partner is HIV-negative, she would also qualify to remain on antiviral therapy as prevention. All postpartum HIV-infected women should be counseled on contraceptive options to prevent unintended pregnancies. Attention should be paid to potential drug interactions between certain antiviral agents and hormonal contraception. If HIV care was provided through a prenatal-care clinic, adequate referral to an HIV clinic should be made.

CONCLUSIONS

Nearly all pediatric HIV infections worldwide occur through mother-to-child transmission of the virus. With implementation of preventive strategies and improved access to antiretroviral therapy during pregnancy and the breast-feeding period, the epidemic of HIV infection in children can be eliminated. Indeed, the Joint United Nations Program on HIV/AIDS (UNAIDS), the World Health Organization (WHO), and the United Nations Children's Fund (UNICEF) announced in 2011 its Countdown to Zero campaign, "a global plan towards the elimination of new HIV infections among children by 2015 and keeping their mothers alive." The goal was to reduce the number of new HIV infections among children by 90 percent and decrease mother-to-child transmission of HIV to 5% by 2015 (UNAIDS 2013). To achieve this goal, routine HIV testing should be performed on all pregnant women. Women infected with HIV should have access to prenatal care, receive effective antiretroviral therapy for their own health and for PMTCT, and be monitored for adherence, toxicity, and response. Women should be counseled about optimal infant feeding in their locale. Breast-feeding mothers should exclusively breast-feed until the infant is six months of age and continue antiviral therapy throughout the breast-feeding period. Infants exposed to HIV should receive antiviral and co-trimoxazole prophylaxis and serial HIV testing. Treatment for HIV should not be limited to the period of MTCT risk, and care for HIV-infected women and their HIV- and antiviral-exposed infants should continue postpartum. While testing and laboratory monitoring protocols, qualifications for therapy, available maternal and infant regimens, and recommendations for infant feeding may vary by local and national HIV program guidelines, the general principles of PMTCT are universal, and if followed, the epidemic of HIV in children will be eliminated.

REFERENCES

Aberg, J., J. E. Gallant, K. G. Ghanem, P. Emmanuel, B. S. Zingman, and M. A. Horberg. 2014. Primary care guidelines for the management of persons infected with HIV: 2013 update by the HIV Medicine Association of the Infectious Diseases Society of America. *Clin Infect Dis* 58 (1): e1–34. doi:10.1093/cid/cit665. Epub 2013 Nov 13.

AIDSinfo. 2014. "Recommendations for Use of Antiretroviral Drugs in Pregnant HIV-1-Infected Women for Maternal Health and Interventions to Reduce Perinatal HIV Transmission in the United States." "Clinical Guidelines Portal." U.S. Department of Health and Human Services. Accessed May 26, 2016. http://aidsinfo.nih.gov/guidelines.

Barret, B., M. Tardieu, P. Rustin, C. Lacroix, B. Chabrol, I. Desguerre, C. Dollfus, M. J. Mayaux, and S. Blanche. 2003. Persistent mitochondrial dysfunction in

HIV-1-exposed but uninfected infants: Clinical screening in a large prospective cohort. *AIDS* 17:1769–1785.

Cohen, M. S., Y. Q. Chen, M. McCauley, T. Gamble, M. C. Hosseinipour, N. Kumarasamy, J. G. Hakim, et al. 2011. Prevention of HIV-1 infection with early antiretroviral therapy. *N Engl J Med* 365:493–505.

Connor, E. M., R. S. Sperling, P. Gelber, P. Kiselev, G. Scott, M. J. O'Sullivan, R. VanDyke, et al. 1994. Reduction of maternal-infant transmission of human immunodeficiency virus type 1 with zidovudine treatment. *N Engl J Med* 331:1173–1180.

Coutsoudis, A., F. Dabis, W. Fawzi, P. Gaillard, G. Haverkamp, D. R. Harris, J. B. Jackson, et al. 2004. Late postnatal transmission of HIV-1 in breast-fed children: An individual patient data meta-analysis. *J Infect Dis* 189:2154.

Davis, John A., and S. Yawetz. 2012. Management of HIV in the pregnant woman. *Clin Obstet Gynecol* 55:531–540.

Ford, N., A. Calmy, I. Andrieux-Meyer, S. Hargreaves, E. J. Mills, and Z. Schubber. 2013. Adverse events associated with nevirapine use in pregnancy: A systematic review and meta-analysis. *AIDS* 27:1135–1143.

Ford, N., A. Calmy, and L. Mofenson. 2011. Safety of efavirenz in the first trimester of pregnancy: An updated systematic review and meta-analysis. *AIDS* 25:2301–2304.

Garcia, P. M., L. A. Kalish, J. Pitt, H. Minkoff, T. C. Quinn, S. K. Burchett, J. Kornegay, et al. 1999. Maternal levels of plasma human immunodeficiency virus type 1 RNA and the risk of perinatal transmission. *N Engl J Med* 341:394–402.

International Perinatal HIV Group. 1999. The mode of delivery and the risk of vertical transmission of human immunodeficiency virus type 1: A meta-analysis of 15 prospective cohort studies. *N Engl J Med* 340:977–987.

Kitahata, M. M., S. J. Gange, A. G. Abraham, B. Merriman, M. S. Saag, A. C. Justice, R. S. Hogg, et al. 2009. Effect of early versus deferred antiretroviral therapy for HIV on survival. *N Engl J Med* 360:1815–1826.

Kourtis, A. P., C. H. Schmid, D. J. Jamieson, and J. Lau. 2007. Use of antiretroviral therapy in pregnant HIV-infected women and the risk of premature delivery: A meta-analysis. *AIDS* 21:607–615.

Lallemant, M., G. Jourdain, S. Le Coeur, S. Kim, S. Koetsawang, A. M. Comeau, W. Phoolcharoen, M. Essex, K. McIntosh, and V. Vithayasai. 2000. A trial of shortened zidovudine regimens to prevent mother-to-child transmission of human immunodeficiency virus type 1. *N Engl J Med* 343:982–991.

Miotti, P. G., T. E. Taha, N. I. Kumwenda, R. Broadhead, L. A. Mtimavalye, L. Van der Hoeven, J. D. Chiphangwi, G. Liomba, and R. J. Biggar. 1999. HIV transmission through breastfeeding: A study in Malawi. *JAMA* 282:744.

Nielsen-Saines, K., D. H. Watts, V. G. Veloso, Y. J. Bryson, E. C. Joao, J. H. Pilotto, G. Gray, et al. 2012. Three postpartum antiretroviral regimens to prevent intrapartum HIV infection. *N Engl J Med* 366:2368–2379.

Parekh, N., H. Ribaudo, S. Souda, J. Chen, M. Mmalane, K. Powis, M. Essex, J. Makhema, and R. L. Shapiro. 2011. Risk factors for very preterm delivery and delivery of very-small-for-gestational-age infants among HIV-exposed and HIV-unexposed infants in Botswana. *Int J Gynaecol Obstet* 115:20–25.

Perinatal Safety Review Working Group. 2000. Nucleoside exposure in the children of HIV-infected women receiving antiretroviral drugs: Absence of clear evidence for mitochondrial disease in children who died before 5 years of age in five United States cohorts. *J Acquir Immune Defic Synd* 25:261–268.

Powis, K. M., D. Kitch, A. Ogwu, M. D. Hughes, S. Lockman, J. Leidner, E. van Widenfelt, et al. 2011. Increased risk of preterm delivery among HIV-infected women randomized to protease versus nucleoside reverse transcriptase inhibitor-based HAART during pregnancy. *J Infect Dis* 204:506–514.

Quinn, T. C., J. M. Mann, J. W. Curran, and P. Piot. 1986. AIDS in Africa: An epidemiologic paradigm. *Science* 234:955–963.

Read, P. J., S. Mandalia, P. Khan, U. Harrisson, C. Naftalin, Y. Gilleece, J. Anderson, D. A. Hawkins, G. P. Taylor, and A. de Ruiter. 2012. When should HAART be initiated in pregnancy to achieve an undetectable HIV viral load by delivery? *AIDS* 26:1095–1103.

Rousseau, C. M., R. W. Nduati, B. A. Richardson, G. C. John-Stewart, D. A. Mbori-Ngacha, J. K. Kreiss, and J. Overbaugh. 2004. Association of levels of HIV-1-infected breast milk cells and risk of mother-to-child transmission. *J Infect Dis* 190:1880.

Shubber, Z., A. Calmy, I. Andrieux-Meyer, M. Vitoria, F. Renaud-Théry, N. Shaffer, S. Hargreaves, E. J. Mills, and N. Ford. 2013. Adverse events associated with nevirapine and efavirenz-based first-line antiretroviral therapy: A systematic review and meta-analysis. *AIDS* 27:1403–1412.

Taylor, G. P., P. Clayden, J. Dhar, K. Gandhi, Y. Gilleece, K. Harding, P. Hay, et al. 2012. Guidelines for the management of HIV infection in pregnant women 2012. *HIV Med* 13 (S2): 87–157. doi:10.1111/j.1468-1293.2012.01030_2.x.

Townsend, C. L., M. Cortina-Borja, C. S. Peckham, A. de Ruiter, H. Lyall, and P. A. Tookey. 2008. Low rates of mother-to-child transmission of HIV following effective pregnancy interventions in the United Kingdom and Ireland, 2000–2006. *AIDS* 22:973–981.

Tubiana, R., J. Le Chenadec, C. Rouzioux, L. Mandelbrot, K. Hamrene, C. Dollfus, A. Faye, C. Delaugerre, S. Blanche, and J. Warszawski. 2010. Factors associated with mother-to-child transmission of HIV-1 despite a maternal viral load < 500 copies/mL at delivery: A case-control study nested in the French Perinatal Cohort (EPF-ANRS CO). *Clin Infect Dis* 50:585–596.

UNAIDS. 2013. *Global Report: UNAIDS Report on the Global AIDS Epidemic*. Geneva: Joint United Nations Programme on HIV/AIDS. Accessed June 4, 2016. http://www.unaids.org/sites/default/files/media_asset/UNAIDS_Global_Report_2013_en_1.pdf.

Wang, L., A. P. Kourtis, S. Ellington, J. Legardy-Williams, and M. Bulterys. 2013. Safety of tenofovir during pregnancy for the mother and fetus: A systematic review. *Clinical Infectious Diseases* 57:1773–1781.

WHO (World Health Organization). 2010a. *Antiretroviral Drugs for Treating Pregnant Women and Preventing HIV Infection in Infants: Recommendations for a Public Health Approach*. Geneva: World Health Organization.

———. 2010b. *WHO Policy on Collaborative TB/HIV Activities: Guidelines for National Programmes and Other Stakeholders.* Geneva: World Health Organization. Accessed May 26, 2016. http://www.who.int/tb/publications/2012/tb_hiv_policy _9789241503006/en/.

———. 2011a. *Guidelines for Intensified Tuberculosis Case-Finding and Isoniazid Preventive Therapy for People Living with HIV in Resource-Constrained Settings.* Geneva: World Health Organization. Accessed May 26, 2016. http://www.who.int/hiv/pub/tb /9789241500708/en/.

———. 2011b. *Guidelines for the Screening, Care and Treatment of Persons with Hepatitis C Infection.* Geneva: World Health Organization. Accessed May 26, 2016. http://www.who.int/hiv/pub/hepatitis/hepatitis-c-guidelines/en/.

———. 2012. *Use of Efavirenz during Pregnancy: A Public Health Perspective; Technical update on treatment optimization.* Geneva: World Health Organization. Accessed May 26, 2016. http://www.who.int/hiv/pub/treatment2/efavirenz/en.

———. 2013. *Consolidated Guidelines on the Use of Antiretroviral Drugs for Treating and Preventing HIV Infection: Recommendations for a Public Health Approach.* Geneva: World Health Organization.

7

Malaria and Pregnancy

BLAIR WYLIE AND JOHANNA DAILY

For obstetrician-gynecologists (ob-gyns) working in malaria-endemic areas with limited resources, the ability to prevent and treat malaria in their patients and themselves is critical. Millions of pregnant women reside in malaria-endemic areas and thus are at risk; pregnancy increases a woman's risk for more severe disease, and rapid treatment is needed to maximize good outcomes. Premature birth and poor fetal outcomes are associated with malarial infection owing to parasitic infection of the placenta. Thus malarial infection can result in adverse consequences for both the mother and fetus. Malarial infection and complications are preventable, and knowledge of practice guidelines to prevent and treat malaria will greatly improve maternal and child health.

Malaria is caused by the protozoan parasite *Plasmodium,* five species of which can infect humans. Each is associated with a geographical area, with some overlap. *P. vivax* is the most prevalent worldwide, though *P. falciparum* is responsible for severe disease, is the most prevalent in Africa, and is often resistant to chloroquine. Knowledge of the local malaria species and antimalarial susceptibilities in the region of practice will dictate treatment.

The life cycle of malaria provides many points at which to intervene and prevent human infection. Infection occurs through the bite of an infected *Anopheles* mosquito, which typically feeds at dusk. The mosquito transmits sporozoites during a blood meal, which invade and silently replicate in the liver for two weeks (depending on the species) before they enter the blood stream and infect erythrocytes. Interventions that target the vector and reduce human contact with mosquitoes are key to preventing infection. The erythrocytic stage may bring clinical symptoms and disease as the parasites replicate, logarithmically increasing pathogen load and inducing inflammation. Patients with partial clinical immunity manifest less inflammation and generate an effective immune response to control the infection. The physiologic changes associated with pregnancy can be accompanied by a temporary lessening of this naturally acquired immunity.

Symptoms associated with malaria infection are highly diverse and nonspecific, rendering a clinical diagnosis inaccurate and thus requiring a diagnostic test. Patients can be asymptomatic carriers or manifest mild symptoms including fever, myalgias, chills, headaches, and malaise. Anemia can accompany malarial infection. More severe disease is rare but includes neurological symptoms such as seizures, mental confusion, coma, and involvement of vital organs resulting in kidney failure, respiratory distress, and death. Immediate treatment in cases of severe disease is critical, as deterioration can occur rapidly and is unpredictable. The risk of severe malaria is higher during pregnancy.

Placental malaria is a central and unique complication of malarial infection during pregnancy. The infected erythrocytes can adhere to the chondroitin sulfate A that lines the intervillous space of the placenta (Figure 7.1). This impairs placental health and increases risk of miscarriage, preterm birth, and stillbirth as well as low birth weight and infant mortality. Measures to prevent placental malaria among women who reside in malaria-endemic areas include administration of antimalarial prophylaxis during the second and third trimesters. Women gain protection from placental malaria through production of antibodies to placental parasites over the course of multiple pregnancies. These antibodies prevent adherence to the placenta and correlate with improved birth outcomes. Vaccines to prevent placental malaria in pregnant women are in development and are based on this natural immunity; however, no pregnancy-specific malaria vaccine is currently available. In summary, malarial infection during pregnancy can have severe consequences for both the mother and the fetus, and obstetricians-gynecologists working in malaria-endemic areas need to know how to prevent and treat it. This chapter reviews the epidemiology, pathogenesis, and treatment of malaria as they pertain to the practice of obstetrics and gynecology in malaria-endemic countries. Table 7.1 highlights the key points of this chapter.

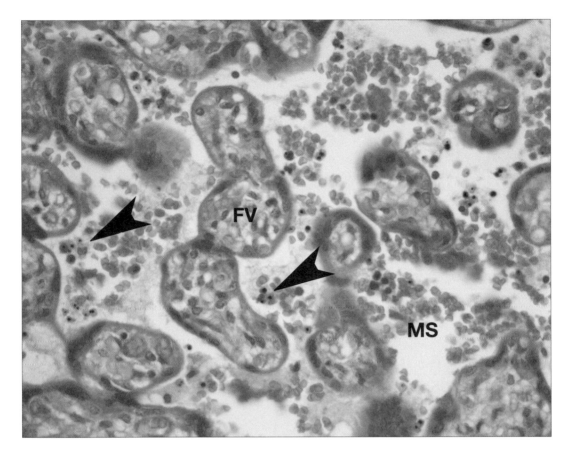

FIGURE 7.1. Placental malaria. Microscopy of a histologic section of placental malaria identifies multiple maternal blood cells containing parasites. Arrows mark *Plasmodium falciparum* parasites. FV=fetal vessel. MS=maternal side. 60x magnification. Hematoxylin and eosin stain.

EPIDEMIOLOGY

Global Epidemiology

Malaria is endemic to many parts of the world including large areas of sub-Saharan Africa, Central and South America, parts of the Caribbean, India, South Asia, Southeast Asia, and the Middle East. Of an estimated 200 to 300 million annual infections, over 500,000 prove fatal (WHO 2012b). In endemic areas, pregnant women, infants, and children are most vulnerable. Fifty million pregnancies occur in malaria-endemic areas annually, resulting in 10,000 maternal deaths, 200,000 cases of severe

Table 7.1   General considerations for malaria during pregnancy

Epidemiology, diagnosis, clinical impact

Malaria requires microscopy or a rapid diagnostic test for diagnosis; clinical diagnosis is often inaccurate.

Malaria during pregnancy has implications for the health of both the mother and the fetus.

Pregnant women from endemic areas who previously acquired disease immunity have reduced immunity during pregnancy.

Pregnant women with malaria are at higher risk of developing hypoglycemia and severe disease.

Plasmodium falciparum can specifically infect the placenta.

Placental malaria can result in low birth weight, fetal loss, and preterm birth.

Repeat pregnancies provide some protection from placental malaria for women who live in endemic areas.

Intermittent preventative therapy is recommended for pregnant women to prevent placental malaria.

Pregnant women suspected of having malaria should receive prompt therapy.

General principles of treatment

Obtain rapid diagnostic test or microscopic diagnosis and identify species of malaria.

Determine whether you are in a chloroquine-sensitive or chloroquine-resistant region and whether this is severe or mild disease.

Rapid initiation of therapy during pregnancy is critical to prevent poor outcomes.

Most *P. falciparum* has become chloroquine resistant thus chloroquine should be used only if the region is known to have chloroquine-sensitive malaria.

Quinine, chloroquine, clindamycin, and proguanil are considered safe during pregnancy.

Artemisinins are not recommended during the first trimester until additional safety data is obtained; however, they are superior to quinine in the setting of severe disease and should be used in severe disease.

Doxycycline, tetracycline, and primaquine should be avoided during pregnancy.

Source: Adapted from WHO (2015), © World Health Organization 2015.

maternal anemia, and 200,000 low-birth-weight infants (Steketee et al. 2001; Guyatt and Snow 2001, 2004).

The five species of malaria that cause human infection are *P. falciparum, P. vivax, P. ovale, P. malariae,* and *P. knowlesi.* The most prevalent human species is *P. vivax,* which is usually not fatal but can result in significant anemia. It can be dormant in the liver and cause relapses months to years later. *P. vivax* can cause more severe disease in pregnant women and neonates, though less often than *P. falciparum* (Nosten et al. 1999).

P. falciparum is the second most prevalent malarial strain and accounts for the majority of severe malaria (Figure 7.1). *P. falciparum* is uniquely virulent through its capacity to generate a high parasite burden and the ability of infected erythrocytes to sequester in tissue microvasculature, including the placenta. *P. malariae* and *P. ovale* are rare and do not cause severe disease.

Recently *P. knowlesi* was identified as infecting humans in Southeast Asia, where it is maintained in macaque (monkey) reservoirs. This species is rare but important, as it can also cause severe and fatal disease (Kantele and Jokiranta 2011). For the remainder of this chapter, we discuss *P. falciparum* unless otherwise stated.

Malarial Infection versus Disease

The clinical presentation of malaria during pregnancy varies according to the level of transmission in a region, known as endemicity. The risk for acquisition of malarial infection depends on the intensity of transmission in the region visited and the season, with increased risk during the rainy season. Although high-transmission regions may result in more total infections, residents gain immunity to disease with each infection. Thus adults in high-transmission regions sustain less severe disease, and during infection they have minimal symptoms or can be asymptomatic. However, this clinical immunity is diminished during pregnancy.

In areas where malaria transmission is unstable, that is, where it occurs episodically and not year-round, women are at risk for more severe illness if they are infected during pregnancy (Desai et al. 2007). Compared with nonpregnant women infected in these areas, those who are pregnant are at elevated risk of severe anemia and serious symptoms, such as cerebral malaria and respiratory distress, and are at heightened risk of mortality (see Chapter 2). Their pregnancies are at risk for miscarriage and preterm birth as well as low birth weight and consequently increased risk of infant mortality. Travelers to malaria-endemic areas with no prior immunity are at risk of severe malaria, as are immigrants who return to these endemic areas, having lost the partial immunity that develops through repeated exposure. Thus understanding transmission intensity and its implications for the population's risk during high and low transmission, combined with assessing an individual's risk for severe disease, will guide interventions and treatment practices.

Unique Epidemiologic Principles of Malaria in Pregnancy

Pregnant women are particularly vulnerable to malarial infection and illness. When compared with nonpregnant adults, pregnant women are more likely to be bitten by mosquitoes. Approximately twice as many *Anopheles* mosquitoes were collected from under the bed nets of pregnant women compared with nonpregnant women in a study from The Gambia (Lindsay et al. 2000). Mosquitoes identify their host through detection of molecules such as carbon dioxide from exhaled breath and body heat, both of which may be increased during pregnancy. Pregnant women sustain more frequent infections and higher parasite loads compared than nonpregnant adults. In a longitudinal study of women from Senegal followed before, during, and after pregnancy, the risk of *P. falciparum* malaria episodes increased significantly during the second and third trimesters when compared with prepregnant women (adjusted relative risk, 95% confidence interval: 2nd trimester 2.5, 1.1 to 5.7; 3rd trimester 2.9, 1.3 to 6.4) (Diagne et al. 2000). This elevated risk persisted for up to sixty days postpartum. The prevalence and density of asymptomatic parasitemia was also higher during pregnancy.

Pregnant women are more likely to have severe malaria than nonpregnant adults. The elevated morbidity and mortality associated with malaria during pregnancy includes increased risk of hypoglycemia, pulmonary edema, acute respiratory distress syndrome, and death (Desai et al. 2007). Notably, the mortality rate of severe malaria during pregnancy is as high as 50% (WHO 2014). In areas where malaria transmission is stable, infection during pregnancy may be associated with lack of clinical illness. Nonetheless, pregnant women are still at increased risk for severe anemia, and their fetuses are at risk for low birth weight owing to placental malaria.

Malaria is more frequent and more severe among nulliparous women compared with multiparous women. Perhaps the most fascinating observation regarding the epidemiology of malaria is that it is both more frequent and more severe among nulliparous women than multiparous women, suggesting parity-specific immunity. During infection, many strains of the parasite are present, each with different tissue-adherence properties. The presence of placental tissue selects for the var2csa expressing strain of malaria, which can adhere to chondroitin sulfate A and replicate in the placenta (Figure 7.1). A nulliparous woman would be exposed to this parasite for the first time and thus not have developed antibodies to this specific strain. With subsequent pregnancies, antibodies to var2csa develop, associated with milder clinical symptoms and less placental malaria. This phenomenon has been demonstrated by showing that antibodies from parous women block binding of parasites to placental cells in culture—including parasites from other regions of the world (Fried and Duffy 1998). This suggests that the mechanism for adherence to the placenta is conserved globally. Given this observation, research groups are actively trying to develop a pregnancy-specific malarial vaccine that targets chondroitin sulfate-binding parasite strains; however, to date none has been fully developed, given the genetic diversity of the surface-expressed erythrocyte membrane proteins that bind chondroitin sulfate A (Duffy et al. 2001; Bordbar et al. 2014). Thus prevention via chemoprophylaxis and bed nets remains the standard of care to prevent placental malaria.

Impact of HIV on malaria in pregnancy. A higher incidence of both malarial infection in the mother and placental malaria can result from HIV infection during pregnancy (ter Kuile et al. 2004). This phenomenon is thought to be secondary to the poor antibody response to malaria antigens in HIV coinfection. The increase in risk of placental malaria among HIV-positive pregnant women is associated with lower levels of antibody to the var2csa strain that is responsible for placental malaria. In addition, with HIV infection, antibodies to var2csa do not increase with each pregnancy; thus all pregnancies, irrespective of parity, are associated with higher risk of placental malaria (Mount et al. 2004). There is conflicting information on whether the presence of placental malaria increases the rate of HIV 1 transmission to the fetus. Nevertheless, women with HIV should take more intensive preventative measures against malaria, including bed nets and chemoprophylaxis (see Chapter 6).

PATHOLOGY AND PATHOPHYSIOLOGY

Malaria Life Cycle

Malaria is caused by a protozoan parasite that is transmitted through the bite of an *Anopheles* mosquito. Like all parasites, *Plasmodium* goes through an elaborate life cycle with multiple hosts. The form injected from the mosquito into the bloodstream is known as a sporozoite. These travel via the bloodstream to the liver, where they infect hepatocytes and mature into liver-stage forms. The patient is clinically asymptomatic during this stage.

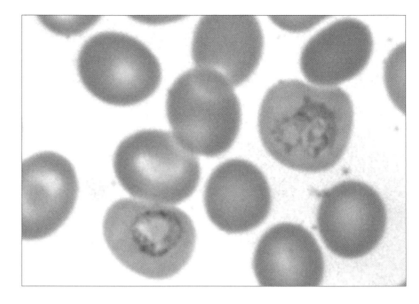

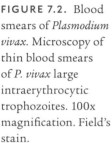

FIGURE 7.2. Blood smears of *Plasmodium vivax*. Microscopy of thin blood smears of *P. vivax* large intraerythrocytic trophozoites. 100x magnification. Field's stain.

After a certain period of time (depending on the species) the parasites exit the liver and enter the bloodstream by the thousands in a form known as merozoites. These immediately infect red blood cells, in which they mature from the ring stage (which circulate in the peripheral blood and are visible under the microscope, Figures 7.2 and 7.3) into trophozoites and divide to become schizonts. Trophozoites sequester out of the circulation into tissue beds, including the placenta. At forty-eight hours, the schizonts release merozoites into the bloodstream and repeat the infection cycle.

Placental Malaria

The placenta is an organ unique to pregnancy and is a target of malarial infection. When an erythrocyte is infected with malaria parasites, it expresses the parasites' proteins on its exterior membrane. The trophozoite-stage proteins transform the red cell surface from smooth to knobby. These parasite proteins can bind to the vascular endothelium throughout the body of the host, blocking microvasculature and causing vascular insufficiency to vital organs. During pregnancy, the placental microvasculature becomes a binding site for parasitized erythrocytes. Infected erythrocytes accumulate in the intervillous spaces, sometimes at high densities (Brabin et al. 2004). Binding is thought to activate the complement cascade, dysregulate angiogenesis, and recruit

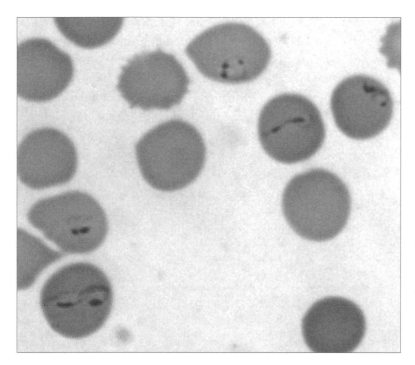

FIGURE 7.3. Blood smears of *Plasmodium falciparum*. Microscopy of thin blood smears of *Plasmodium falciparum* with small intraerythrocytic ring forms. 100x magnification. Field's stain.

cytokines and an inflammatory infiltrate that can lead to placental dysfunction, impaired fetal growth, and fetal loss (Silver et al. 2010; Conroy et al. 2011).

Binding of infected erythrocytes in the placenta appears to be localized to the fibrinoid strands within the intervillous space. Researchers systematically searched for the parasite receptor and ultimately discovered that chondroitin sulfate A (CSA), a component of the extracellular matrix, supported parasite binding to placentas (Fried and Duffy 1998). In addition, these parasitized erythrocytes from the placenta that bind CSA did not bind CD36, an endothelial component that commonly binds isolates from nonpregnant individuals. It is important to note that individuals are often infected with not one but a range of parasite strains, each with differing binding properties, including the expression of different proteins allowing sequestration. The presence of placental tissue selects for CSA-binding parasites, which survive in the placenta, replicate, and expand a placental-adherent strain. In fact, a placenta is required for selection and expansion of this parasite. This lends credence to the observation that the phenotype of placental parasites differs from that of nonpregnant isolates.

Based on these data, a pregnancy-specific malaria vaccine may one day be feasible (Duffy et al. 2001). Parasites isolated from the placentas of Kenyan women were incubated with sera from primigravid women, multigravid women, and men. Sera from secundigravid and multigravid women inhibited binding of parasites to immobilized CSA, whereas sera from males and primigravid women did not. Sera from Malawi and Thai-Burmese primigravids, secundigravids, and multigravids demonstrated similar results. This pioneering work underscores the hope that a pregnancy-specific malaria vaccine is plausible and that it would have widespread efficacy. Var2csa, which is responsible for placental adherence, is the primary vaccine candidate. The task of creating a pregnancy-specific vaccine is not trivial, as this gene is polymorphic across malarial strains despite a conserved binding site.

GLOBAL IMPACT OF THE DISEASE

Travelers to malarious areas with no prior immunity to malaria are at high risk of developing the disease. As stated above, immigrants who return to endemic areas after living in nonendemic areas lose the partial immunity they developed through repeated exposure to malarial parasites. The risk for acquisition depends on the intensity of transmission in the region visited and the season, with increased transmission during the rainy season. Updated information about malaria endemicity can be found online through the Centers for Disease Control (www.cdc.gov /malaria/map). These interactive maps display information on malarial prevalence in specific geographic locations as well as recommended prophylactic medications.

Malaria in pregnancy is an important cause of both morbidity and mortality to the mother and the baby. For the mother, the primary effect is anemia, which can be severe. For the baby, the biggest consequence of infection is poor intrauterine growth, leading to low birth weight, growth restriction, and consequently increased risk for death in infancy. Prevention of malaria during pregnancy in endemic areas could save the lives of 10,000 mothers, prevent 200,000 cases of severe anemia, and prevent cases of low birth weight in 200,000 infants each year. It is important to keep in mind that these numbers are likely gross underestimations owing to underreporting (Desai et al. 2007; Guyatt 2004; Steketee 2001).

PREVENTION AND TREATMENT

Prevention

Prevention of infection during pregnancy is important to avert potentially severe complications. Two major control strategies are emphasized for the prevention of malaria among pregnant women living in endemic areas: vector control and chemoprophylaxis (see Table 7.2).

Vector Control

A key prevention strategy revolves around reducing exposure to *Anopheles,* the mosquito vector that carries malaria, which feeds at dusk and during the night. Therefore, pregnant women living in endemic areas are instructed to sleep under an insecticide-treated bed net (ITN). A Cochrane review of the efficacy of ITNs for the prevention of pregnancy malaria found reduced placental malaria in all pregnancies (RR 0.79, 95% CI 0.63–0.98) compared with no nets in African trials (Gamble, Ekwaru, and ter Kuile 2006). Insecticide-treated bed nets also reduced the risk of low birth weight (RR 0.77, 95% CI 0.61–0.98) and fetal loss in the first through fourth pregnancies (RR 0.67, 95% CI 0.47–0.97) but not among later pregnancies. For anemia and clinical malaria, the effects of ITNs were insignificant although trended toward improvement.

While these results suggest improvement in pregnancy outcomes for women sleeping under bed nets, there are major challenges to ITN use and adherence during pregnancy. While some antenatal clinics in endemic areas provide ITNs to their pregnant patients, ITNs are not universally available and may be too expensive for mothers to purchase. Even in households where an ITN is available, pregnant women may not be the ones to sleep under the net and may defer to the head of the household or prefer protecting their children. Furthermore, ITNs require ongoing maintenance, such as repairing holes and reapplication of insecticide, to sustain their effectiveness.

Reduction of vectors near the home is also a key intervention. The elimination of standing water, the use of window screens, and indoor residual spraying to reduce mosquito populations are additional effective interventions.

Chemoprophylaxis and Intermittent Preventive Treatment in Pregnancy

In addition to vector control, chemoprophylaxis is recommended for prevention of malaria during pregnancy, a strategy similar to that prescribed

Table 7.2 Prevention of malaria in pregnancy

Chemoprophylaxis for pregnant non-immune travelers

Travel should be deferred until after delivery if risk is high for malaria, if at all possible. If not, chemoprophylaxis outlined below is recommended.

For pregnant non-immune women:

Mefloquine (chloroquine-resistant regions)	• Mefloquine hydrochloride 250 mg salt q week; start 2–3 weeks prior to travel and continue 4 weeks post travel.
Chloroquine (chloroquine-sensitive regions)	• Chloroquine phosphate 500 mg salt q week, start 1–2 weeks prior to travel and continue q week for 4 weeks post travel.
Hydroxychloroquine sulfate (alternative for chloroquine-sensitive regions)	• Hydroxychloroquine sulfate 400 mg salt q week, start 1–2 weeks prior to travel and continue q week for 4 weeks post travel.

Intermittent preventive therapy of pregnancy for residents of endemic areas

Low-transmission areas: IPTp-SP dose in second trimester, and again in third trimester	• Sulfadoxine/pyrimethamine (SP) 500 mg/25 mg tablets; administer 3 tablets for total required dosage of 1500 mg/75 mg; first dose early in second trimester; repeat in third trimester; doses administered as directly observed therapy.
Moderate to high transmission: IPTp-SP second trimester and at each scheduled antenatal visit	• SP 500 mg/25 mg tablets; administer 3 tablets for total required dosage of 1500 mg/75 mg; doses should be repeated at monthly intervals at each antenatal visit until delivery.
HIV-infected	• If not using co-trimoxazole prophylaxis, then monthly doses of SP as outlined above; if on co-trimoxazole, additional SP is not needed.

Vector avoidance/control for both travelers and residents

Reduce exposure between dusk and dawn
Screened homes
Sleep under insecticide-treated bed-nets
Use of insect repellants
Reduce skin exposure (long-sleeved clothing, long pants)
Indoor residual spraying
Eliminate standing water near homes

Source: Adapted from WHO (2015), © World Health Organization 2015.
IPTp = Intermittent preventive therapy in pregnancy.
IPTp-SP = intermittent preventive therapy in pregnancy with sulfadoxine-pyrimethamine.

to travelers visiting malaria-endemic areas. Initially, policy makers recommended that pregnant women receive weekly chloroquine; however, resistance to chloroquine has become widespread except for areas in the Caribbean, Central America, and the Middle East.

The World Health Organization currently recommends that pregnant women living in areas of moderate to high transmission receive chemoprophylaxis with intermittent preventive (or presumptive) treatment during pregnancy (IPTp). Curative doses of an antimalarial are administered during the latter half of pregnancy. This strategy assumes that in endemic areas the majority of women may be harboring undetectable parasites in the placenta. Indeed, a number of studies have demonstrated the presence of placental parasitemia in the absence of peripheral parasites (Ismail 2000).

There have been a number of investigations into the efficacy of IPTp. In randomized trials involving over 14,481 pregnant women, IPTp significantly decreased the risk of severe anemia by 40% (RR 0.6, 95% CI 0.5–0.8), and low birth weight by 27% (RR 0.7, 95% CI 0.6.–0.9) (Radeva-Petrova D. et al. 2014).

In Africa, the medication recommended for IPTp is sulfadoxine-pyrimethamine (SP) (Table 7.2) (WHO 2012b). One dose (1,500/75 mg) is administered after the onset of fetal movement to avoid administration during the first trimester. Ideally, IPTp should be administered under direct observation and can be given with or without food. This dose is repeated at each antenatal visit until delivery but no more often than monthly in moderate- to high-transmission areas. In low-transmission areas, IPTp is administered only twice, starting in the second trimester.

Co-trimoxazole prevents HIV-related opportunistic infections and is routinely given to HIV-infected individuals who are immunosuppressed. Pregnant women who are HIV-positive with a low CD4+T cell count or clinical features of immunosuppression should continue cotrimoxazole during pregnancy. This prevents malaria infection, making additional sulfadoxine/pyrimethamine (SP)-based IPTp for malaria unnecessary (WHO 2006). For HIV-infected women who are not on co-trimoxazole and are living in high- or moderate-transmission areas, the guidelines for IPTp are the same as for HIV-negative women.

Because sulfadoxine/pyrimethamine is a folate antagonist, high doses of folate (greater than or equal to 5 milligrams) should be avoided, as they may negate the protective mechanism of action of SP.

Sulfadoxine/pyrimethamine has a long half-life and thus can be dosed infrequently, making it an ideal prophylactic drug. There are few pharmacokinetic studies of SP during pregnancy. It is not known whether the efficacy of IPTp-SP is related to clearance of an infected placenta, prophylaxis against future infections, or both. Research is under way to determine whether SP remains the best drug for prevention of pregnancy malaria, how frequently it should be administered, and whether the current timing of administration is optimal. SP drug resistance has arisen in many regions, though in general, it continues to provide protection against placental malaria. Alternative IPTp regimens, including use of artemisinin-based combination therapy, are also being considered and studied owing to SP resistance. Nonetheless, SP remains a cornerstone of IPTp for malaria.

As with ITN use, there are a number of challenges to widespread adherence to IPTp guidelines. The medicine may not always be available and can be expensive to purchase, and pregnant women may be hesitant to use medications during pregnancy for fear of harming the baby. Resistance to SP is increasing, although the WHO continues to recommend SP administration as the IPTp of choice.

Recommendations for Those Working in Endemic Areas

Obstetrician-gynecologists working in malarious areas should pay particular attention to protecting themselves against malaria. Chemoprophylaxis appropriate to the geographic location should be faithfully taken, and an insecticide-treated bed net should be used at nighttime, carefully tucked under the mattress. The outdoors should be avoided at dusk and at night; if that is not possible, permethrin-embedded clothing that minimizes skin exposure (long sleeves, long pants) should be worn at high-risk times. An effective insect repellant should be applied to exposed skin. Available data on the use of N,N-Diethylmetatolumide (DEET) appears reassuring even in pregnancy (McGready et al. 2001). From limited data, it seems that maternal toxic effects are not apparent until orders of magnitude greater than the typical human exposure.

Diagnosis

In endemic areas, malaria should be included in differential diagnosis in a pregnant woman who complains of headaches, fatigue, fever, or anemia.

Severe malaria should be strongly entertained in the differential of seizures and loss of consciousness during pregnancy, alongside other considerations such as preeclampsia/eclampsia or meningitis.

Bloodstream Infection

Diagnosis of malaria from clinical signs and symptoms alone is not reliable, as there is great overlap between malaria and other infections; a laboratory diagnosis is required. Detection of malarial parasites from a blood smear by microscopy is the gold standard for malaria diagnosis; it can confirm the presence of parasites, quantify the degree of parasitemia, and identify the species, all of which are useful for prognosis and informing treatment (Figures 7.2 and 7.3). Malaria microscopy requires a health-care infrastructure with supplies, reagents, working microscopes, and electricity (Kilian et al. 2000). A high level of expertise is required of the microscopist to properly stain the slide and obtain an accurate result. It is difficult to have sufficient expertise and equipment to achieve the necessary level of diagnostic accuracy by microscopy in all clinics, particularly in rural areas.

An excellent alternative to microscopy is a rapid diagnostic test (RDT) that detects various malaria-specific antigens in blood using a simple point-of-care platform. This has become the standard of care for diagnosis in most rural clinics, and in some regions the RDT outperforms microscopy (Harchut et al. 2013). The RDT detects the presence of parasite antigens (HRP-2 and parasite-specific LDH) in a blood sample obtained from a finger-stick capillary tube. The serum is loaded into the RDT cassette, buffer is added to the cassette, and within about fifteen minutes a result is obtained. These tests provide on average 95% sensitivity (Abba et al. 2011). The RDT strip contains a control antigen to confirm that the test strip is functioning properly.

The advantages of RDTs over conventional microscopy include the ease of performance and interpretation and the availability of the information at the point of care. Test kits can be stored at room temperature, and electricity is not required. Individuals with little or no formal medical training can be taught how to use and interpret an RDT.

However, there are also some limitations with RDTs. First, they may be more expensive than standard microscopy. They also give only qualitative information and cannot be used to quantify the degree of parasitemia. Because tests can remain positive for several weeks after treatment, the

RDT cannot differentiate between ongoing infection and successfully treated infection. In these situations, microscopic examination of a blood smear will be needed to detect an active malaria infection. In areas where microscopy is substandard, an RDT is the test of choice and has become a much-needed tool for the diagnosis of malaria to guide proper treatment.

Placental Infection

Placental infection can be a diagnostic challenge in areas of stable malaria transmission. Pregnant women have partial immunity and can clear the bloodstream parasites to produce negative blood smears; however, their placentas may still be harboring infected erythrocytes adherent to the synctiotrophoblast (Figure 7.1). A representative study from Tanzania demonstrated that approximately half of women with placental parasites found at the time of delivery had no parasites visible on peripheral blood smear (Ismail et al. 2000). These occult placental infections compromise the function of the placenta and fetal health. There is no reliable biomarker that identifies placental infection when the peripheral blood smear is negative. Ongoing research seeks to identify a biomarker of placental malaria; this could be a constellation of biomarkers such as complement by-products or angiogenic markers that distinguish between women with and without placental infection. Thus targeted treatment for occult placental malaria is not possible; therefore all pregnant women living in endemic areas should be instructed to receive IPTp. Alternatively some experts have suggested intermittent screening and treatment in pregnancy (ISTp) as an alternative to IPTp. Under this strategy, an RDT is administered at each antenatal visit, and those who test positive are treated for malaria. While at any single time point peripheral blood smears may be negative despite placental infection, repeated testing increases the likelihood of detecting asymptomatic placental infections. This strategy may be particularly appealing in areas of lower transmission (where prevalence is low) to reduce unnecessary exposure to medications during pregnancy. In a randomized trial from Ghana comparing standard IPTp with ISTp, the authors found no significant difference in maternal severe anemia or low birth weight (Tagbor et al. 2010). These results are encouraging and warrant further investigation. The guidelines of the regional ministry of health and WHO can be used by obstetrician-gynecologists to inform the proper IPTp practice in each area.

Treatment

Uncomplicated Malaria

Malaria is considered uncomplicated when there is no clinical or laboratory evidence of end-organ dysfunction. Uncomplicated malaria can be caused by any of the five *Plasmodium* strains. Signs and symptoms are nonspecific and often include fever. A woman with malaria should be treated promptly with effective antimalarial medications. The World Health Organization publishes and updates guidelines, available online, for the treatment of uncomplicated and severe malaria with specific recommendations for pregnant women (WHO 2015). Oral quinine and clindamycin are administered for seven days for uncomplicated malaria during the first trimester (Table 7.3). Artemisinin-based combination therapies (ACTs) are typically avoided in the first trimester, particularly early in gestation, pending sufficient evidence regarding safety. At the time of this writing, ACTs are considered only if no other treatment is available or if the woman has previously failed quinine and clindamycin treatment. In the second and third trimesters, ACTs are increasingly used as first-line treatment for uncomplicated malaria because of their effectiveness. Practitioners should refer to country-specific guidelines to determine which ACT is available and effective for the local population and which is recommended during pregnancy.

Antimalarial treatment is focused on clearing the parasites from the maternal bloodstream. Symptoms such as fever and myalgia can be treated with acetaminophen or paracetamol.

Severe Malaria

Severe malaria is diagnosed when there is evidence of end-organ dysfunction such as coma, seizure, respiratory distress, hypoglycemia, or severe anemia (Hgb < 5 g/dL) (WHO 2015). The mortality associated with severe malaria during pregnancy can be as high as 50%. Because clinical deterioration can occur rapidly, parenteral antimalarials should be initiated even before diagnostic confirmation with microscopy or RDT. Furthermore, medications should not be withheld secondary to concerns about potential or unknown medication risks to the developing fetus.

The World Health Organization recommends intravenous artesunate as the treatment of choice for severe malaria irrespective of the stage of pregnancy, due to the survival benefit as compared to quinine alone (WHO 2015) (Table 7.3). Intravenous quinine with clindamycin is an

Table 7.3   Treatment guidelines for malaria in pregnancy

Treatment recommendations[a]	Dosing[a]
Uncomplicated malaria, first trimester	
Chloroquine-resistant	
Quinine plus clindamycin for 7 days (quinine monotherapy if clindamycin unavailable)	Quinine sulfate 542 mg base po tid x 7 days Clindamycin 20 mg base/kg/day po divided tid x 7 days
ACT if this is the only treatment available, if treatment with 7-day quinine plus clindamycin fails, or if uncertainty of compliance with 7-day course	ACT known to be effective in country or region
Chloroquine-sensitive	
Chloroquine	Chloroquine 600 mg base po followed by 300 mg base at 6, 24, and 48 hours
Hydroxychloroquine (alternative)	Hydroxychloroquine 620 mg base followed by 310 mg at 6, 24, and 48 hours
Uncomplicated malaria, second and third trimesters	
ACTs known to be effective in the country/region	ACT known to be effective in country/region
Artesunate plus clindamycin for 7 days (if ACT treatment fails)	artesunate (2mg/kg once per day) plus clindamycin 10 mg base/kg/day po bid x 7 days (maximum 1800 mg)
Quinine plus clindamycin for 7 days (alternative)	Quinine sulfate 542 mg base po tid x 3 days (7 days if in Southeast Asia) Clindamycin 20 mg base/kg/day po divided tid x 7 days (maximum 1,800 mg)
Severe malaria	
Chloroquine resistant	
IV artesunate is first-line therapy	Artesunate 2.4 mg/kg as 1st dose, then 2.4 mg/kg at 12 and 24 hours, followed by 2.4 mg/kg daily; minimum of 24 hours; and when able to take po to complete a standard course with po regimen as above
Alternative: IV quinine dihydrochloride (plus clindamycin[b] po)	Quinine dihydrochloride[c] 16.7 mg base/kg in 5% dextrose loading dose over 4 hours, followed by 25 mg base/kg/day divided bid to tid in equal administrations of 8.35 mg base/kg over 2 hours at 8- or 12-hour intervals (maximum 1800 mg salt/day) when able to take po to complete a standard course with po regimen as above.
Alternative: IV quinidine gluconate (requires ECG monitoring) (plus clindamycin po)	Quinidine gluconate 6.25mg base/kg IV loading in normal saline over 1–2 hours, followed by 0.0125mg salt/kg/minute continuous infusion for at least 24 hours. Needs ECG monitoring. When able to take po to complete a standard course with po regimen as above.

Table 7.3 (continued)

Treatment recommendations[a]	Dosing[a]
	Alternate dosing: Quinidine gluconate 15mg base/kg IV loading in normal saline over 4 hours followed by 7.5mg base/kg infused over 4 hours, then every 8 hrs starting 8 hrs after the beginning of the loading dose. Needs ECG monitoring. When able to take po to complete a standard course with po regimen as above.
Clindamycin po (to add to IV quinine or quinidine dose outlined above)	Clindamycin 20 mg base/kg/day orally (maximum 1800 mg) divided into 3 equal doses; when able to take po to complete a standard course with po regimen as above.
Chloroquine-sensitive IV quinidine, quinine, or artemisinin	See dosing above under chloroquine-resistant section.

Other

Pre-referral treatment for moderate to severe malaria (or if not taking po)

Rectal artesunate, quinine[c] IM, artesunate IM, artemether IM	Several rectal dosing formulations available; refer to local availability

Lactating women

Standard antimalarial treatment (including ACTs) should be administered except for primaquine and tetracycline	Primaquine should not be used unless breastfed infant determined not to be G6PD-deficient.

Species other than Plasmodium falciparum

P. vivax, P.ovale, P. knowlesi, P. malariae are generally chloroquine sensitive[d]	Mild malaria: Treat with chloroquine or oral ACT in second and third trimester Severe malaria: treat as for severe *P. falciparum* doses as above
P. vivax or P. ovale, in addition to above, need to eradicate liver stage (typically done with primaquine), however primaquine should not be used during pregnancy.	Suppression with chloroquine 500 mg q week until delivery, then complete course of primaquine 30 mg base po qd x 14 days to eradicate potential liver stages after delivery.

Source: Adapted from WHO (2015), © World Health Organization 2015.

ACT = artemisinin combination therapy; ECG = electrocardiogram; G6PO = glucose-6-phosphate dehydrogenase; IM = intramuscular; IV = intravenous; po = by mouth.

a. Treatment recommendations and dosing summarized from WHO (2015). Practitioners are strongly encouraged to check for any updates (available online), as specific recommendations may have changed since publication of this chapter.

b. If clindamycin is unavailable or unaffordable, then the monotherapy should be given.

c. Monitor blood glucose frequently; recurrent hypoglycemia associated with IV quinine use.

d. Exception: *P. vivax* in Papua New Guinea or Indonesia is considered chloroquine resistant.

alternative. Quinine has been associated with an increased risk of hypoglycemia, and thus blood glucose levels should be monitored routinely for women on intravenous quinine.

If possible, pregnant women with severe malaria should be admitted to an intensive-care setting with frequent monitoring of their vital signs and blood glucose levels. Intravenous dextrose should be administered in the event of hypoglycemia. Respiratory status should be carefully watched, as pulmonary edema can develop suddenly, even after delivery. Packed red blood cells, if available, should be transfused if there is evidence of severe anemia (Hgb < 5 g/dL). Repeated blood smears are useful in documenting improvement in parasite density and eventual clearance.

Plasmodium vivax

Chloroquine is the drug of choice for treatment of *P. vivax* in the first trimester in chloroquine-sensitive regions. During the second or third trimester, ACT is recommended. Owing to the prolonged liver stage, primaquine is used to eradicate the hypnozoite; however, primaquine should not be used during pregnancy but should instead be deferred until postpartum. Thus pregnant women should be treated for the active malaria infection, continue on a chloroquine preventative regimen, and then be treated with primaquine after delivery. Primaquine should be avoided in individuals with G6PD.

PREGNANCY MANAGEMENT

Malaria infection increases the risk for both preterm delivery and impaired fetal growth. Management recommendations are based primarily on expert opinion rather than clinical trials. In general, a preterm delivery should not be induced in the setting of diagnosed malaria, as adequate antimalarial treatment should clear parasites from the placenta. The exception may be severe malaria syndromes in which maternal health is compromised, although there is a lack of data to guide whether evacuation of the uterus with an induced delivery or dilation and extraction will improve maternal outcome. The patient should be monitored for signs of miscarriage or preterm labor. If possible, fetal assessment is recommended to rule out worrisome fetal heart rate tracings and depleted amniotic fluid volume. For women who remain pregnant after an episode of malaria, it is reasonable to obtain fetal growth ultrasounds. The placenta should be examined after delivery for evidence of residual parasites and an infant blood smear sent to rule out congenital malarial infection (which is rare). These recommendations must be tailored to the availability of such testing in resource-limited settings. In the case of severe malaria, emphasis should first be placed on care of the mother. Fetal decelerations in the setting of acidosis can resolve with improved maternal status. The surgical stress of a cesarean to an already compromised mother may substantially increase the risk to her health and thus should be performed only after careful consideration.

SUMMARY

Malaria during pregnancy poses substantial risks to both mother (anemia, acute respiratory distress, coma, death) and fetus (stillbirth, preterm delivery, impaired fetal growth). Prompt recognition and treatment of malaria are critical to reduce the burden of disease. While malaria prevalence has declined in sub-Saharan Africa over the past decade following intensification of malaria control efforts, malaria is far from eliminated. The standard malaria prevention package for pregnant women in areas of moderate to high transmission includes both vector control (sleeping under an insecticide-treated bed net, eliminating standing water, using screens in the home) and chemoprophylaxis (intermittent preventive therapy, typically with sulfadoxine-pyrimethamine). Bloodstream malaria requires a diagnostic test, either RDT or microscopy, owing to the nonspecificity of the clinical symptoms. Occult placental malaria remains a diagnostic challenge, as women in endemic areas may harbor parasites in the placenta without either overt symptoms or peripheral parasitemia. There is hope that a pregnancy-specific malaria vaccine may one day prevent adherence of parasitized erythrocytes to the placenta. Clinicians caring for pregnant women in malaria-endemic areas should become well versed in the prevention, recognition, and treatment of the disease to maximize health outcomes.

USEFUL RESOURCES

For those practicing obstetrics in resource-limited settings, the following resources may be useful to have on hand or via the Internet.

CDC Yellow Book (Health Information for International Travellers). For access information, go to: http://wwwnc.cdc.gov/travel/page/yellowbook-home-2014.

Centers for Disease Control. CDC Malaria Map Application. Accessed May 13, 2016. http://www.cdc.gov/malaria/map.

Roll Back Malaria Toolbox. Accessed May 13, 2016. http://www.rollbackmalaria.org /toolbox/index.html. Designed to help policymakers and program managers effectively deploy and evaluate strategies to reduce malaria.

REFERENCES

Abba K., J. J. Deeks, P. Olliaro, C. M. Naing, S. M. Jackson, Y. Takwoingi, S. Donegan, and P. Garner. 2011. Rapid diagnostic tests for diagnosing uncomplicated P. falciparum malaria in endemic countries. *Cochrane Database Syst Rev.* 7:CD008122.

Bordbar, B., N. Tuikue Ndam, E. Renard, S. Jafari-Guemouri, L. Tavul, C. Jennison, S. Gnidehou, et al. 2014. Genetic diversity of VAR2CSA ID1-DBL2Xb in worldwide Plasmodium falciparum populations: Impact on vaccine design for placental malaria. *Infect Genet Evol* 25:81-92. doi:10.1016/j.meegid.2014.04.010. Epub 2014 Apr 21.

Brabin, B. J., C. Romagosa, S. Abdellgalil, C. Menendez, F. H. Verhoeff, R. McGready, K. A. Fletcher, et al. 2004. The sick placenta: The role of malaria. *Placenta* 25 (5): 359–378.

Conroy, A. L., C. R. McDonald, K. L. Silver, W. C. Liles, and K. C. Kain. 2011. Complement activation: A critical mediator of adverse fetal outcomes in placental malaria? *Trends Parasitol* 27 (7): 294–299.

Desai, M., F. O. ter Kuile, F. Nosten, R. McGready, K. Asamoa, B. Brabin, and R. D. Newman. 2007. Epidemiology and burden of malaria in pregnancy. *Lancet Infect Dis* 7 (2): 93–104.

Diagne, N., C. Rogier, C. S. Sokhna, A. Tall, D. Fontenille, C. Roussilhon, A. Spiegel, and J. F. Trape. 2000. Increased susceptibility to malaria during the early postpartum period. *N Engl J Med* 343 (9): 598–603.

Duffy P. E., A. G. Craig, and D. I. Baruch. 2001. Variant proteins on the surface of malaria-infected erythrocytes—developing vaccines. *Trends Parasitol* 17 (8): 354–356.

Fried, M., and P. E. Duffy. 1998. Maternal malaria and parasite adhesion. *J Mol Med* 76 (3–4): 162–171.

Fried, M., F. Nosten, A. Brockman, B. J. Brabin, and P. E. Duffy. 1998. Maternal antibodies block malaria. *Nature* 395:851–852.

Gamble, C., J. P. Ekwaru, and F. O. ter Kuile. 2006. Insecticide-treated nets for preventing malaria in pregnancy. *Cochrane Database Syst Rev* 2:CD003755.

Garner P. and A. M. Gülmezoglu. 2006. Drugs for preventing malaria in pregnant women. *Cochrane Database Syst Rev* 18 (4): CD000169.

Gething, P. W., A. P. Patil, D. L. Smith, C. A. Guerra, I. R. F. Elvazar, G. I. Johnston, A. J. Tatem, and S. A. Hay. 2011. A new world malaria map: *Plasmodium falciparum* endemicity in 2010. *Malar J* 10:378.

Guyatt, H. L., and R. W. Snow. 2001. The epidemiology and burden of Plasmodium falciparum-related anemia among pregnant women in sub-Saharan Africa. *Am J Trop Med Hyg* 64 (S1-2): 36–44.

———. 2004. Impact of malaria during pregnancy on low birth weight in sub-Saharan Africa. *Clin Microbiol Rev* 17 (4): 760–769.

Harchut, K., C. Standley, A. Dobson, B. Klaassen, C. Rambaud-Althaus, F. Althaus, and K. Nowak. 2013. Over-diagnosis of malaria by microscopy in the Kilombero Valley, Southern Tanzania: An evaluation of the utility and cost-effectiveness of rapid diagnostic tests. *Malar J.* 12:159.

Ismail, M. R., J. Ordi, C. Menendez, P. J. Ventura, J. J. Aponte, E. Kahigwa, R. Hirt, A. Cardesa, and P. L. Alonso. 2000. Placental pathology in malaria. A histological, immunohistochemical, and quantitative study. *Hum Pathol* 31 (1): 85–93.

Kantele, A., and T. S. Jokiranta. 2011. Review of cases with the emerging fifth human malaria parasite, Plasmodium knowlesi. *Clin Infect Dis* 52 (11): 1356–1362.

Kilian, A. H., W. G. Metzger, E. J. Mutschelknauss, G. Kabagambe, P. Langi, R. Korte, and F. von Sonnenburg. 2000. Reliability of malaria microscopy in epidemiologic studies: Results of quality control. *Trop Med Int Health* 5 (1): 3–8.

Lindsay, S., J. Ansell, C. Selman, V. Cox, K. Hamilton, and G. Walraven. 2000. Effect of pregnancy on exposure to malaria mosquitoes. *Lancet* 355:1972.

McGready, R., K. A. Hamilton, J. A. Simpson, T. Cho, C. Luxemburger, R. Edwards, S. Looareesuwan, N. J. White, F. Nosten, and S. W. Lindsay. 2001. Safety of insect repellant N, N-dietyl-M-toluamide (DEET) in pregnancy. *Am J Trop Med Hyg* 65 (4): 285–289.

Mount, A. M., V. Mwapasa, S. R. Elliot, J. G. Beeson, E. Tadesse, V. M. Lema, M. E. Molyneaux, S. R. Meschnick, and S. J. Rogerson. 2004. Impairment of humoral immunity to Plasmodium falciparum malaria in pregnancy by HIV infection. *Lancet* 363: 1860–1867.

Nosten, F., R. McGready, J. A. Simpson, K. L. Thwai, S. Balkan, T. Cho, L. Hkirijaroen, S. Looareesuwan, and N. J. White. 1999. Effects of Plasmodium vivax malaria in pregnancy. *Lancet* 354:546–549.

Radeva-Petrova D., K. Kayentao, F. O. ter Kuile, D. Sinclair, and P. Garner. 2014. Drugs for preventing malaria in pregnant women in endemic areas: Any drug regimen versus placebo or no treatment. *Cochrane Database Syst Rev.* 10:CD000169. doi:10.1002/14651858.CD000169.pub3.

Silver, K. L., K. Zhong, R. G. Leke, D. W. Taylor, and K. C. Kain. 2010. Dysregulation of angiopoietins is associated with placental malaria and low birth weight. *PLoS One* 5 (3): e9481. doi:10.1371/journal.pone.0009481.

Steketee, R. W., B. L. Nahlen, M. E. Parise, and C. Menendez. 2001. The burden of malaria in pregnancy in malaria-endemic areas. *Am J Trop Med Hyg* 64 (S1-2): 28–35.

Tagbor, H., J. Bruce, M. Agbo, B. Greenwood, and D. Chandramohan. 2010. Intermittent screening and treatment versus intermittent preventive treatment of malaria in pregnancy: A randomised controlled non-inferiority trial. *PloS One* 5 (12): e14425.

Ter Kuile, F. O., M. E. Parise, F. H. Verhoeff, V. Udhayakumar, R. D. Newman, A. M. van Eijk, S. J. Rogerson, and R. W. Steketee. 2004. The burden of co-infection with human immunodeficiency virus type 1 and malaria in pregnant women in sub-Saharan Africa. *Am J Trop Med Hyg* 71 (S2): 41–54.

WHO (World Health Organization). 2006. *Guidelines on Co-trimoxazole Prophylaxis for HIV-Related Infections among Children, Adolescents and Adults: Recommendations for a Public Health Approach.* Geneva: World Health Organization. Accessed May 13, 2016. http://www.who.int/hiv/pub/guidelines/ctx/en/.

———. 2012. *World Malaria Report.* Geneva: World Health Organization. Accessed May 13, 2016. http://www.who.int/malaria/publications/world_malaria_report _2012/en/index.html.

———. 2013. *WHO Policy Brief for the Implementation of Intermittent Preventive Treatment of Malaria in Pregnancy Using Sulfadoxine-Pyrimethamine (IPTp-SP).* Geneva: World Health Organization. Accessed May 13, 2016. http://www.who.int/malaria /publications/atoz/iptp-sp-updated-policy-brief-24jan2014.pdf?ua=1.

2014. Severe malaria. *Trop Med Int Health* 19 (S1): 7–131. doi:10.1111/tmi.12313.

———. 2015. *Guidelines for the Treatment of Malaria.* 3rd ed. Geneva: World Health Organization. Accessed May 13, 2016. http://apps.who.int/iris/bitstream/10665 /162441/1/9789241549127_eng.pdf?ua=1&ua=1.

———. 2015. *Malaria Treatment Guidelines.* 3rd ed. Geneva: World Health Organization. Accessed May 13, 2016. http://www.who.int/malaria/publications/atoz /9789241549127/en/.

PART THREE

Gynecologic Challenges

8

Contraception

MARIA I. RODRIGUEZ

Contraceptive information and services are fundamental to health, human rights, and development (WHO 2014). Ensuring that contraceptive services are available, accessible, and acceptable to all individuals has exceptional health, social, and economic benefits. The advantages of family planning extend far beyond the individuals who directly use the services; couples, families, communities, and entire countries benefit (Dehlendorf et al. 2010; WHO 2014). However, limited choice and restricted access to family planning remains a pervasive problem globally (Darroch 2012; WHO 2014; WHO and Johns Hopkins Bloomberg School of Public Health 2007).

Barriers to contraception exist at the policy, community, facility, and individual levels. At the policy level, some state actors limit the availability of particular contraceptive methods such as emergency contraception, or they may fail to keep and distribute regular stocks of contraceptives at an affordable price throughout the country (WHO 2014). States and the international donor community may not have invested adequate resources to create good-quality contraceptive services, including appropriately trained staff offering a full range of methods within easy reach of the entire population (WHO 2014). In some areas, spousal or parental consent may be needed for individuals to access services. Other barriers within the community include misconceptions regarding the risk of pregnancy and the safety of contraceptives. Stigma regarding sexual activity and contraceptive use by unmarried individuals represents an additional obstacle for adolescents seeking services (WHO 2014; Chandra-Mouli, Camacho, and Michaud 2013). At the facility level, the severe shortage of skilled health-care workers trained in providing contraceptive services is a key constraint to improving access (Darroch et al. 2013). The current network of health-care providers fails to reach some of the most vulnerable groups: the unmarried, the young, the poor, migrants, and rural women (WHO 2014; Chandra-Mouli, Camacho, and Michaud 2013).

Addressing these barriers through the provision of equitable, quality contraceptive information and services is essential to improving health and development (WHO 2014). Though modern contraception is safe and effective in preventing unintended pregnancy (WHO and Johns Hopkins Bloomberg School of Public Health 2007), it must actually be used. Among reproductive-age women who are sexually active, 85% will become pregnant within one year if they are not using a method of contraception (WHO and Johns Hopkins Bloomberg School of Public Health 2007). Contraception is an essential, but underutilized, strategy to prevent maternal mortality and morbidity, as it prevents unintended pregnancy and lowers the likelihood of unsafe abortion. Providing universal access to women in developing countries who currently have an unmet need for modern methods of contraception would prevent 54 million unintended pregnancies, 26 million abortions (of which 16 million would be unsafe), and 7 million miscarriages; this would also prevent 79,000 maternal deaths and 1.1 million infant deaths (Singh and Darroch 2012b).

Unsafe abortion is defined by the World Health Organization (WHO) as a procedure for terminating an unintended pregnancy that is carried out either by persons lacking the necessary skills or in an environment that does not conform to minimal medical standards or both (WHO 2012). Standards for the provision of safe surgical and medical abortion have been established, including WHO's (2012) second edition of *Safe Abortion: Technical and Policy Guidance for Health Systems*. However, unsafe abortion remains endemic in many settings. In 2008, approximately 47,000 pregnancy-related deaths resulted from complications of unsafe abortion worldwide; moreover, it is estimated that 5 million women suffer short- and long-term disability as a result of complications owing to unsafe abortion annually (WHO 2008b). Each year, an estimated 22 million unsafe abortions occur, 98% of which are in developing countries (WHO 2008b). Depending on the context, multiple barriers prevent women from accessing information and services for safe abortion, including legal restrictions, inability to pay, lack of social support, delays in seeking health care, providers' negative attitudes, and poor quality of services (WHO 2008b) (see Chapter 2).

The wide range of modern methods of contraception includes steril-ization, intrauterine devices, implants, injectable drugs, contraceptive pills, condoms, and other supply methods such as vaginal spermicides. How-ever, the contraceptive choices available to an individual will vary greatly on her context. Addressing the barriers to contraception described above and ensuring universal access to reproductive health is the focus of sev-eral key global initiatives, and coordinated efforts across multiple sectors will be needed (WHO 2006; ICPD 1994).

The rapid scale-up of health systems and services is essential to elimi-nating unmet needs for contraception and achieving international goals for reproductive health (ICPD 1994; WHO 2011b). At the same time, it is critical that scale-up not compromise the commitment to the rights-based approach to family planning articulated in Cairo at the 1994 International Conference on Population and Development (ICPD 1994). The application of numeric targets to family planning programs in the 1960s and 1970s produced some cases of human rights infringements, with documented cases of clients who were uninformed or even unwilling to receive the con-traceptive method they were given (WHO 2014).

This chapter reviews key elements for the safe and effective provision of contraception in a range of settings. We focus on the most common methods of modern contraception, including discussion of mechanism of action, common side effects, contraceptive eligibility, and important coun-seling messages.

EPIDEMIOLOGY

Unintended pregnancy resulting from unmet need for contraception threatens the lives and well-being of women, girls, and their families glob-ally (WHO 2014). The latest estimates are that 222 million women have an unmet need for modern contraception, and the need is greatest where the risks of maternal mortality are highest (Singh and Darroch 2012a). In the least developed countries, six out of ten women who do not want to get pregnant, or want to delay the next pregnancy, are not using any method of contraception (Singh and Darroch 2012a). In some areas of Africa, where maternal mortality rates remain among the highest in the world, the pro-portion of women who express a need to stop or delay childbearing but are not using a contraceptive method remains over 20% (Darroch, Singh, and Nadeau 2008; WHO 2008b).

Significant changes in the world's population affect not only which contraceptive services are needed but also how they are delivered. The number of women wanting to avoid pregnancy and in need of effective contraception has increased substantially from 2003 (54% of 1.32 billion) until 2012 (57% of 1.52 billion) (Darroch and Singh 2013). Promisingly, there has also been a decrease in unmet need for modern contraception among women wishing to avoid pregnancy: from 29% (210 million) in 2003 to 26% (222 million) in 2012 (Darroch and Singh 2013). However, significant inequalities in access to contraception exist both within countries and across regions (WHO 2014). Unmet need for modern contraception remained very high in 2012, especially in sub-Saharan Africa (60%), western Asia (50%), and south Asia (34%) (Darroch and Singh 2013).

Demographic changes in recent decades have led to the largest generation of adolescents in the world today, with unique needs and priorities. Unintended pregnancy among adolescents is a common public health problem globally that is associated with significant health risks and social costs (WHO 2011a). Infants born to adolescent mothers account for roughly 11% of all births worldwide, with 95% occurring in developing countries (WHO 2011a). Childbirth at an early age is associated with increased health risks for both the mother and the infant. In low- and middle-income countries, complications from pregnancy and childbirth are the leading cause of death for adolescents aged fifteen to nineteen (WHO 2008a).

Historically, contraception has been promoted within family-planning programs, whose efforts centered on the need of married couples to space children and limit family size. However, such programs may not meet the needs of adolescents and young people, particularly those who are unmarried or not in a formal union. While some barriers to obtaining contraceptives are shared by adults and adolescents, others are specific to this younger population (Chandra-Mouli et al. 2014; WHO 2014). In many places, contraceptives are simply not available at all, owing to sporadic supply or lack of providers or facilities. Where contraceptive services are available, restrictive laws and policies may make them unavailable to adolescents. Even if adolescents are able to obtain contraceptive services, they may not do so because of fear that their privacy may not be respected or that health-care workers may be judgmental (Chandra-Mouli et al. 2014; WHO 2014). Providers may not be willing to offer adolescents methods other than condoms, owing to misperceptions of risk in nulliparous women

(Chandra-Mouli et al. 2014). Adolescents may not use contraceptives correctly and consistently because of limited understanding, misperceptions about their effects, and fears of the reactions of others.

The selection of contraceptive methods available varies considerably by location. Of the many modern methods, the majority of facilities may have only a few options available, and supplies are frequently limited (see Table 8.1). For methods such as the condom or pill, which require a frequent supply, this poses a significant challenge. In the past decade, there has been a shift away from sterilization, one of the most effective methods of contraception, toward injectables and barrier methods (Darroch and Singh 2013). This trend toward less effective methods may contribute to rates of unintended pregnancy. Strengthening and maintaining the quality of family-planning programs is key to both efficacy and acceptability. A critical area for quality improvement is broadening the selection of contraceptive methods available (WHO 2014); the most effective methods are frequently the least available. Long-acting and permanent methods include the intrauterine device (IUD) and the progestin implant as well as male and female sterilization. The IUD and implant are reversible and may also be referred to as long-acting reversible contraception (LARC). These methods are useful for couples wishing to space pregnancies. Male and female sterilization are permanent methods for couples who have completed childbearing.

GLOBAL IMPACT OF DISEASE

Women with unintended pregnancies that are continued to term are more likely to receive inadequate or delayed prenatal care and have poorer health outcomes than women with planned pregnancies, such as low infant birth weight, infant mortality, and maternal mortality and morbidity (Kost, Landry, and Darroch 1998; Hook 1963; Najman et al. 1991; Cheng et al. 2009; Gipson, Koenig, and Hindin 2008). These risks of unintended pregnancy are higher for adolescents and girls (WHO 2011a; Cook et al. 2001). Compared with adults, adolescents are at greater risk for medical complications with pregnancy and are often forced to make compromises in education and employment that may subsequently lead to poverty and lower educational attainment (WHO 2011b; Chen et al. 2007; Klepinger, Lundberg, and Plotnick 1995; Boden, Ferguson, and Horwood 2008).

Table 8.1   Mechanism of action and efficacy of common methods of modern contraception

Contraceptive method	Failure rates % perfect use (typical use)	Mechanism of action
Barrier method		
Diaphragm	6 (16)	Mechanical barrier to prevent sperm from reaching egg.
Female condom	5 (21)	
Male condom	2 (15)	
Combined hormonal contraception		
Pill	0.3 (8)	Suppresses the release of an egg from the ovary (ovulation).
Patch	0.3 (8)	
Injectable		
Ring	0.3 (8)	
Progestin-only contraception		
Progestin-only pill	0.3 (8)	Suppresses the release of an egg from the ovary (ovulation) and thickens cervical mucus, which acts as a mechanical barrier to sperm.
Progestin injectable	0.3 (3)	
Long-acting reversible contraception		
Implant	0.05 (0.05)	The implant works by suppressing ovulation.
Copper intrauterine device	0.6 (0.8)	The Copper IUD works by damaging the sperm and egg before they meet.
Levonorgestrel intrauterine device	0.2 (0.2)	The LNG IUD works by thickening the cervical mucus and acting as a barrier method to sperm, as well as affecting sperm capacitation. The progestin thins the endometrium, which impacts implantation.
Permanent contraception		
Permanent methods		Permanently occluding the tubes that allow sperm (vas deferens) or egg (fallopian tube) to meet.
• Female (tubal occlusion)	0.5 (0.5)	
• Male (vasectomy)	0.15 (0.10)	

Source: Adapted from WHO (2011) and Hatcher (2007).

Providing high-quality contraceptive care requires a range of elements, including informed choice of methods, technically competent providers, adherence to medical standards of care, and provider-client relationships based on respect. In the next section, we review for providers key elements of the most common methods of contraception including mechanism of action, common side effects, contraceptive eligibility, and counseling messages.

GUIDELINES FOR CARE

Screening for Contraceptive Use

A focused and accurate medical history is essential to enabling a client to pick a method of contraception that is safe and meets her needs. Contraception should be routinely discussed with all women of reproductive age, including adolescents. In the medical history, clients should be asked about their pregnancy intentions; are they actively planning a pregnancy, or seeking to limit or space births? The medical history should also include past experience with contraceptive use, age, tobacco use, risk factors for sexually transmitted infections, history of migraines with neurologic symptoms, breast-feeding, recent pregnancy (including possibility of current pregnancy), and any major medical illness.

The World Health Organization produces several key guidelines on contraceptive provision. An important resource for providers is the WHO's (2010) *Medical Eligibility Criteria for Contraceptive Use*, which offers evidence-based guidance on the safety of different methods for women and men with specific characteristics or known medical conditions. A range of medical conditions is covered, and the recommendations are based on systematic reviews of clinical and epidemiological research. Examples of health conditions covered include postpartum or postabortion state, obesity, living with HIV, deep venous thrombosis, pulmonary embolus, and liver disease including cirrhosis and viral hepatitis. The safety of each type of contraception with the associated condition is assigned a rating of 1 to 4, based on available evidence. A rating of 1 would be given to a condition for which there is no restriction for the use of the contraceptive method. Category 2 would apply to a condition for which the advantages of using the method generally outweigh the theoretical or proven risks. Category 3 indicates a condition for which the theoretical or proven risks usually outweigh

Table 8.2   Pregnancy checklist

No	Question	Yes
	Did you have a baby less than six months ago, are you fully or nearly fully breast feeding, and have you had no monthly bleeding since then?	
	Have you abstained from sexual intercourse since your last monthly bleeding or delivery?	
	Have you had a baby in the last four weeks?	
	Did your last monthly bleeding start within the past seven days (or within the past twelve days if the client is planning to use an IUD)?	
	Have you had a miscarriage or abortion in the last seven days (or within the past twelve days if the client is planning to use an IUD)?	
	Have you been using a reliable contraceptive method consistently and correctly?	

Source: Reprinted from WHO and Johns Hopkins Bloomberg School of Public Health (2011) Pregnancy Checklist, p. 372. © 2007, 2008, 2011 World Health Organization and Johns Hopkins Bloomberg School of Public Health/Center for Communication Programs.

the advantages of the method, and category 4 is a condition for which the contraceptive method poses an unacceptable health risk (WHO 2010).

The *Medical Eligibility Criteria for Contraceptive Use* is a companion guideline to WHO's *Selected Practice Recommendations for Contraceptive Use.* The guideline addresses ongoing controversies and inconsistencies related to maximizing the effectiveness of contraceptive methods and how to manage their side effects or other problems during use. Both documents are available online, in a range of languages (http://www.who.int/reproductivehealth/publications/family_planning/en/).

A critical component of evaluating a client for contraceptive use is determining the possibility of current pregnancy. Where pregnancy tests are not readily available, screening questions can be used instead. The World Health Organization has created a checklist to safely rule out pregnancy and confirm that a woman may safely begin the method of her choice (see Table 8.2). If the client answers no to all questions, then pregnancy cannot be ruled out. Either a pregnancy test should be administered or the client should abstain from intercourse (or use a barrier method) while waiting for her next menses to begin the method. If she answers yes to at least one of the questions and has no signs or symptoms of pregnancy (for example, nausea, emesis, amenorrhea, breast tenderness), she may begin the method of her choice.

Contraceptive Counseling

Good contraceptive counseling is essential for informed decision making and helping a client find a contraceptive method that meets her needs (WHO and Johns Hopkins Bloomberg School of Public Health 2007; WHO 2014). As side effects contribute significantly to discontinuation of contraception, explaining these up front and discussing where follow-up can be obtained are essential to acceptability. Counseling needs to be tailored to the individual client. A women's fertility preferences as well as overall health influence her choice of method (WHO and Johns Hopkins Bloomberg School of Public Health 2007). Many myths exist around contraception, and dispelling these is an important part of client education, as is discussing management of side effects for each method.

The WHO identifies these core components of contraceptive counseling (WHO and Johns Hopkins Bloomberg School of Public Health 2007):

- Show every client respect, and help each client feel at ease.
- Encourage clients to explain needs, express concerns, ask questions.
- Let the client's wishes and needs guide discussion.
- Listen carefully. It is as important as giving correct information.
- Give key information and instructions. Use words clients know.
- Respect and support clients' decisions. Unless a medical reason prevents it, give clients the methods that they want.
- Bring up side effects, if any, and take concerns seriously.
- Check understanding.
- Invite clients to come back any time for any reason.

CONTRACEPTIVE METHODS

Barrier Methods

All barrier methods act by physically preventing the union of sperm and egg. An advantage to barrier methods is their dual function: both contraception and protection from sexually transmitted infections (STIs) (Darney and Speroff 2011; Cates and Stone 1992). Barrier methods (condoms and diaphragms) provide protection (about a 50% reduction) against STIs and pelvic inflammatory disease. This includes infections owing to chlamydia, gonorrhea, trichomonas, herpes simplex, cytomegalovirus, and human immunodeficiency virus (HIV) (Darney and Speroff 2011). However, it is important to note that only the condom has been proved to prevent HIV infection (Darney and Speroff 2011). Women at risk of HIV acquisition or transmission should be encouraged to use condoms with every act of intercourse. In 2012, barrier methods accounted for 13% of modern contraception in developing countries (Darroch and Singh 2013).

Consistent (with every act of intercourse) and correct use of barrier methods is essential to contraceptive efficacy. Male and female condoms, the diaphragm, and cervical caps are all examples of barrier methods. Use of the male or female condom can be initiated at any time. If a woman requests a diaphragm or cervical cap and has recently been pregnant (within six weeks), she should receive a backup method and return for a fitting six weeks postpartum, when the uterus and cervix have returned to normal size (WHO and Johns Hopkins Bloomberg School of Public Health 2007; WHO 2010).

Barrier methods can be used safely by nearly all couples (WHO 2010). Couples with a severe allergy to latex should not use male condoms or diaphragms. Use of the cervical cap is not recommended for women with cervical intraepithelial neoplasia or cervical cancer (WHO 2010).

Combined Hormonal Contraception

Combined hormonal contraceptives (CHC) consist of low doses of two hormones, a progestin and an estrogen. Combined hormonal contraceptives prevent ovulation by inhibiting gonadotropin secretion by an effect on both the pituitary and hypothalamic centers. The progestin primarily suppresses secretion of luteinizing hormone, the signal for ovulation, while the estrogen component has several effects. Estrogen primarily suppresses follicle-stimulating hormone secretion, preventing a dominant follicle from developing on the ovary. Estrogen also stabilizes the endometrium to minimize irregular bleeding with CHC and potentiates the impact of the progestin component (Darney and Speroff 2011).

Though the most commonly used form of CHC is the pill, a monthly injectable, a patch, and ring format also exist. Use of oral contraception accounts for 13% of modern contraception in developing countries (Darroch and Singh 2013). Contraindications and side effects are similar across all formulations, but the patch, ring, and injectable are not widely available in developing countries. Therefore, we focus here on use of the pill.

The CHC pill is typically available in a packet of twenty-eight. The first twenty-one pills contain both estrogen and progestin, and the last seven pills are placebo. During the hormone-free week, a withdrawal bleed occurs. Common misconceptions about the pill are that it builds up in a woman's body and that a "rest" from the pill is needed, that it may affect sexual behavior, cause infertility, or disrupt an existing pregnancy (WHO and Johns Hopkins Bloomberg School of Public Health 2007).

Consistent use of the method is essential to ensuring effective protection against pregnancy. This means a pill every day and starting each new pack of pills on time. The risk of pregnancy is greatest when three or more days of pills are missed (especially at the start or end of the pack) or a pill pack is started three or more days late (WHO and Johns Hopkins Bloomberg School of Public Health 2007). Counseling a client regarding strategies to help remember to take the pill daily, such as linking it with a daily event, like brushing her teeth, may help reduce the likelihood of missed pills. If a woman misses one or two pills, taking them immediately keeps the risk of pregnancy low. If three or more pills are missed, she should take a hormonal pill as soon as possible, and finish all of the hormonal pills in her current pack. She should not take the placebo pills but should throw them away and begin another pack. A backup method of contraception is advised for seven days after missing three or more pills (WHO and Johns Hopkins Bloomberg School of Public Health 2007). The injectable, patch, and ring have the advantage of being dosed differently (monthly for the injectable and ring, weekly for the patch), which may make it easier for some women to use them correctly.

A woman can start using CHC whenever she is reasonably certain she is not pregnant (Table 8.2). Side effects with all types of CHC are similar and may include changes in bleeding patterns (such as lighter bleeding, irregular bleeding, infrequent bleeding, no menses), headaches, dizziness, breast tenderness, weight change, mood change, and acne (WHO and Johns Hopkins Bloomberg School of Public Health 2007; Hatcher 2007). It is important to reassure the client that side effects are not a sign of illness.

While CHC is a safe and appropriate method of contraception for most women, there are several clinical situations that require caution and clinical judgment in prescribing. Such common conditions include hypertension, tobacco use, history of a blood clot or breast cancer, and age over

Table 8.3   Contraceptive options for clients with common medical conditions

Client	Contraceptive options
Adolescence through menopause without any medical conditions	CHC, progestin injectable, progestin implant, IUD
Smoker younger than thirty-five	CHC, progestin injectable, progestin implant, IUD
Smoker older than thirty-five	Progestin-only pill, progestin injectable, progestin implant, IUD Contraindicated: estrogen-containing methods (CHC)
Breast-feeding mother	Less than twenty-one days postpartum Progestin-only pill, progestin injectable, progestin implant, IUD Contraindicated: estrogen-containing methods More than six weeks and less than six months postpartum Progestin-only pill, progestin injectable, progestin implant, IUD. CHC can be initiated with clinical judgment. More than six months postpartum No restrictions based on postpartum or breast-feeding status.
Migraines without aura or neurologic symptoms, younger than thirty-five	CHC, progestin injectable, progestin implant, IUD
Migraines with aura or known vascular complication, any age	Progestin-only pill, progestin injectable, progestin implant, IUD Contraindicated: estrogen-containing methods (CHC)
Migraines of any type, thirty-five and older	Progestin-only pill, progestin injectable, progestin implant, IUD Contraindicated: estrogen-containing methods (CHC)

Source: Adapted from WHO (2010), © World Health Organization 2010.

thirty-five. Table 8.3 summarizes different contraceptive options for clients with common conditions.

Progestin-Only Contraception

Contraceptive methods containing only the hormone progestin include a pill, injectable, implant, or an intrauterine device (discussed in next section). The progestin-only pill (POP) along with the CHC pill account for 13% of modern contraceptive use in developing countries (Darroch and Singh 2013). The injectable and implant account for 9% of contraceptive use; the injectable accounts for most of this use (Darroch and Singh 2013).

Progestin-only pills contain 35 to 75% of the progestin dose in CHC pills, but they are taken continuously without a pill-free interval. The low dose of progestin acts by thickening the cervical mucus, making penetration by sperm difficult, and causing the endometrial lining to thin and be unsuitable for implantation. However, the low dose of progestin in the POP does not consistently inhibit ovulation, which will occur approximately 40% of the time (Darney and Speroff 2011). To maximize efficacy, the POP must be taken at the same time daily.

With perfect use, the pregnancy rate for POP users is only slightly higher than that with perfect use of CHC pills (0.5% versus 0.2 to 0.3%). For typical use, the effectiveness rate is generally 92 to 95%, although wide variations are reported. These differences may reflect the difficulty in taking the pill at the same time daily. The POP has the advantage of being safe for use by women for whom estrogen is contraindicated.

The category of long-acting reversible contraceptives encompasses injections, IUDs, and subdermal implants. Because they do not rely on compliance, they are the most effective reversible types of contraception over an extended period and are much more cost-effective than condoms or birth-control pills.

The progestin-only injectable contraceptives depot medroxyprogesterone acetate and norethisterone enanthate have effects on the endometrial lining and cervical mucus similar to those of POP, but also block ovulation. This is because the circulating level of progestin is high enough to inhibit luteinizing hormone and prevent the release of an egg.

The injectable is highly effective at preventing pregnancy when used correctly. The biggest risk factor for contraceptive failure is a missed or delayed injection. Depot medroxyprogesterone acetate is given by intramuscular injection every three months (thirteen weeks) and norethisterone enanthate every two months (eight weeks). The injection can be given two weeks before or after the scheduled date (WHO and Johns Hopkins Bloomberg School of Public Health 2007).

Among the progestin implant systems in use worldwide are Implanon, Nexplanon, Norplant, and Jadelle (formerly called Norplant-2). Implanon and Nexplanon are both single-rod systems containing 68 milligrams of etonogestrel that are designed for up to three years of use (Darney and Speroff 2011). Jadelle and Sinoplant (a Chinese version of the drug) are two-rod systems that combined contain 150 milligrams levonorgestrel and can be used for five years (WHO and Johns Hopkins Bloomberg School of Public Health 2007; Darney and Speroff 2011). In many parts of the world, Jadelle has replaced Norplant; however, Norplant is still used worldwide. Norplant is a six-rod system that also contains levonorgestrel and is labeled for five years of use, though large studies have indicated continued efficacy for seven years (WHO and Johns Hopkins Bloomberg School of Public Health 2007).

For all implants, a specially trained provider performs a minor surgical procedure to place the implants under the skin on the inside of a woman's upper arm. The implants steadily release a very low dose of progestin. The implants work by blocking ovulation and thickening cervical mucus to act as a barrier to sperm. A woman can start using implants whenever it is reasonably certain she is not pregnant (Table 8.1). No breast, cervical, or laboratory exams are required (WHO and Johns Hopkins Bloomberg School of Public Health 2007).

The most common side effect noted with all progestin methods is a change in menstruation. This may present as lighter bleeding and fewer days of menses, prolonged bleeding at irregular intervals, infrequent bleeding, or amenorrhea. The etonorgestrel implants (Implanon and Nexplanon) cause less prolonged or irregular bleeding than the levonorgestrel implants (Norplant and Jadelle). Etonorgestrel implant users are more likely to have infrequent or no monthly bleeding.

Contraindications to progestin-only methods include active thrombophlebitis or thromboembolic disease, undiagnosed genital bleeding, acute liver disease, benign or malignant liver tumors, and known or suspected breast cancer.

Intrauterine Devices

Intrauterine devices, which also fall into the LARC category, are a highly effective, reversible form of contraception that remains underutilized globally. While IUDs account for 28% of all modern contraceptive use in developing countries, large variations exist (Darroch and Singh 2013). High uptake of the IUD in Asia accounts for the relatively high global prevalence; in most regions of Africa, IUD use is under 5% (Darroch et al. 2013). Two basic types of IUDs are marketed globally: a copper-containing IUD and a progestin IUD. Both are highly effective at preventing pregnancy, with failure rates comparable to sterilization. Both methods are immediately reversible, with no delay in return to fertility.

The copper IUD is a small, flexible device that is placed by a trained provider at the uterine fundus. It protects against pregnancy for up to twelve years, primarily by causing a chemical change that damage sperm and egg before they meet.

The progestin IUD constantly releases a small amount of levonorgestrel that is absorbed mainly at the level of the uterus, though it prevents pregnancy by several means. The progestin IUD also has a spermicidal effect, and it thickens cervical mucus to act as a barrier against sperm and renders the endometrial lining thin and inhospitable to implantation (Darney and Speroff 2011). Ovulation is not reliably affected by either IUD, and as important to keep in mind, the IUD is not an abortifacient (Darney and Speroff 2011).

While different brands of IUDs vary in design, all are small, flexible plastic frames. The copper IUD contains copper sleeves or wire around it. A specially trained health-care provider inserts it into a woman's uterus through her vagina and cervix. Almost all types of IUDs have one or two strings, or threads, tied to them to facilitate removal. The user can check that the IUD is still in place by touching the strings, which hang through the cervix into the vagina. A provider can easily remove the IUD by pulling gently on the strings with forceps (WHO and Johns Hopkins Bloomberg School of Public Health 2007).

The IUD is a safe and appropriate method for a wide range of women, including adolescents and women who have never had a child. It may be safely used by women who are breast-feeding, have just had an abortion or miscarriage (if no there is no evidence or risk of infection), have just given birth, have a history of ectopic pregnancy or pelvic inflammatory disease, or have vaginal infections or STIs other than purulent cervicitis, chlamydia, or gonorrhea and are infected with HIV (WHO and Johns Hopkins Bloomberg School of Public Health 2007). Helping a woman decide if the IUD is right for her requires careful attention to menstrual history and risk of STI.

The levonorgestrel IUD produces serum levels in the nanogram range, and thus the systemic side effects experienced with other progestin-only methods are not applicable. The changes in menstrual bleeding are similar to those seen with other progestin-only methods. A trend toward amenorrhea has been noted with longer use.

The symptoms most often responsible for copper IUD discontinuation are increased uterine bleeding and increased menstrual pain (Darney and Speroff 2011). Women with prolonged, heavy menstrual bleeding or significant menstrual cramps may not be able to tolerate a copper IUD. Smaller copper and progestin IUDs reduce the incidence of pain and bleeding considerably, but a careful menstrual history is still important in helping a woman consider an IUD. Because bleeding and cramping are most severe in the first few months after IUD insertion, treatment with a nonsteroidal anti-inflammatory drug during the first several menstrual periods can reduce bleeding and cramping (Darney and Speroff 2011).

The LARC methods are also very effective in postabortion and postpartum applications; offering women these options at those important times is useful in preventing future pregnancies. For LARC methods that involve the insertion of foreign bodies—IUDs and implants—advising patients regarding availability of removal services is an essential component of method counseling (WHO 2014).

Permanent Contraception

Female and male sterilization are permanent contraceptive methods for couples who have completed childbearing. Sterilization accounts for 38% of modern contraceptive use in developing countries, with the vast majority attributable to female sterilization (Darroch and Singh 2013). The many misconceptions women may have about sterilization include possible changes in menstrual cycles, lasting pain in back or low abdomen, decreased libido, or overall weakness (WHO and Johns Hopkins Bloomberg School of Public Health 2007).

Female sterilization is referred to by many names: tubal ligation, tubal sterilization, tubectomy, voluntary surgical contraception, mini-lap, "the operation," and tying or cutting tubes. It is one of the most effective forms of contraception, with a failure rate of less than one pregnancy per hundred women in the first year of use (WHO and Johns Hopkins Bloomberg School of Public Health 2007). It works by blocking the fallopian tubes and preventing an egg from meeting sperm. A small risk of pregnancy remains after the first year of use and persists until the woman undergoes menopause. Over ten years of use, failure rates are about two pregnancies per 100 women (WHO and Johns Hopkins Bloomberg School of Public Health 2007). There are many different techniques for performing female sterilization, and the one selected affects contraceptive efficacy.

Female sterilization can be performed immediately after a delivery or outside of pregnancy. It can be performed abdominally by a mini-laparotomy or laparoscopy. Using hysteroscopy, sterilization can be accomplished transcervically as well, with placement of implants in the ostia of the fallopian tubes. In this section, we focus on abdominal techniques.

With proper counseling and informed consent, any woman can have permanent contraception. It is safe for women who are breast-feeding, young, have few or no children, are infected with HIV, are unmarried, or do not have their husband's permission (WHO and Johns Hopkins Bloomberg School of Public Health 2007). While no medical conditions prohibit sterilization, it is a major surgery, and the difficulty and risks associated with the procedure will vary. A preoperative evaluation should consider the woman's overall medical condition, including blood pressure, heart disease, diabetes, or infection (including possibility of HIV or viral hepatitis). To assess surgical difficulty, it is important to evaluate clients for acute pelvic infections, unexplained bleeding suggesting a gynecologic cancer, hernia, and symptoms of endometriosis or a fixed uterus owing to previous surgery or infection (WHO and Johns Hopkins Bloomberg School of Public Health 2007).

Using proper technique to prevent infection is essential. Female sterilization is a pelvic surgery that can be performed under local anesthesia, which is safer than general anesthesia. Using sterile technique and a two- to three-centimeter skin incision, a mini-laparotomy is made. If a woman has not recently been pregnant, it is made at the pubic line. For women who have just given birth, the incision is usually made infraumbilically, as the uterine fundus will be abdominal. The fallopian tubes are visualized, grasped with an atraumatic clamp, and walked to the fimbriated end to ensure correct anatomy. A three-centimeter section of the tube is then ligated with plain suture and transected. The same procedure is repeated on the contralateral side. Female sterilization can also be accomplished laparoscopically, with clips, rings, or coagulation used to occlude the fallopian tubes (WHO and Johns Hopkins Bloomberg School of Public Health 2007; Hatcher 2007).

Counseling should emphasize that this is a permanent, irreversible form of contraception, and ensuring client understanding is essential. It is important to discuss the fact that, until menopause, a small risk of method failure and subsequent pregnancy persists. While a woman may discuss sterilization with her partner or others, the decision must be hers alone. Providers have a responsibility to ensure that the woman is making the decision freely, without coercion. The WHO emphasizes six key points to obtaining informed consent for female sterilization (WHO and Johns Hopkins Bloomberg School of Public Health 2007).

- Offer alternative methods of contraception that are reversible.
- Explain that sterilization is a surgical procedure.
- Discuss the benefits as well as the risks of the surgery.
- Emphasize that if successful, the surgery will prevent the woman from ever having more children.
- The procedure is permanent and can not be reversed.
- The woman has the right to decide against the procedure at any point before it takes place, without losing access to any other services.

The surgery can be performed whenever it is reasonably certain the woman is not pregnant. The procedure can be safely performed following an uncomplicated birth or an abortion if the woman has given informed consent in advance. If the pregnancy was complicated by infection or hemorrhage, the surgery should be delayed and reversible contraception given (WHO and Johns Hopkins Bloomberg School of Public Health 2007).

The most common complications of the procedure are skin infection or abscess, though proper infection control technique can limit these risks. Women should be instructed to seek care if they have pain at the site, a fever, or notice redness or drainage coming from the incision. Hemorrhage or anesthetic complications are unlikely, but if a woman experiences light-headedness or dizziness or faints, she should seek medical attention promptly for evaluation of acute anemia and ectopic pregnancy.

CONCLUSION

Contraceptive information and services are crucial strategies to improve health and development globally. Concerted efforts by all stakeholders are needed to improve the range of choices available to women and the quality of services.

At the system level, identifying opportunities to integrate contraceptive services within the existing health system is essential for expanding access to care and reducing the number of unintended pregnancies. The provision of postpartum, postabortion, and longer-acting contraceptive methods to women accessing emergency contraception are examples of opportunities for integrating contraceptive services (WHO 2014).

Family planning helps reduce the risk of maternal and child morbidity and mortality if couples space their pregnancies at least two years apart (WHO 2014). However, on average, two-thirds of women who have not yet completed one year since their last delivery have an unmet need for contraception. Nearly 40% report they intend to use a method during the next twelve months but are not currently doing so (WHO 2010). Women presenting for abortion and postabortion care, as well as for emergency contraception, have a demonstrated unmet need for contraception. During such contact with the health system women may be motivated to initiate contraception. These opportunities should be used to provide contraceptive information and services.

For providers working to improve contraceptive care for women and girls globally, ensuring informed consent and method acceptability through comprehensive counseling is key to protecting human rights and promoting contraceptive continuation (WHO 2014). The World Health Organization offers many valuable guides for providers to evidence-based contraceptive service delivery (WHO 2014, 2010; WHO and Johns Hopkins Bloomberg School of Public Health 2007). These resources are available in a range of formats (print, electronic, toolkits) and languages to enable providers to care for women in all settings.

REFERENCES

Boden, J. M., D. M. Fergusson, and L. John Horwood. 2008. Early motherhood and subsequent life outcomes. *J Child Psychol Psychiatry* 49 (2): 151–160. doi:JCPP1830 [pii]10.1111/j.1469-7610.2007.01830.x.

Cates, W., Jr., and K. M. Stone. 1992. Family planning, sexually transmitted diseases and contraceptive choice: A literature update; Part I." *Fam Plann Perspect* 24 (2): 75–84.

Chandra-Mouli, V., A. V. Camacho, and P. A. Michaud. 2013. WHO guidelines on preventing early pregnancy and poor reproductive outcomes among adolescents in developing countries. *J Adolesc Health* 52 (5): 517–522. doi:10.1016/j.jadohealth.2013.03.002.

Chandra-Mouli, V., D. R. McCarraher, S. J. Phillips, N. E. Williamson, and G. Hainsworth. 2014. Contraception for adolescents in low and middle income countries: Needs, barriers, and access. *Reprod Health* 11 (1): 1. doi:10.1186/1742-4755-11-1.

Chen, X. K., S. W. Wen, N. Fleming, K. Demissie, G. G. Rhoads, and M. Walker. 2007. Teenage pregnancy and adverse birth outcomes: A large population based retrospective cohort study. *Int J Epidemiol* 36 (2): 368–373. doi:dyl284 [pii]10.1093 /ije/dyl284.

Cheng, D., E. B. Schwarz, E. Douglas, and I. Horon. 2009. Unintended pregnancy and associated maternal preconception, prenatal and postpartum behaviors. *Contraception* 79 (3): 194–198. doi:S0010-7824(08)00457-5 [pii] 10.1016/ j.contraception.2008.09.009.

Cook, R., O. A. Wilson, S. Scarrow, and B. Dickens. 2001. *Advancing Safe Motherhood through Human Rights*. Geneva: World Health Organization.

Darney, P. D., and L. Speroff. 2011. *A Clinical Guide to Contraception*. 5th ed. Philadelphia: Lippincott.

Darroch, J. E. 2012. Trends in contraceptive use. *Contraception*. doi:10.1016/ j.contraception.2012.08.029.

Darroch, J. E., and S. Singh. 2013. Trends in contraceptive need and use in developing countries in 2003, 2008, and 2012: An analysis of national surveys. *Lancet* 381:1756–1762. doi:10.1016/S0140-6736(13)60597-8.

Darroch, J. E., S. Singh, and J. Nadeau. 2008. Contraception: An investment in lives, health and development. *Issues in Brief,* no. 5: 1–4.

Dehlendorf, C., M. I. Rodriguez, K. Levy, S. Borrero, and J. Steinauer. 2010. Disparities in family planning. *Am J Obstet Gynecol* 202 (3): 214–220. doi:10.1016/j. ajog.2009.08.022.

Gipson, J. D., M. A. Koenig, and M. J. Hindin. 2008. The effects of unintended pregnancy on infant, child, and parental health: A review of the literature. *Studies in Family Planning* 39 (1): 18–38.

Hatcher, R. A. 2007. *Contraceptive Technology*. 19th rev. ed. New York: Ardent Media.

Hook, K. 1963. Refused abortion: A follow-up study of 249 women whose applica- tions were refused by the National Board of Health in Sweden. *Acta Psychiatr Scand Suppl* 39 (168): 1–156.

International Conference on Population and Development (ICPD). 1994. *Program of Action: Report of the International Conference on Population and Development*. Cairo: ICPD.

Klepinger, D. H., S. Lundberg, and R. D. Plotnick. 1995. Adolescent fertility and the educational attainment of young women. *Fam Plann Perspect* 27 (1): 23–28.

Kost, K., D. J. Landry, and J. E. Darroch. 1998. Predicting maternal behaviors during pregnancy: Does intention status matter? *Fam Plann Perspect* 30 (2): 79–88.

Najman, J. M., J. Morrison, G. Williams, M. Andersen, and J. D. Keeping. 1991. The mental health of women 6 months after they give birth to an unwanted baby: A longitudinal study. *Social Science & Medicine* 32 (3): 241–247.

Singh, S., and J. E. Darroch. 2012a. *Adding It Up: The Costs and Benefits of Contraceptive Services; Estimates for 2012*. New York: Guttmacher Institute and United Nations Population Fund.

———. 2012b. *Adding It Up: The Costs and Benefits of Investing in Family Planning and Newborn and Maternal Health; Estimates for 2012*. New York: Guttmacher Institute.

WHO (World Health Organization). 2006. *Accelerating Progress towards the Attainment of International Reproductive Health Goals: A Framework for Implementing the WHO Global Reproductive Health Strategy.* Geneva: World Health Organization.

———. 2008a. "Trends in Maternal Mortality: 1990 to 2008." In *Estimates Developed by WHO, UNICEF, UNFPA and the World Bank.* Geneva: World Health Organizaiton.

———. 2008b. *Unsafe Abortion: Global and Regional Estimates of the Incidence of Unsafe Abortion and Associated Mortality in 2008.* Geneva: World Health Organization.

———, ed. 2010. *Medical Eligibility Criteria for Contraceptive Use.* Geneva: World Health Organization.

———. 2011a. *Preventing Early Pregnancy and Poor Reproductive Health Outcomes among Adolescents in Developing Countries.* Geneva: World Health Organization.

———. 2011b. *Universal Access to Reproductive Health: Accelerated Actions to Enhance Progress on Millennium Development Goal 5 through Advancing Target 5B.* Geneva: World Health Organization.

———. 2012. *Safe Abortion: Technical and Policy Guidelines.* Geneva: World Health Organization.

———. 2014. *Ensuring Human Rights in the Provision of Contraceptive Information and Services.* Geneva: World Health Organization.

World Health Organization Department of Reproductive Health and Research (WHO/RHR) and Johns Hopkins Bloomberg School of Public Health/Center for Communication Programs (CCP), Knowledge for Health Project. 2011. *Family Planning: A Global Handbook for Providers.* Baltimore and Geneva: CCP and WHO.

9

Cervical Cancer

RENGASWAMY SANKARANARAYANAN

Cervical cancer is the fourth most common cancer in the world, with disproportionately high incidence in developing countries. Of the estimated 527,624 new cases and 265,653 cervical cancer deaths in the world annually, developing countries account for 444,546 new cases and 230,158 deaths (Ferlay et al. 2013). Persistent infection with one of the high-risk human papillomaviruses (HPV) causes virtually all cervical cancers. Large-scale, population-based cervical cytology screening programs, in which women are repeatedly screened by Pap smear every three to five years (or even more often in some countries), are responsible for a significant reduction in cervical cancer incidence and mortality in high-resource countries in Europe and North America as well as Australia. This reduction in cervical cancer burden is a major achievement in cancer prevention. However, more than 60% of cervical cancer cases in high-resource countries occur in women belonging to the medically underserved, poorer socioeconomic categories of the population, as part of a complex of diseases linked to poverty, low household income, race, and ethnicity, resulting in inequalities in health-care access and health disparities.

Cervical cancer is a major public health problem in many low- and middle-income countries (LMICs) in Asia, sub-Saharan Africa, Central America, South America, and the Caribbean, with age-standardized incidence rates exceeding 20 per 100,000 women in most of these areas (Forman et al. 2013) (Figure 9.1). Likely explanations for the high burden of cervical cancer in LMICs include lack of effective prevention and screening programs, suboptimal performance of existing cytology screening programs, the high prevalence of HPV infection in the general population, and human immunodeficiency virus (HIV) infection in certain populations. In this chapter we discuss the epidemiology, pathology, prevention, early detection, and treatment of cervical neoplasia, with particular reference to LMICs.

EPIDEMIOLOGY

Etiology

As stated above, the etiology of cervical cancer worldwide has been linked to persistent infection with one of the high-risk HPV infections. A working group of the International Agency for Research on Cancer concluded that there is sufficient evidence to indicate that persistent infection with one of the high-risk carcinogenic types of HPV (HPV 16, 18, 31, 33, 35, 39, 45, 51, 52, 56, 58, 59, or 68) is a necessary cause for cervical precancerous lesions and cancer; of these types, HPV 16 and 18 are associated with 70 to 75% of the cervical cancer cases across the world (International Agency for Research on Cancer, 2007). Integration of HPV viral DNA into the cellular genomes of cervical cancer and the reduction in high-grade cervical intraepithelial neoplasia (CIN3) following HPV vaccination support the causal role of HPV infection. The type HPV 16 accounts for 20% of HPV infections but causes 40% of CIN3 and 50 to 60% of cervical cancers; HPV 18 is responsible for most adenocarcinomas. While the entire anogenital epithelium in women can be infected by HPV, the cervical transformation zone (TZ) is particularly susceptible to carcinogenesis induced by HPV infection.

Early age at first sexual intercourse and at first childbirth, a high number of lifetime sexual partners for women and their male partners, and having nonmonogamous male partners are the main risk factors for genital HPV infection in women. Peak HPV acquisition occurs in adolescence and early adulthood. The most important biomarker of HPV infection is the presence of HPV DNA or mRNA. Although a woman's lifetime probability of being infected with HPV is as high as 80 to 90%, 90% of infections become undetectable within two years of acquisition. In 5 to 10% of women the infection is persistently detectable on repeated testing, indicating elevated risk for cervical cancer. It is not clear to what extent undetectability indicates resolution of the infection or the persistence of a latent stage; the underlying mechanisms of clearance or persistence are not known. Since only a small proportion of women with HPV infections

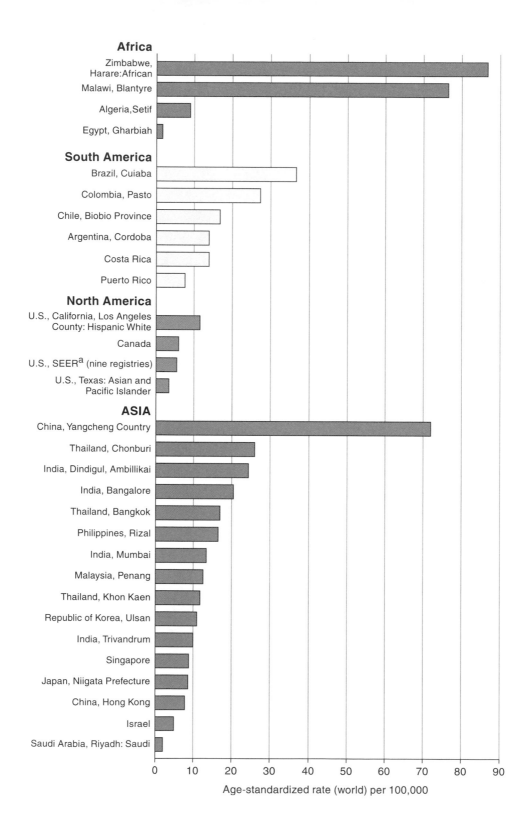

Africa

Zimbabwe, Harare:African
Malawi, Blantyre
Algeria,Setif
Egypt, Gharbiah

South America

Brazil, Cuiaba
Colombia, Pasto
Chile, Biobio Province
Argentina, Cordoba
Costa Rica
Puerto Rico

North America

U.S., California, Los Angeles County: Hispanic White
Canada
U.S., SEER[a] (nine registries)
U.S., Texas: Asian and Pacific Islander

ASIA

China, Yangcheng Country
Thailand, Chonburi
India, Dindigul, Ambillikai
India, Bangalore
Thailand, Bangkok
Philippines, Rizal
India, Mumbai
Malaysia, Penang
Thailand, Khon Kaen
Republic of Korea, Ulsan
India, Trivandrum
Singapore
Japan, Niigata Prefecture
China, Hong Kong
Israel
Saudi Arabia, Riyadh: Saudi

0   10   20   30   40   50   60   70   80   90

Age-standardized rate (world) per 100,000

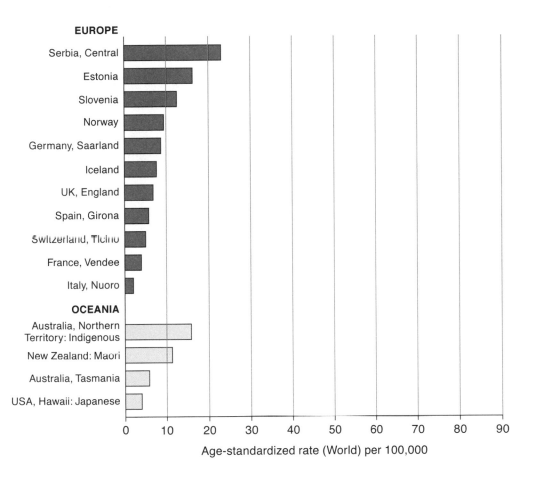

FIGURE 9.1. Age-standardized incidence rates of cervical cancer, by country, 2003 to 2007.

a. SEER-Surveillance, Epidemiology and End Results Program.

progress to invasive cancer, other factors such as the type and duration of HPV infection, immune-compromised states such as HIV infection, poor nutritional status, and smoking may contribute to cervical carcinogenesis. The HPV types 16 and 18 are more likely to persist than other high-risk HPV infections, which tend to resolve spontaneously.

Women infected with HIV are at elevated risk for cervical neoplasia owing to a high frequency of incident, persistent, and progressive HPV infection. Immune restoration associated with antiretroviral therapy (ART) seems to have little impact on the high risk of HPV infection and the cumulative incidence of cervical cancer among HIV-infected women. In fact, the increased survival of HIV-infected women in a moderately immunocompromised state, through use of ART, seems to increase the risks of persistent HPV infection and the development of cervical neoplasia.

Factors such as multiparity, early age at first full-term pregnancy, having a nonmonogamous male partner, long-term oral contraceptive use, poor sanitation and hygiene, coinfection with other agents (for example, herpes simplex virus 2, *Chlamydia trachomatis*), and smoking may potentiate the progression of HPV infection to cervical neoplasia and are associated with an increased risk of cervical cancer, even after adjusting for HPV infection. Multiparity probably explains the highest proportion of cervical cancer among HPV-infected women, while a general decline in parity contributes to the declining trends in cervical cancer incidence in countries with no screening programs. Male circumcision and barrier protection during sexual intercourse may reduce the risk of HPV infection and cervical cancer.

Natural History of Cervical Neoplasia

The natural history of cervical cancer is the most understood among all cancers, based on several prospective studies, and offers several opportunities for prevention of invasive cancer. The long natural history involves four distinct stages: HPV infection of the metaplastic epithelium of the TZ, long-term HPV-infection persistence, clonal progression of HPV-infected epithelium to high-grade cervical-cancer precursor lesions (CIN3), and progression of CIN3 to invasive cancer. If infection is not prevented in the first place by interventions such as HPV vaccination, the progression from HPV infection to cancer takes two to three decades, providing a wide window of opportunity to prevent invasive cancer by screening. The knowledge of cervical cancer's natural history helps identify appropriate age groups to screen and the optimal frequency of screening.

As stated above, HPV infection is ubiquitous among women of reproductive age. The peak incidence is among women below twenty-five years of age, followed by a decline that plateaus around thirty to thirty-five years, and in some low-resource countries a second peak is observed in women over fifty. Since the rate of incident infections declines steadily with age, infections acquired at a young age contribute to most cervical cancers. Among HPV-infected women, the most important determinant of cancer risk is persistence of infection, particularly of HPV 16. A minority of women may demonstrate minor cellular abnormalities such as atypical squamous cells of undetermined significance (ASCUS) and low-grade squamous intraepithelial lesions (LSIL) on cytology or CIN1 on histology within months or years following incident and transient HPV infections. Both LSIL and CIN1 are poorly reproducible cytological and histological manifestations of incident and transient HPV infections, and more than 90% regress. In a great majority of women (approximately 90%), infection clears within two years and the low-grade lesions eventually resolve. The frequency of redetection after clearance ranges from 5 to 20% depending on age and length of follow-up; sexual behaviors are associated with redetection, but most redetections clear rapidly. Reactivation of latent infections could also account for re-detection.

Persistent HPV infections may progress to high-grade squamous intraepithelial lesions (HSIL) or CIN2 and 3. It is not clear whether CIN2 is a heterogeneous intermediary step between CIN1 and 3 with its own progression and regression dynamics or is a misclassification of CIN1 or CIN3; thus the very existence of CIN2 is increasingly being questioned. Diagnosis of CIN2 is less reproducible and more likely to regress spontaneously than CIN3; around 70% of CIN2 lesions in women under twenty-five years and around 40 to 50% in older women regress. Currently, CIN3 is considered to be the real precursor of cervical cancer, although 20 to 30% of cases regress. It takes less time for an HPV infection to develop into CIN3 than it takes for CIN3 to develop into invasive cancer. Peak occurrence of CIN3 is between twenty-five and thirty-five years of age, and it is the most reproducible histological diagnosis along the spectrum of CIN. Repeated HPV positivity conveys substantially more risk of CIN3 than a single positive test. Among women with two positive HPV tests two years apart, 19.3% had an absolute risk of CIN3 or worse lesions (CIN 3+) at twelve years; for HPV 16, the risk of CIN 3+ at three, five, and twelve years of follow-up was 8.9%, 23.8%, and 47.4%, respectively. The same cofactors for cervical cancer (multiparity, HIV infection, long-term hormonal contraceptive use, and smoking) may also increase the risk of progression to CIN3. Of untreated CIN3 lesions, 10 to 20% may progress to invasive cancer in five years, and 40 to 50% progress within thirty years; whereas only 0.7% of adequately treated CIN3 progresses to cancer (McCredie et al. 2008).

The risk of CIN3 or worse lesions and cervical cancer is extremely low for several years following one or two negative HPV tests (Schiffman et al. 2011; Sankaranarayanan et al. 2009). Women who are HPV negative include those who were once positive but whose infections cleared and those who never acquired HPV infection; however, it is not possible to distinguish between those two groups serologically. The low risk of CIN3+ in HPV-negative women indicates that once cleared, infections rarely reappear and do not cause substantial CIN3 lesions.

Trends in Cervical Cancer Incidence and Mortality

The age-standardized incidence rates of cervical cancer among different populations in the world as reported by cancer registries are shown in Figure 9.1. The rates vary between 1.6 in Gharbiah, Egypt, to 86.7 in Harare, Zimbabwe. The incidence of cervical cancer is high in sub-Saharan Africa, particularly in eastern, western, and southern Africa, Central and South America, the Caribbean, and South and Central Asia (Forman et al. 2013). Incidence rates exceed 30 per 100,000 women in sub-Saharan Africa. The lowest rates are found in western Asia, Australia, New Zealand, and North America. Incidence rates are lower than 10 per 100,000 women in high-resource countries in Europe, North America, Australia, and New Zealand, where cytology screening programs have existed for over three decades. Incidence rates vary from 7 to 25 per 100,000 in India, which contributes one-fifth of the global burden. While rates are above 20 per 100,000 in Eastern European countries, notably lower rates (less than 7 per 100,000) are found in the eastern Mediterranean countries including Israel. The large global variation reflects geographical differences in HPV prevalence and the availability of successful and effective cytology screening programs. For instance, the prevalence of cervical HPV infection is highest in sub-Saharan Africa (24%), Eastern Europe (21%), Latin America (16%), and Southeast Asia (14%) and lowest in western Asia (1.7%). The low risk of cervical cancer in Middle East reflects the low prevalence of HPV infection in the general population, whereas the high rates in sub-Saharan Africa, particularly in eastern Africa, reflect the high prevalence of HPV (greater than 30%) and HIV infections. However, the disproportionately high burden of cervical cancer in de-

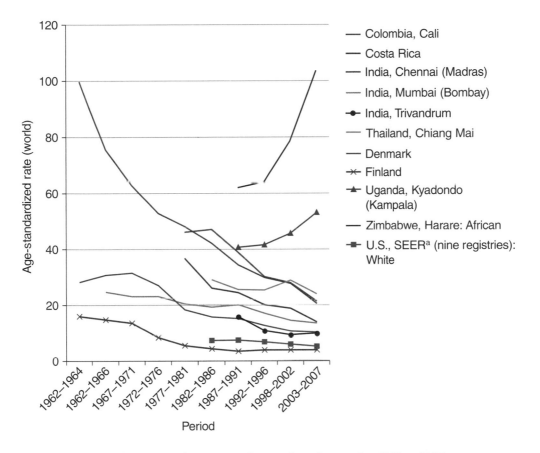

FIGURE 9.2. Trends in cervical cancer incidence, selected countries, 1962 to 2007.
a. SEER-Surveillance, Epidemiology and End Results Program.

veloping countries and among disadvantaged populations elsewhere is predominantly is attributable to lack of screening.

Trends in cervical cancer incidence in selected high-, middle-, and low-resource countries are shown in Figure 9.2. In several high-resource Western countries and in Australia and New Zealand, where cervical screening programs have long been in place, cervical cancer incidence and mortality rates have declined more than 70% over the past forty years. However, cervical cancer incidence is increasing among younger generations in high-income countries such as Finland, the United Kingdom, Denmark, and China, possibly owing to changing sexual behaviors. Incidence rates have declined in many LMICs in Asia and Latin America, in part owing to improved socioeconomic conditions, better education, fewer childbirths, advances in family planning, and later age at marriage, although the decreases

Table 9.1   Global incidence, mortality, and prevalence of cervical cancer[a]

Population	Incidence		Mortality		Prevalence	
	Number	ASR (W)	Number	ASR (W)	Number	Five-year
World	527,624	14	265,653	6.8	527,459	1,547,161
More developed regions	83,078	9.9	35,495	3.3	83,071	288,967
Less developed regions	444,546	15.7	230,158	8.3	444,388	1,258,194
WHO Africa region	92,340	33.4	56,601	21.5	92,282	236,199
WHO Americas region	83,195	14.9	35,673	5.9	83,177	279,242
WHO East Mediterranean region	14,861	6.4	7,791	3.6	14,861	42,080
WHO Europe region	67,355	11.2	27,984	3.8	67,350	225,187
WHO South-East Asia region	175,229	20.5	94,294	11.3	175,213	465,485
WHO Western Pacific region	94,442	8.5	43,220	3.6	94,374	298,590
Africa	99,038	27.6	60,098	17.5	98,980	254,152
Latin America and Caribbean	68,818	21.2	28,565	8.7	68,803	227,273
Asia	284,823	12.7	144,434	6.4	284,738	806,714
Europe	58,373	11.4	24,385	3.8	58,369	199,817
Oceania	2,195	10.2	1,063	4.5	2,195	7,236

Data sources: Ferlay et al. (2013); Bray et al. (2013).

a. World Health Organization Geographic Classification.

in proportionate terms have been much smaller than in developed countries. However, cervical incidence rates have shown an increasing or stable trend in sub-Saharan African countries such as Uganda and Zimbabwe, in Asian countries such as Thailand, and in Eastern European populations.

Global Burden of Disease

The most recent estimates of incident and prevalent cervical cancer cases and deaths in the world and for specific regions in 2012 are given in Table 9.1 (Ferlay et al. 2013). As stated above, cervical cancer is the fourth most-common cancer; it is also the fourth most common cause of cancer death in women in the world after breast, colorectal, and lung cancers. The figures indicate a disproportionately high burden of cervical cancer in developing countries, and more than 90% of cases in Africa occur in sub-Saharan Africa. The worldwide number of new cases and cervical cancer deaths projected for 2025 are 659,000 and 348,500, respectively.

Survival from Cervical Cancer in LMICs

Population-based five-year survival rates for cervical cancer in selected LMICs and high-income countries in Asia and Latin America are given in Table 9.2 for two different time periods; they indicate little change in survival rates from cervical cancer over time in LMICs (Sankaranarayanan, Swaminathan, and Parkin 1998; Sankaranarayanan and Swaminathan 2011). In these areas, five-year survival seldom exceeds 50%, indicating advanced clinical stages at presentation and poor access to effective treatment, owing to fragmented and underdeveloped health services and the necessity of paying out of pocket for health care.

PATHOLOGY

Histologically, the most frequent type of cervical cancer is squamous cell carcinoma arising from squamous intraepithelial precursor lesions; it accounts for 80 to 90% of cases worldwide; adenocarcinoma and its subtypes developing from glandular precursor lesions account for 10 to 20% of cases (Forman et al. 2013). Rare types of cervical cancers include adenoid cystic carcinoma, adenoid basal and small cell carcinoma, and carcinosarcoma, which are not known to have precursor lesions; other rare cervical cancers include sarcoma, melanoma, and primary lymphoma.

Squamous cell carcinoma develops from precancerous lesions designated as CIN, which is categorized into three grades (CIN1, 2, and 3) based on the degree of involvement of atypical, dysplastic basaloid cells in the cervical epithelium. The atypical cells involve the basal third of the epithelium in CIN1, whereas in CIN2 and 3 the middle and superficial thirds are involved, respectively. The Bethesda system for cervical cytology designates two categories of precursor lesions: low-grade squamous intraepithelial lesions (LSILs) and high-grade squamous intraepithelial lesions (HSILs) (see Table 9.3). Low-grade squamous intraepithelial lesions are characterized by extensive HPV-related cellular changes such as koilocytosis with mild atypia and mitosis, while HSILs are characterized by small to medium-sized atypical cells that lack HPV-related cytological changes; CIN1 relates to LSIL, and CIN2 and 3 relate to HSIL.

Squamous cell carcinoma consists of nests and irregular clusters of tumor cells often with keratinization, which is a sign of good differentiation, and may be subdivided into well (grade 1), moderately (grade 2), and

Table 9.2 Five-year survival in selected countries in Asia, Africa, and Latin America

Country and registry	Registration period	Total number	Five-year relative survival (%)	Registration period	Total number	Five-year relative survival (%)
China - Hong Kong SAR				1996–2001	2,624	76.8
China - Qidong	1982–1991	200	33.6	1992–2000	144	39.4
China - Shanghai	1988–1991	619	51.9	1992–1995	548	60.1
China - Tianjin				1991–1999	567	62.4
Costa Rica				1995–2000	1,485	53.8
Cuba	1988–1989	1,531	55.9	1994–1995	1,221	58.1
The Gambia				1993–1997	202	23.6
India - Bangalore	1988–1992	2,155	40.4			
India - Barshi	1988–1992	247	33.3	1993–2000	406	35.1
India - Bhopal				1991–1995	332	35.4
India - Chennai	1984–1989	3,289	60.0	1990–1999	4,438	59.4
India - Karunagappally				1991–1997	170	56.3
India - Mumbai	1982–1986	2,354	50.0	1992–1994	4,436	46.1
Philippines - Manila				1994–1995	377	36.3
Philippines - Rizal	1987	181	29.0			
Singapore				1993–1997	984	63.5
Republic of Korea - Busan				1996–2001	2,264	76.3
Republic of Korea - Incheon				1997–2001	1,298	78.9
Republic of Korea - Seoul				1993–1997	5,357	78.7
Thailand - Chiang Mai	1983–1992	1,555	68.2	1993–1997	885	60.2
Thailand - Khon Kaen	1985–1992	820	57.5	1993–1997	554	54.5
Thailand - Lampang				1990–2000	1,079	64.3
Thailand - Songkhla				1990–1999	780	61.8
Turkey - Izmir				1995–1997	246	62.3
Uganda - Kampala				1993–1997	283	19.8

Data sources: Sankaranarayanan and Swaminathan (2011); Sankaranarayanan, Swaminathan, and Parkin (1998).

Table 9.3 FIGO stages, treatment policies, and survival rates, by stage

Stage	Criteria	Treatment	Five-year survival (%)
I	Tumor confined to the cervix		
IA	Invasive carcinoma diagnosed only by microscopy. Stromal invasion with a maximal depth of five millimeters measured from the base of the epithelium and a horizontal spread of seven millimeters or less	Radical hysterectomy or total hysterectomy or conization or intracavitary radiotherapy	>95
IB	Clinically visible lesion confined to the cervix or microscopic lesion greater than 1A	Radical hysterectomy with bilateral pelvic lymphadenectomy or radical radiotherapy (external-beam therapy plus intracavitary radiation) or radical radiotherapy plus concurrent cisp atinum-based chemotherapy	80–90
II	Tumor invades beyond uterus but not to pelvic wall or to lower third of vagina		
IIA	Tumor without parametrial invasion	Radical hysterectomy with bilateral pelvic lymphadenectomy or radical radiotherapy (external-beam therapy plus intracavitary radiation) with concurrent cisplatinum-based chemotherapy	60–70
IIB	Tumor with parametrial invasion	Radical radiotherapy (external-beam therapy plus intracavitary radiation) with concurrent cisplatinum-based chemotherapy	50–60
III	Tumor extends to pelvic wall, involves lower third of vagina, causes hydronephrosis or nonfunctioning kidney		
IIIA	Tumor involves lower third of vagina		40–50
IIIB	Tumor extends to pelvic wall, causes hydronephrosis or nonfunctioning kidney		40–50
IVA	Tumor invades mucosa of the bladder or rectum or extends beyond true pelvis		15–20
IVB	Distant metastasis	Palliative radiotherapy, palliative chemotherapy, comprehensive palliative care including opioid and nonopioid analgesics	<5

Data source: Sobin, Gospodarowicz, and Wittekind (2009).

poorly differentiated (grade 3) cancers. However, neither grading nor keratinization influences prognosis. Microinvasive cancer is defined by a maximum horizontal dimension of seven millimeters in the absence of clinically visible tumor and is subdivided into two categories by maximal vertical depth: three millimeters (Ia1) and five millimeters (Ia2).

The precursor lesion of adenocarcinoma, adenocarcinoma in situ (AIS), is not further subdivided. Adenocarcinoma shows a variety of histological patterns, the most common being endocervical, mucinous, and endometrioid.

Cervical cancer may exhibit an ulcerative, exophytic, or infiltrative appearance and spread locally or via lymphatic and hematogenous routes. Local extension involves endocervix, vaginal fornices, and epithelium, followed by progressive infiltration of parametrium, uterine corpus, bladder, and rectum. Involvement of the bladder may lead to ureteric obstruction, hydroureter, and hydronephrosis. Lymphatic spread occurs in a stepwise fashion, first involving pelvic nodes followed by common iliac and para-aortic nodes. Spread to the pelvic nodes is observed in 15, 30, or 50% of cases confined to the cervix, extending to the parametrium, or involving the pelvic side wall (respectively); the corresponding para-aortic nodal involvement is 5, 15, and 30%. Blood-borne spread may result in distant metastasis in the lungs, bone, and liver.

PREVENTION

The discovery that high-risk HPV infections cause almost all cervical cancers has led to two new approaches to cervical cancer prevention: HPV vaccination to prevent infections in younger women (less than or equal to eighteen years) and HPV testing in older women (older than thirty years). However, significant barriers in policy development, resource allocation, and organization of programs to improve access, awareness, and acceptability all need to be addressed to successfully utilize these promising new tools for cervical-cancer prevention in LMICs.

Primary Prevention

Primary prevention of cervical cancer is based on creating healthier lifestyles; improved socioeconomic status, education, and empowerment of women; male circumcision; improved hygiene; increasing awareness of the risks of infection; and HPV vaccination. The slow decline in cervical cancer incidence (Figure 9.2) in many LMICs that lack screening programs, such as India, results from socioeconomic development, improvements in education and awareness, better sanitation, and increasing family planning practices.

Prophylactic HPV vaccination has emerged as a major strategy for cervical cancer prevention. The currently available bivalent vaccine covers HPV 16 and 18, while the quadrivalent vaccine targets oncogenic HPV 16 and 18 as well as HPV 6 and 11, which are responsible for genital warts and respiratory papillomatosis. Efficacy of both vaccines against HPV type-related CIN3 in HPV-naïve populations in phase 3 clinical trials exceeded 99%. Protection also extends prevention of vulvar, vaginal, and anal precancerous lesions associated with vaccine-covered HPV types; the quadrivalent vaccine provides significant protection against genital warts (greater than 95%). However, the vaccines have no impact on prevalent HPV infections and disease (Schiller et al. 2012; Palefsky et al. 2011).

Vaccination against HPV has the potential to prevent 70% of cervical cancers in adequately vaccinated populations and 75 to 80% of cases if cross-protection is taken into account. The evidence to date strongly not only supports the value of HPV vaccination as an important public health intervention against cervical cancer but also makes a strong case for its introduction in national immunization programs. These vaccines are now licensed in more than 130 countries, and more than 180 million vaccine doses have been used so far with excellent safety and tolerability profiles. Mild to moderate injection-site symptoms, headache, and fatigue were the most common adverse events following HPV vaccination.

Vaccination against HPV is currently part of national immunization programs (NIPs) in more than fifty countries targeting preadolescent and adolescent girls and part of "catch-up" immunization of older cohorts with variable upper age limits. Six years after the introduction of HPV vaccination in Denmark in 2006, there was a significant 44% reduction in CIN2–3 lesions among vaccinated women in the 1991 to 1992 birth cohort and a significant 73% reduction in CIN2–3 lesions in the 1993 to 1994 birth cohort (Baldur-Felskov et al. 2014). In April 2007, Australia introduced quadrivalent HPV vaccination for girls twelve to thirteen years old through schools in an NIP, followed by a catch-up vaccination for girls and women thirteen to twenty-six years old, also via schools, community-based programs, and general practices from July to December 2009. Third-dose coverage among the primary target group of twelve- and thirteen-year-olds exceeded a modest 70%, reflecting real-world experience. Signs of vaccine effectiveness have already emerged in the targeted age group, including a 77% fall in prevalence of HPV infections with the strains covered, 90% reduction in genital warts, and 48% reduction in CIN3/AIS lesions (Garland 2014). It is hoped that these early findings will encourage LMICs to roll out HPV vaccination programs to prevent cervical cancer.

Among LMICs, fourteen countries have implemented HPV vaccination as part of NIPs with very high coverage of the target populations (greater than 90% third-dose coverage) and excellent safety profile: Argentina, Bhutan, Brazil, Colombia, Fiji, Malaysia, Mexico, Panama, Paraguay, Peru, Rwanda, South Africa, Uruguay, and Zambia. The major barriers to HPV vaccination include high costs, significant antivaccine propaganda, political and media frenzies spreading misinformation and exaggerated coverage of adverse events, and the logistical difficulties of finding suitable health-service platforms and vaccinating preadolescent and adolescent girls. Factors critical to the introduction of HPV vaccination in LMICs through NIPs include government commitment, procuring HPV vaccines at affordable prices through tiered pricing, Global Alliance for Vaccines and Immunisation (GAVI) and negotiated pricing, education of the community at large, and specific education about vaccine safety and efficacy.

Fewer than three doses of HPV vaccine have recently been shown to be immunogenic and protect against infection with the HPV strains included in the vaccine (Lazcano-Ponce et al. 2014; Safaeian et al. 2013; Kreimer et al. 2011). Reducing the number of doses from the current three-dose schedule will lower costs and increase both accessibility and compliance with vaccine schedules. Based on findings that the immunogenicity of two doses is comparable to three doses in girls nine to fourteen years old, the European Medical Agency for the EU and ten countries in Central and North America, Africa, and Asia licensed (and some are already implementing) two-dose schedules in their NIPs (Romanowski et al. 2014).

Screening

It is well established that screening asymptomatic, apparently healthy women with cervical screening tests such as conventional cytology (Pap smear), liquid-based cytology, and HPV testing and visual inspection with acetic acid (VIA) to detect (and subsequently treat) precancerous lesions are effective means of preventing cervical cancer. Currently the most widely used test is the Pap smear. High-resource countries have integrated cytology screening into medical and public health services and have achieved high coverage rates by screening women at frequent intervals (two to five years), investigating screen-positive women with colposcopy and directed biopsies, and treating women found to have CIN2–3 and AIS, leading to substantial declines in cervical cancer incidence and mortality. With limited health services, competing priorities, lack of resources, and suboptimal commitment to preventive health for women, most LMICs do not have the capacity to initiate and sustain quality-assured cytology screening programs. Moreover, large-scale cytology screening in several Latin American and Asian middle-income countries was largely ineffective in reducing cervical cancer burden owing to poor coverage, treatment, and follow-up care and lack of quality assurance (Murillo et al. 2008; Sankaranarayanan et al. 2012). The high risk of cervical cancer, the difficulty of introducing quality-assured cytology screening, and the need for affordable and simple tests have motivated the evaluation of innovative approaches for cervical cancer prevention in LMICs.

Visual inspection with acetic acid (VIA), the most feasible test that can be provided by health workers, nurses, and doctors after a brief period of training, is the most widely evaluated Pap smear alternative in LMICs. It gives immediate results, allowing investigation and treatment in a single visit; and the sensitivity and specificity of a single, quality-assured VIA in detecting CIN2–3 lesions are around 50 and 85%, respectively (Sankaranarayanan et al. 2012). Visual inspection with acetic acid involves naked-eye visualization of the cervix under bright light one minute after the application of 5% acetic acid; detection of dense acetowhitening in the cervix abutting the squamocolumnar junction constitutes a positive test outcome. Visual inspection with Lugol's iodine (VILI; if positive, acetowhite lesions turn yellow) may be used as a second test following VIA to clarify equivocal results or to confirm a positive VIA test. However, the accuracy of VIA in detecting CIN2–3 lesions in postmenopausal women is not satisfactory owing to the inability to visualize the TZ.

The visual tests seem to perform better in HIV-infected women than in the general population, owing to the increased prevalence of large high-grade lesions in the former (Joshi et al. 2013). Considering the challenges in implementing cytology and HPV screening, VIA is more feasible as a point-of-care screening test in low-resource settings, given its limited consumable and infrastructure requirements, immediate results allowing one-visit investigation and treatment, and the ease with which providers can be trained, despite the variation in accuracy and reproducibility owing to the subjective nature of the test. In two randomized trials in India, VIA screening was associated with 30 to 35% reduction in cervical cancer mortality (Sankaranarayanan et al. 2007; Shastri et al. 2014). The safety, acceptability, and effectiveness of a single-visit "screen-and-treat" approach, in which VIA-positive women eligible for cryotherapy are treated in the same sitting, has been well established (Mwanahamuntu et al. 2011). Women with precancerous lesions who are ineligible for cryotherapy may be referred for excisional methods such as Loop electrosurgical-excision procedure (LEEP) for diagnosis and treatment. This paradigm represents a major innovation for scaling up cervical cancer screening in LMICs and has been adopted by many countries in sub-Saharan Africa and Asia (Sankaranarayanan et al. 2012). There are validated resources available for training providers in VIA screening. Primary-care practitioners should use every opportunity in routine health-care interactions to screen women aged thirty and above with VIA and investigate and screen-and-treat positive women (Sankaranarayanan et al. 2013). Despite all its limitations, implementing VIA screening in low-income countries is a realistic approach to building up infrastructure and human resources that may facilitate the future introduction of affordable HPV screening (Sankaranarayanan et al. 2012). Screen-and-treat programs based on VIA have been implemented through HIV care services in sub-Saharan African countries (Mwanahamuntu et al. 2011).

Testing for HPV involves detecting HPV DNA or mRNA in cervical cell samples collected by pelvic examination or by self-sampling. Since a negligible minority of women in LMICs have ever been screened, collecting cervical samples by pelvic examination is preferable, as it provides an opportunity to visually inspect for cancer. The testing is the most reproducible, provider-independent cervical screening test and also the most biologically relevant, since virtually all cervical cancers are caused by persistent HPV infection. Testing for HPV is more sensitive but less specific than cytology for the detection of precancerous lesions and cancer, including a demonstration that one-time HPV-based screening is superior to Pap smears and VIA for reducing cervical cancer mortality and significantly lowering cumulative incidence of CIN3+ lesions or cancer in women aged thirty or above who were HPV-negative compared with those who were cytologically negative (Sankaranarayanan et al. 2009; Ronco et al. 2014). The accuracy of HPV testing in detecting CIN2+ lesions exceeds 90% and for CIN3+ exceeds 95%; although the specificity is lower than cytology, the difference was not always significant.

A pooled 53% reduction in CIN3+ lesions was found in HPV-negative women compared with cytology-negative women at enrollment in four randomized trials; moreover, in three trials, the detection rate of cervical cancer in round 2 of testing was 87% lower in HPV-negative women at recruitment (Ronco et al. 2014). Following a single round of HPV testing, the incidence of advanced-stage cancer (stage II+) was reduced a significant 53%, and cervical cancer mortality was reduced 48% compared with the control arm, who received routine care (Sankaranarayanan et al. 2009). The evidence base for HPV testing suggests that it is more effective than cytology as a primary screening test for women aged thirty and above, and the screening intervals for HPV-negative women can be extended to five years or more; a recent WHO guidance note even recommends a ten-year interval (WHO 2013). Reflex cytology testing or genotyping for HPV 16 or 18 can be used to triage HPV-positive women. The Netherlands has now introduced primary HPV screening in its national screening program. Women in LMICs who are HPV-positive may be triaged by VIA screening to permit a two-visit screen-and-treat approach.

There are still considerable challenges in introducing HPV screening programs and fulfilling the promise of a feasible point-of-care screening test in LMICs unless more affordable and rapid tests become widely available. Even the currently available careHPV test has limitations in LMICs in terms of costs and scaling up to higher-volume screening. Nevertheless, HPV testing is the promise of the future in all settings (including high-resource countries), given that widespread HPV vaccination will significantly reduce HPV infections and CIN lesions. A pragmatic way of introducing HPV testing in LMICs would be to offer it once at thirty or thirty-five years of age and (resources permitting) repeating it at ten-year intervals, assuming the eventual wider availability of several affordable and rapid HPV tests. Primary-care practitioners in LMICs may prescribe HPV testing for women aged thirty or older years if affordably available; women with a negative test may be advised to repeat the test after five to ten years, and those with a positive test may be triaged with VIA in a screen-and-treat approach or cytology or colposcopy.

Treatment of Cervical Precancerous Lesions

The aim of treatment of CIN 2–3/AIS is to prevent progression to cancer by destroying or removing the entire TZ. Women with CIN1 may be followed for two years and should continue to be if it persists or progresses; alternatively, women in LMICs age thirty years and older with CIN 1 may be treated if there is a high probability of loss to follow-up. Treatment of young women and adolescents with any grade of CIN should be discouraged to avoid pregnancy-related risks such as abortion, preterm labor, and premature rupture of membranes. Therefore, to avoid detection and treatment of transient CIN in young women, screening in LMICs should commence only in women over thirty.

Ablative treatments for CIN include cryotherapy, cold coagulation, and laser vaporization. Excisional methods include LEEP, laser excision, and cold-knife conization (CKC). The choice between ablative or excisional treatment depends upon the type of TZ, size and clinical extent of the lesion, whether the lesion is CIN or AIS, and the need to rule out microinvasive cancer. The treatment options must be discussed with the woman, and her informed consent should be obtained beforehand. Ablation may be used for treating ectocervical, fully visible CIN lesions if: (1) they involve less than three-fourths of the TZ in a fully visible type 1 TZ; (2) there is no extension to vagina or ectocervix; and (3) invasive cancer has been ruled out (Sankaranarayanan 2014). Ablative cryotherapy and cold coagulation can be performed by trained nurses, midwives, and doctors as an outpatient procedure, without local anesthesia.

Cryotherapy, which destroys neoplastic tissues by freezing the TZ to below −20°C and induces cryonecrosis, is the most widely used ablative treatment in LMICs. Nitrous oxide or carbon dioxide refrigerant is used to cool a metallic cryoprobe to below −20°C, which is then applied to the cervix to freeze the TZ; a "double-freeze" technique of three minutes freeze, five minutes thaw, and three minutes freeze is used. Adequate freezing will result in an ice ball extending four to five millimeters from the outer edge of the probe. Cure rates for CIN2–3 lesions following cryotherapy exceed 90% (Sauvaget, Muwonge, and Sankaranarayanan2013).

Cryotherapy or cold coagulation may be used in a single-visit screen-and-treat approach in LMICs, where it is provided to VIA-positive women with ectocervical lesions involving less than three-fourths of the cervix and without any clinical evidence of cancer, without colposcopy or biopsy triage (Mwanahamuntu et al. 2011). In settings with capacity for colposcopy and histology, a "see-and-treat" approach may be used, that is, cryotherapy or cold coagulation may be offered during a colposcopy visit after taking biopsies, with histology available a posteriori.

Cold coagulation involves applying a heated metallic probe (up to 120°C using a Semm electrical machine) to the cervix for twenty to forty-five seconds to destroy the TZ. Multiple overlapping applications may be used to cover the entire TZ adequately. More than 90% of women with CIN2–3 lesions are cured following cold coagulation (Dolman et al. 2014).

Owing to its easy portability, shorter treatment time, and absence of the need for refrigerants, cold coagulation may be a more feasible ablative treatment option in LMICs.

Excisional treatments such as LEEP, laser excision, and CKC require much more sophisticated surgical skills and equipment infrastructure than cryotherapy or cold coagulation. They are mostly delivered by doctors, though in some settings trained nurses may provide LEEP. Side-effects like bleeding and complications such as late miscarriages, preterm deliveries, premature rupture of membranes, and cervical stenosis are more likely following excisional treatments than following ablation. Excisional treatment is used for treating larger CIN lesions, lesions extending to the cervical canal, lesions in the partially visible or invisible TZ, AIS, and when microinvasive cancer is suspected.

The Loop electrosurgical-excision procedure, which involves electrosurgery to cut tissue and achieve hemostasis under local anesthesia, is the most widely used excisional treatment for CIN and yields cervical-tissue specimens for histological diagnosis. An electrically activated tungsten loop electrode is used to excise the TZ; then a three- or five-millimeter ball electrode is used to coagulate the bleeding points, the cut edges, and the floor of the wound under colposcopic control. It is important that all LEEP providers (including doctors) be adequately trained. A single-pass LEEP using a single cut is used to excise an ectocervical lesion not extending into the canal, and larger lesions may be removed using multiple cuts. The most common side effect (in 4 to 6% of women) following LEEP is bleeding, and cure rates following LEEP are in the range 80 to 95%.

Laser excision under local anesthesia uses a highly focused CO_2 laser spot to excise a cylindrical cervical specimen encompassing the abnormal TZ to a depth of 1 to 1.5 centimeters. The advantages of laser excision include less trauma and blood loss. However, the surgical skills required for laser excision are much more advanced than those necessary for LEEP.

Cold-knife conization is now restrictedly used when microinvasive cancer is suspected and colposcopic-directed biopsy indicates AIS. The procedure provides the cleanest cervical specimen for histological purposes but is associated with more bleeding and adverse pregnancy outcomes than LEEP or laser excision.

After treatment for CIN, women should be advised to obtain follow-up care and to seek prompt medical attention in case they experience symptoms possibly signaling adverse events. Women may be assessed six to twelve months after treatment to evaluate lesion clearance or progression.

Since women treated for CIN are at high risk for cancer, they may be followed up for several years.

DIAGNOSIS, STAGING, AND TREATMENT OF CERVICAL CANCER

Women with early cervical cancer are mostly asymptomatic and may have a normal-looking cervix or a small ulcerated lesion resembling benign inflammation. Thus VIA, cervical smears, and colposcopy are effective in detecting preclinical asymptomatic cervical cancer. As the disease progresses, the cervix becomes abnormal with erosion, ulceration, or ulceroproliferative growth, which may extend to the vagina. Patients with locally advanced disease present with irregular vaginal bleeding, postcoital bleeding, vaginal discomfort, malodorous yellow or serosanguinous vaginal discharge, and pain in the lower abdomen or back. Hematuria, dysuria, fistula, constipation, and rectal bleeding may occur if bladder and rectum are involved. Rectal examination may reveal a mass or gross blood from tumor extension, and leg edema suggests that the tumor is causing lymphatic or vascular obstruction. Punch biopsies from cervical growth will confirm diagnosis.

Cervical cancer is staged using the International Federation of Gynecology and Obstetrics (FIGO) clinical staging system (Table 9.3) after a thorough pelvic examination; bimanual palpation; perrectal examination for thorough evaluation of the cervix, vagina, and parametrium; physical examination of extrapelvic regions to detect spread to abdomen, chest, and supraclavicular nodes; and internationally accepted investigative procedures under clinical staging guidelines such as chest x-ray, intravenous pyelography (as part of imaging investigations), cystoscopy, and proctoscopy to document extent of tumor spread. Other investigations such as computed tomography scan, magnetic resonance imaging, and positron emission tomography scan are used in advanced health-care systems to plan treatment, but these are not widely available in public health services in LMICs. It should be emphasized that findings from these advanced investigations are not permissible under FIGO staging guidelines.

Treatment for cervical cancer involves surgery, radiotherapy, and chemotherapy, and the choice of treatment in LMICs depends upon the stage of the disease, general condition of the patient, and treatment facilities available. For early disease (stages I and IIA), surgery is the treatment of choice, although surgery and radiotherapy are equally effective for early-stage, small-volume disease. However, the decision to use surgery or radio-therapy for early-stage disease depends on several issues. Patients who are in poor general health or have serious comorbidities may not be good surgical candidates. A significant survival advantage following cisplatinum-based chemotherapy administered concurrently with radiotherapy (compared with radiotherapy alone) for locally advanced cervical cancers has been shown in randomized trials (Loizzi et al. 2003). Radiotherapy with concurrent cisplatinum-based chemotherapy is the current standard of care for locally advanced cases (stages IIB to IVA). Palliative radiotherapy or palliative chemotherapy is used for stage IVB disseminated disease.

Patients with stage IA disease may be treated with conization, total hysterectomy, or radical hysterectomy, and five-year survival exceeds 95%. Selected patients with a depth of invasion less than three millimeters (stage IA1) but no lymphovascular space invasion and who desire to remain fertile may be treated with CKC with close follow-up. Those who do not wish to preserve fertility may be treated with total hysterectomy and oophorectomy, which should be deferred in young patients. For those with tumor invasion between three and five millimeters, radical hysterectomy with pelvic node dissection is the treatment of choice. Patients in poor general health with comorbid medical conditions may be treated with intracavitary radiotherapy alone to deliver 7,500 to 8,000 cGy to the cervix.

Patients with stage IB and IIA disease may be treated with radical hysterectomy with bilateral pelvic lymph node dissection or with radical radiotherapy, producing cure rates exceeding 85%. Those with bulky tumors exceeding four centimeters should be treated with radiotherapy consisting of external beam radiotherapy directed to the pelvis; intracavitary radiation with intrauterine and vaginal placement of radioactive sources to deliver a standard dose to the tumor with less irradiation of the surrounding tissues; and concurrent cisplatinum-based chemotherapy.

Patients with stages IIB, III, and IVA are treated with radiotherapy (external beam therapy and intracavitary radiation) concurrent with cisplatinum-based chemotherapy; five-year survival ranges from 20 to 60% depending on the stage. Results from randomized clinical trials have demonstrated significant improvement in survival when cisplatinum alone or cisplatinum plus 5-fluorouracil are combined with radiotherapy. Consequently, concurrent chemoradiotherapy has become the standard of care for locally advanced cervical cancer. Radiotherapy consists of external-beam radiotherapy to reduce tumor mass, enabling intracavitary radiotherapy delivered using a weekly high-dose after loading technique.

Patients with stage IVB cervical cancer are treated with palliative radiotherapy to shrink the tumor and control bleeding and pain, reduce discharge, and help relieve bone pain from skeletal metastasis. Those with disseminated disease are treated with palliative chemotherapy. Palliative care to control pain using opioid and nonopioid analgesics as per the WHO ladder method has a major role in improving quality of life for these advanced patients. Poor prognostic factors for cervical cancer include advanced clinical stage, large tumor volume, bilateral parametrial involvement, para-aortic lymph node involvement, old age, and poor general health.

For recurrent disease, treatment will depend upon previous therapy. Treatment of pelvic recurrences after primary surgical management may include cisplatinum chemotherapy and radiation. Central pelvic recurrences smaller than two centimeters after radical radiotherapy may be treated by modified radical hysterectomy. For large-volume disease recurring fifteen months after concurrent chemoradiotherapy, combination chemotherapy with paclitaxel and cisplatinum may be used. However, recurrences within fifteen months are less likely to respond to further treatment and are candidates for palliative care with adequate pain control.

Recovery from surgery and its complications occurs relatively quickly, whereas the acute and chronic effects of radiation last for years. The complications of radical hysterectomy include hemorrhage, urinary dysfunction, bowel obstruction, and stricture of the rectosigmoid colon. During and soon after radiotherapy, side effects such as abdominal cramps, rectal discomfort, rectal bleeding, diarrhea, dysuria, frequency of urination, and nocturia can be symptomatically treated. Proper skin hygiene should prevent perineal desquamation. Late sequelae of radiotherapy may include rectal or vaginal stenosis, chronic cystitis, and radiation enteritis.

CONCLUSIONS

There is an urgent need for governments in LMICs to invest in HPV vaccination and early detection of cervical cancer through public health services. Both vaccination and HPV testing, used appropriately, have the potential to eliminate cervical cancer. Vaccinating girls nine to thirteen years of age with HPV vaccine (for example, choosing a single age group such as twelve-year-olds) and providing at least one HPV test for thirty- or thirty-five-year-old women (repeated after ten years if resources permit) seems to be a pragmatic approach to prevent cervical cancer in LMICs and in underserved populations.

Whereas HPV vaccination may be incorporated into NIPs and administered through school health services, integrating early detection into underdeveloped public health services will be a major challenge, particularly in LMICs. In such areas there are frequently no adequate facilities for pelvic examination in the primary-care setting, and diagnostic and treatment services for both precancer and cancer are very limited in secondary and tertiary care. For instance, the infrastructure, consumables, and human resources for delivering biopsy, histopathology, cryotherapy, cold coagulation, LEEP, radical surgery, radiotherapy, and chemotherapy are largely inadequate in many countries. Unless governments commit to implementing pragmatic policies and strengthening health services within a specified time frame as part of national cancer-control initiatives, introduction and scaling up of early detection of cancer will remain a distant, abstract goal.

While waiting for government investment, the least that primary-care practitioners in LMICs can do is vaccinate preadolescent girls, screen women above the age of thirty years with whatever method is affordable and feasible, and ensure treatment of screen-positive women (Sankaranarayanan, Ramadas, and Qiao 2013). There is a significant need for strong advocacy from women and society at large for an effective political agenda and government investment in cervical cancer prevention.

REFERENCES

Baldur-Felskov, B., C. Dehlendorff, C. Munk, and S. K. Kjaer. 2014. Early impact of human papillomavirus vaccination on cervical neoplasia: Nationwide follow-up of young Danish women. *J Natl Cancer Inst* 106 (3): djt460. doi:10.1093/jnci/djt460. Epub 2014 Feb 19.

Bray, F., J. S. Ren, E. Masuyer, and J. Ferlay. 2013. Estimates of global cancer prevalence for 27 sites in the adult population in 2008. *Int J Cancer* 132 (5): 1133–1145.

Dolman, L., C. Sauvaget, R. Muwonge, and R. Sankaranarayanan. 2014. Meta-analysis of the efficacy of cold coagulation as a treatment method for cervical intraepithelial neoplasia: A systematic review. *BJOG*. 121 (8): 929–942.

Ferlay, J., I. Soerjomataram, M. Ervik, R. Dikshit, S. Eser, C. Mathers, M. Rebelo, D. M. Parkin, D. Forman, and F. Bray. 2013. *GLOBOCAN 2012 v1.0, Cancer Incidence and Mortality Worldwide: IARC CancerBase 11*. Lyon, France: IARC. Accessed April 4, 2014. http://globocan.iarc.fr.

Forman, D., F. Bray, D. H. Brewster, C. Gombe Mbakawa, B. Kohler, M. Piñeros, E. Steliarova-Foucher, R. Swaminathan, and J. Ferlay. 2013. *Cancer Incidence in*

Five Continents. Vol. X (electronic version). Lyon, France: IARC. Accessed April 4, 2014. http://www.iarc.fr/en/publications/pdfs-online/epi/sp164/.

Garland, S. M. 2014. The Australian experience with the human papillomavirus vaccine. *Clin Ther* 36 (1): 17–23.

International Agency for Research on Cancer (IARC). 2007. *IARC Monographs on the Evaluation of Carcinogenic Risks to Human*. Vol. 90. *Human papillomaviruses*. Lyon, France: IARC.

——. n.d. *Cancer Incidence in Five Continents*. Vol. I-X (electronic version). Lyon, France: IARC. Accessed April 4, 2016.

Joshi, S., R. Sankaranarayanan, R. Muwonge, V. Kulkarni, T. Somanathan, and U. Divate. 2013. Screening of cervical neoplasia in HIV-infected women in India. *AIDS* 27 (4): 607–615.

Kreimer, A. R., A. C. Rodriguez, A. Hildesheim, R. Herrero, C. Porras, M. Schiffman, P. Gonzalez, et al. 2011. Proof-of-principle evaluation of the efficacy of fewer than three doses of a bivalent HPV16/18 vaccine. *J Natl Cancer Inst* 103 (19): 1444–1451.

Lazcano-Ponce, E., M. Stanley, N. Munoz, L. Torres, A. Cruz-Valdez, J. Salmeron, R. Rojas, R. Herrero, and M. Hernández-Ávila. 2014. Overcoming barriers to HPV vaccination: Non-inferiority of antibody response to human papilloma-virus 16/18 vaccine in adolescents vaccinated with a two-dose vs. a three-dose schedule at 21 months. *Vaccine* 32 (6): 725–732.

Loizzi, V., G. Cormio, G. Loverro, L. Selvaggi, P. J. Disaia, and F. Cappuccini. 2003. Chemoradiation: A new approach for the treatment of cervical cancer. *Int J Gynecol Cancer* 13 (5): 580–586.

McCredie, M. R., K. J. Sharples, C. Paul, J. Baranyai, G. Medley, R. W. Jones, and D. C. Skegg. 2008. Natural history of cervical neoplasia and risk of invasive cancer in women with cervical intraepithelial neoplasia 3: A retrospective cohort study. *Lancet Oncol* 9 (5): 425–434.

Murillo, R., M. Almonte, A. Pereira, E. Ferrer, O. A. Gamboa, J. Jerónimo, and E. Lazcano-Ponce. 2008. Cervical cancer screening programs in Latin America and the Caribbean. *Vaccine* 26 (S11): L37–48.

Mwanahamuntu, M. H., V. V. Sahasrabuddhe, S. Kapambwe, K. S. Pfaendler, C. Chibwesha, G. Mkumba, V. Mudenda, et al. 2011. Advancing cervical cancer prevention initiatives in resource-constrained settings: Insights from the Cervical Cancer Prevention Program in Zambia. *PLoS Med* 8 (5): e1001032.

Palefsky, J. M., A. R. Giuliano, S. Goldstone, E. D. Moreira, Jr., C. Aranda, H. Jessen, R. Hillman, et al. 2011. HPV vaccine against anal HPV infection and anal intraepithelial neoplasia. *N Engl J Med* 365:1576–1585.

Romanowski, B., T. F. Schwarz, L. M. Ferguson, M. Ferguson, K. Peters, M. Dionne, L. Schulze, et al. 2014. Immune response to the HPV-16/18 AS04-adjuvanted vaccine administered as a 2-dose or 3-dose schedule up to 4 years after vaccination: Results from a randomized study. *Hum Vaccin Immunother* 10 (5): 1155–1165.

Ronco, G., J. Dillner, K. M. Elfstrom, S. Tunesi, P. J. Snijders, M. Arbyn, H. Kitchener, et al. 2014. Efficacy of HPV-based screening for prevention of invasive cervical cancer: Follow-up of four European randomised controlled trials. *Lancet* 383:524–532.

Safaeian, M., C. Porras, Y. Pan, A. Kreimer, J. T. Schiller, P. Gonzalez, D. R. Lowy, et al. 2013. Durable antibody responses following one dose of the bivalent human papillomavirus L1 virus-like particle vaccine in the Costa Rica Vaccine Trial. *Cancer Prev Res (Phila)* 6 (11): 1242–1250.

Sankaranarayanan, R. 2014. "Treatment of Precancerous Cervical Lesions." Chapter 8 in *Advances in Cervical Cancer Management* [e-book]. *Future Science Group*, edited by P. W. Grigsby, 100–120. EISBN: 978-1-78084-450-3.

Sankaranarayanan, R., P. O. Esmy, R. Rajkumar, R. Muwonge, R. Swaminathan, S. Shanthakumari, J. M. Fayette, and J. Cherian. 2007. Effect of visual screening on cervical cancer incidence and mortality in Tamil Nadu, India: A cluster-randomised trial. *Lancet* 370:398–406.

Sankaranarayanan, R., B. M. Nene, S. S. Shastri, K. Jayant, R. Muwonge, A. M. Budukh, S. Hingmire, et al. 2009. HPV screening for cervical cancer in rural India. *N Engl J Med* 360 (14): 1385–1394.

Sankaranarayanan, R., A. Nessa, P. O. Esmy, and J. M. Dangou. 2012. Visual inspection methods for cervical cancer prevention. *Best Pract Res Clin Obstet Gynaecol* 26 (2): 221–232.

Sankaranarayanan R., K. Ramadas, and Y. L. Qiao. 2013. "Early Detection of Cancer in Primary Care in Less-Developed Countries." In *Cancer Control 2013: Cancer Care in Emerging Health Systems,* edited I. Magrath, 68–72. Brussels: International Network for Cancer Treatment and Research.

Sankaranarayanan, R., and R. Swaminathan. 2011. *Cancer Survival in Africa, Asia, the Caribbean and Central America.* IARC Scientific Publication 162. Lyon, France: IARC.

Sankaranarayanan, R., R. Swaminathan, and D. M. Parkin. 1998. *Cancer Survival in Developing Countries.* IARC Scientific Publication 145. Lyon, France: International Agency for Research on Cancer.

Sauvaget, C., R. Muwonge, and R. Sankaranarayanan. 2013. Meta-analysis of the effectiveness of cryotherapy in the treatment of cervical intraepithelial neoplasia. *Int J Gynaecol Obstet* 120 (3): 218–223.

Schiffman, M., A. G. Glass, N. Wentzensen, B. B. Rush, P. E. Castle, D. R. Scott, J. Buckland, et al. 2011. A long-term prospective study of type-specific human papillomavirus infection and risk of cervical neoplasia among 20,000 women in the Portland Kaiser Cohort Study. *Cancer Epidemiol Biomarkers Prev* 20 (7): 1398–1409.

Schiller, J. T., X. Castellsague, and S. M. Garland. 2012. A review of clinical trials of human papillomavirus prophylactic vaccines. *Vaccine* 30 (S5): F123–138.

Shastri, S. S., I. Mittra, G. A. Mishra, S. Gupta, R. Dikshit, S. Singh, and R. A. Badwe. 2014. Effect of VIA screening by primary health workers: Randomized controlled study in Mumbai, India. *J Natl Cancer Inst* 106 (3): dju009.

Sobin, L. H., M. Gospodarowicz, and C. Wittekind, eds. 2009. *International Union against Cancer (UICC): TNM Classification of Malignant Tumours.* 7th ed. Hoboken, NJ: Wiley-Blackwell.

World Health Organization (WHO). 2013. *WHO Guidance Note: Comprehensive cervical cancer prevention and control; A healthier future for girls and women.* Geneva: World Health Organization.

10

Gender-Based Violence in Resource-Limited Settings

ROSE LEONARD MOLINA AND JENNIFER SCOTT

Addressing gender inequality and violence against women is central to advancing women's health on a global level. Global efforts to promote gender equality and to eliminate violence against women are at the core of the Millennium Development Goals and international policy and programming. The United Nations has described gender-based violence (GBV) as "a pandemic in diverse forms" (UN Women n.d.), highlighting its prevalence as a global disease process that takes a myriad of overt to subtle forms, ranging from sexual violence to economic exclusion to political oppression.

The United Nations Declaration on the Elimination of Violence against Women defines violence against women as "any act of gender-based violence that results in, or is likely to result in, physical, sexual or psychological harm or suffering to women, including threats of such acts, coercion or arbitrary deprivations of liberty, whether occurring in public or in private life" (United Nations 1993, 3). Furthermore, the Beijing Declaration and Platform for Action described GBV as "an obstacle to the achievement of the objectives of equality, development and peace" and a violation of human rights and fundamental freedoms (United Nations 1995). Globally, GBV presents a critical public health challenge with significant health, social, and economic consequences for individuals, families, and societies (United States Agency for International Development 2012).

In general, GBV is any violence directed against a person on the basis of gender. It reflects and reinforces underlying inequalities between women and men (European Institute for Gender Equality n.d.). As with any type of interpersonal violence, it is important to note that GBV affects women, men, girls, and boys. Forms of GBV are commonly categorized based on the type of violence (physical, sexual, or emotional violence), the perpetration of violence (partner or nonpartner violence), or the context of violence (conflict related or politically motivated). The terms *gender-based violence* and *violence against women* are often used interchangeably, given that the majority of violence is directed against women. For the purposes of this chapter, the term *gender-based violence* is primarily used and can manifest as any of the following forms, which are not mutually exclusive (European Institute for Gender Equality n.d.; United States Agency for International Development 2012):

- sexual harassment, domestic violence, intimate-partner violence (physical or sexual violence, or both), and rape
- trafficking of women, forced labor, and forced prostitution
- systematic rape, sexual slavery, and forced pregnancy as seen in conflict settings
- gender-inequitable traditional practices such as female genital cutting, forced and early marriages, bride dowry, widow inheritance, and honor crimes, and
- forced sterilization, forced abortion, reproductive and contraceptive coercion, female infanticide, and prenatal sex selection

The manifestation of GBV in private and public life varies depending on the specific local context. It is important to understand the gender, social, and cultural norms relevant to the local setting that contribute to gender inequality and to GBV. Gender-based violence is challenging and complex and requires heightened sensitivity and awareness from health-care providers. This chapter provides an overview of GBV for the health-care provider working internationally and in resource-limited settings. It is not a comprehensive review of all forms of violence against women, but it highlights important considerations, which need to be adapted to the local context. We offer both evidence-based recommendations and suggestions based on field experience to support a health-care provider working in various international settings.

EPIDEMIOLOGY

Globally, it is estimated that 30% of women aged fifteen years or older have experienced intimate-partner violence in their lifetimes, and there is substantial geographic variation, from 16% in East Asia to 66% in central sub-Saharan Africa (Devries et al. 2013) (Figure 10.1). In a multicountry study of violence, 26 to 80% of men surveyed disclosed perpetration of physical or sexual violence against an intimate partner, which varied by site and country (Jewkes et al. 2013). Additionally, 7% of women aged fifteen years or older reported nonpartner sexual violence during their lifetimes, also with substantial geographic variation (Abrahams et al. 2014). Worldwide, one in seven homicides (14%) is committed by an intimate partner, and the proportion of women killed by their partners is six times higher than the proportion of men killed by their partners (39% and 6%, respectively) (Stockl et al. 2013). Furthermore, the United Nations estimates that 600 million women live in countries where domestic violence is not a crime (Devries et al. 2013). Though variations in the legal definitions and cultural perceptions of violence make it challenging to measure, worldwide data indicate that GBV is widely prevalent.

Studies measuring the incidence and prevalence of GBV vary according to setting, study design, and definitions of violence. These data also reflect only those who are willing to disclose their experiences of violence, and multiple barriers may limit the measurement of GBV. Barriers to reporting GBV include shame and stigma, perceived impunity for perpetrators, lack of awareness of services, financial limitations to seeking services, cultural beliefs, fear of losing children, distrust of health-care workers, fear of retaliation, and normalization of violence (Palermo, Bleck, and Peterman 2014). Additionally, there remains a significant discrepancy between reporting to informal sources, such as family or friends, and to formal sources, such as the police. Globally, the formal reporting rate is approximately 7%, which indicates that the estimates of violence in the literature may be underestimates of the true problem (Palermo, Bleck, and Peterman 2014). Sexual violence is more commonly reported to formal authorities than physical violence. Other attributes associated with formal reporting of violence include marital status, older age, higher education attainment, increasing wealth, and urban residence (Palermo, Bleck, and Peterman 2014). As a result of gender, social, and economic inequalities and discrimination, women who endure GBV may face challenges in seeking safety, justice, and treatment. Consideration of such challenges emphasizes the importance of collaboration among medical, judicial, and law enforcement sectors to document and provide appropriate services for GBV survivors. It is important for health-care providers to gain knowledge of the

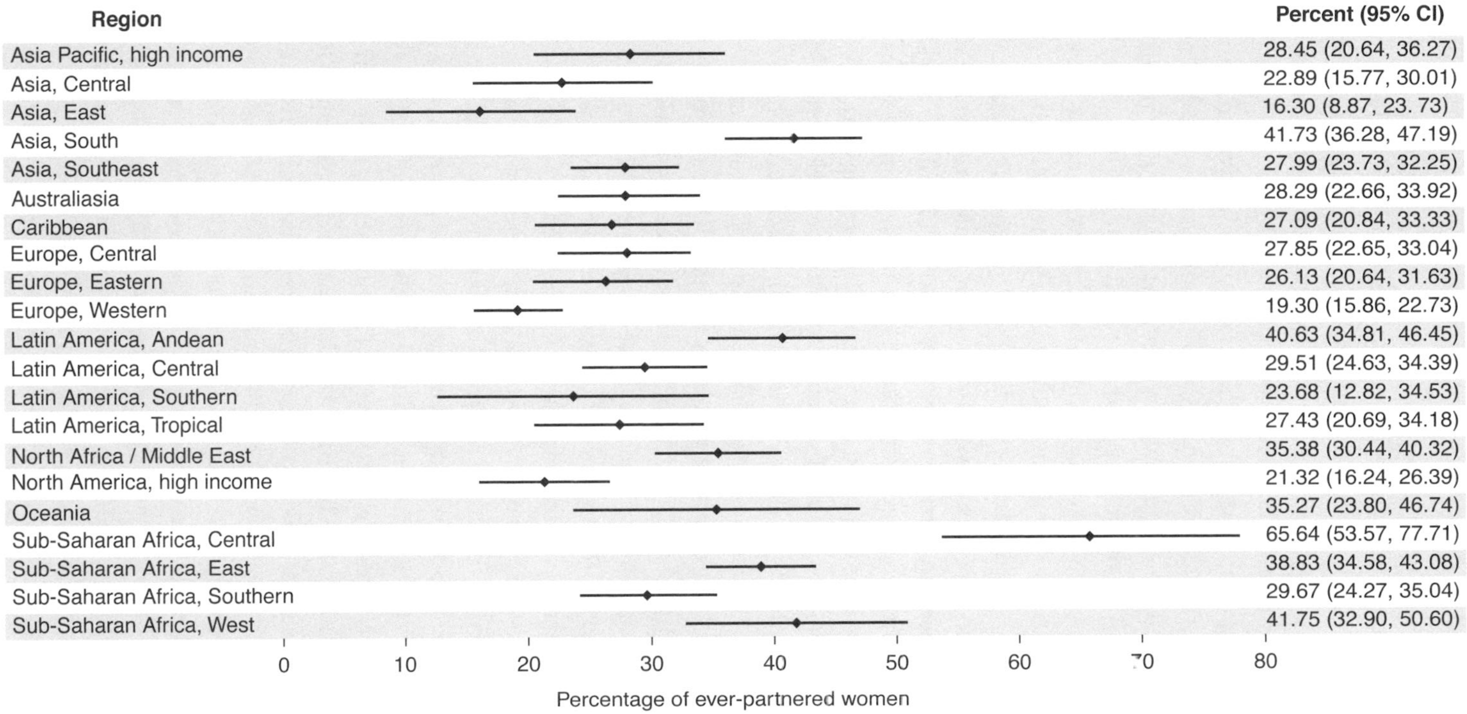

Region	Percent (95% CI)
Asia Pacific, high income	28.45 (20.64, 36.27)
Asia, Central	22.89 (15.77, 30.01)
Asia, East	16.30 (8.87, 23. 73)
Asia, South	41.73 (36.28, 47.19)
Asia, Southeast	27.99 (23.73, 32.25)
Australiasia	28.29 (22.66, 33.92)
Caribbean	27.09 (20.84, 33.33)
Europe, Central	27.85 (22.65, 33.04)
Europe, Eastern	26.13 (20.64, 31.63)
Europe, Western	19.30 (15.86, 22.73)
Latin America, Andean	40.63 (34.81, 46.45)
Latin America, Central	29.51 (24.63, 34.39)
Latin America, Southern	23.68 (12.82, 34.53)
Latin America, Tropical	27.43 (20.69, 34.18)
North Africa / Middle East	35.38 (30.44, 40.32)
North America, high income	21.32 (16.24, 26.39)
Oceania	35.27 (23.80, 46.74)
Sub-Saharan Africa, Central	65.64 (53.57, 77.71)
Sub-Saharan Africa, East	38.83 (34.58, 43.08)
Sub-Saharan Africa, Southern	29.67 (24.27, 35.04)
Sub-Saharan Africa, West	41.75 (32.90, 50.60)

Percentage of ever-partnered women

FIGURE 10.1. Prevalence of intimate-partner violence, by region.

local systems and processes that exist for a survivor of GBV to report violence and to seek justice and care.

Violence against women occurs across their life cycles and spans multiple special populations that require disaggregated analysis, as they are at particular risk for different forms of violence and subsequent health, social, legal, and economic consequences. Examples include child brides, girls who undergo genital cutting, trafficked girls and women, immigrant and displaced persons, women in humanitarian crises or conflict settings, women with disabilities, pregnant women, the lesbian, gay, bisexual, and transgender (LGBT) community, and sex workers. It is critical that healthcare providers working internationally recognize who is at risk for violence and where and when women may be most vulnerable to GBV.

Sex workers are particularly vulnerable to violence. Police are often reported as perpetrators themselves and may not register reports of violence against sex workers in settings where sex work is criminalized (Deering et al. 2014). Overall prevalence of violence against sex workers at any time throughout their lives is estimated at 41 to 65% (Deering et al. 2014). Variables that influence patterns of violence against sex workers include work environments (public versus private locations), education level, social networks (group or coalition of sex workers versus solo practice), autonomy around the decision to engage in sex work (as opposed to trafficked or forced sex work), and use of alcohol or drugs (Deering et al. 2014). The World Health Organization and the United Nations advocate for decriminalization of sex work, as it is paramount to avert violence that stems from the legal setting in which sex work is practiced.

While GBV occurs around the world, it is especially prevalent during humanitarian crises, including natural disasters and political conflicts. A systematic review of GBV in complex emergencies notes an increase in GBV during crises, with an elevation in intimate-partner violence, suggesting that women encounter the greatest risk for violence in their own homes (Stark and Ager 2011). The lifetime prevalence of sexual assault in humanitarian settings varies, with estimates of 17% of internally displaced persons in Sierra Leone (Amowitz et al. 2002) to nearly 40% of female household respondents in eastern Democratic Republic of Congo (Johnson et al. 2010), as examples. Estimates of GBV tend to be generated from nonprobability samples (facility data, organizational data, or police data), and population-based assessments are needed to understand the prevalence of GBV. When comparing incidence and prevalence of GBV between different countries and populations, it is important to understand the methodology used to estimate GBV, including the inherent limitations and biases, to inform policy and programming.

PATHOLOGY AND PATHOPHYSIOLOGY

At the international level, the general consensus is that GBV is inextricably linked to gender-based inequalities. Gender equality is defined as the "equal enjoyment by women and men of socially valued goods, opportunities, resources, and rewards" (United Nations Population Fund 2005, 1; OECD Development Assistance Committee 1998). The United Nations Millennium Development Goal 3 aims to promote gender equality and empower women by creating targets to eliminate gender disparities in education, promote women's participation in the labor market, and increase parliamentary representation by women (United Nations 2013). Similarly, Goal 5 of the United Nations 2030 Agenda for Sustainable Development aims to achieve gender equality and empower all women and girls (United Nations 2016, 20). Achieving gender equality requires women's empowerment to ensure that they have equal decision-making power in the private and public sectors and equal access to resources.

To understand the numerous factors that contribute to GBV, various conceptual frameworks have been proposed, including an ecological framework as described by the World Health Organization (see Figure 10.2). This framework includes complex interactions at multiple levels: the individual, the relationship, the community, and the society (Krug et al. 2002). At the individual perpetrator level, risk factors include young age, alcohol abuse, depression, personality disorders, low academic achievement, low income, and having witnessed or experienced violence as a child. At the relationship level, risk factors include marital conflict or instability, male dominance in the family, economic stress, and familial dysfunction. At the community level, risk factors include weak community sanctions against domestic violence, poverty, and low social capital. At the societal level, risk factors include traditional gender norms and social norms supportive of violence (Krug et al. 2002). Another lens through which violence can be understood includes identification of various institutional influences, such as those influences from schools, religions, and media (Crowell and Burgess 1996).

Researchers have also considered whether some women may have individual risk factors for victimization, such as number of sexual partners,

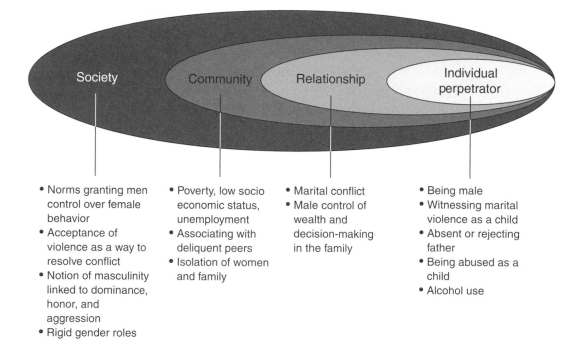

- Norms granting men control over female behavior
- Acceptance of violence as a way to resolve conflict
- Notion of masculinity linked to dominance, honor, and aggression
- Rigid gender roles

- Poverty, low socio economic status, unemployment
- Associating with deliquent peers
- Isolation of women and family

- Marital conflict
- Male control of wealth and decision-making in the family

- Being male
- Witnessing marital violence as a child
- Absent or rejecting father
- Being abused as a child
- Alcohol use

FIGURE 10.2. Ecological framework of factors contributing to gender-based violence.

alcohol use, and lower education attainment. However, one challenge in examining this question is distinguishing between traits and behaviors evident before victimization and those that manifest afterward. One common risk factor for victimization of women demonstrated in several studies is their exposure to childhood violence, which is also a risk factor for perpetrating violence (Crowell and Burgess 1996). Factors associated with male perpetration of intimate-partner violence relate to gender and relationship practices, experiences of childhood trauma, alcohol misuse, depression, low education, poverty, and involvement with gangs and weapons, among others (Jewkes et al. 2013). When providing clinical services or resources to a GBV survivor, the focus is on providing direct care and identifying potential factors that put an individual at risk for future acts of violence.

Many women and girls are at risk for GBV based on circumstances related to humanitarian crises, such as in the aftermath of a natural disaster, in conflict and postconflict settings, and in crises related to political violence. In any crisis setting, all forms of GBV can occur, but sexual violence is particularly common. In the early stages of an emergency, families and communities are disrupted, populations are displaced, and social protection mechanisms are interrupted (Inter-Agency Standing Committee 2015). As an emergency situation stabilizes, there may be an increase in domestic violence and harmful traditional practices such as forced marriages, female genital cutting, and honor killings (Inter-Agency Standing Committee 2015).

Chronic humanitarian crises can be more complex. Over recent decades, civilians have become the target in conflicts, as seen in Bosnia, Rwanda, Darfur, Sierra Leone, Liberia, Democratic Republic of Congo, and Syria, and sexual violence has been used as a strategy of war in these conflict zones. Women and girls are particularly vulnerable to sexual violence, as it is used as "a tactic of war to humiliate, dominate, instill fear in, disperse and/or forcibly relocate civilian members of a community or ethnic group" (United Nations 2008, 1) The United Nations has passed security resolutions to protect civilians and to constitute rape and other forms of sexual violence in conflict as crimes against humanity and war crimes (Overstreet and Quinn 2013).

When working internationally, a health-care provider must consider gender dynamics and gender-related variables when developing and implementing programs. Women and men have unique concerns, and it is important to overcome underlying systematic gender inequalities when implementing a program, providing clinical services, or conducting research (United Nations Population Fund 2005). It can be helpful to obtain knowledge of country-specific gender disparities in economic, education, social, and health indicators before working in a setting; these can be identified from various sources, including demographic health survey data by country and data collected by the World Health Organization, the United Nations, and other international organizations (United Nations Population Fund 2005). It is important to be aware of the forms of violence that women may experience in a particular community, but it can take time to develop an understanding of the unique cultural structures that promote violence. This awareness can be fostered through dialogue with local partners or can be formally assessed as part of program research or implementation. Furthermore, whether developing a clinical program or designing research, it is critical to work with local partners and community organizations to outline a conceptual framework to identify the individual, relational, and community-level risk factors for violence that are relevant to that setting. Outlining a theoretical framework in advance of program or research implementation and revisiting the framework throughout the course of a program or research study may allow for a more comprehensive, yet targeted, approach.

GLOBAL IMPACT OF DISEASE

Violence against women creates immediate health risks and carries long-term consequences for women, families, and communities. Additionally, GBV can occur multiple times throughout a woman's life, leading to cumulative physical, psychological, and social consequences. Data collection on the global impact of GBV is challenging, as it relies on women's access to reporting mechanisms and their willingness to report and requires sufficient resources to document, analyze, and interpret data.

The World Health Organization outlines various consequences of violence including physical (acute injuries and chronic pain syndromes), psychological and behavioral (depression, anxiety, post-traumatic stress disorder, substance abuse), and sexual and reproductive (poor pregnancy outcomes and sexually transmitted infections), as well as fatal consequences; many of these are intertwined (Table 10.1). Women who have experienced violence are twice as likely to suffer from depression (Krug et al. 2002). Those who have experienced sexual violence, in particular, have nearly twice the risk of acquiring HIV or syphilis (Krug et al. 2002).

Pregnancies can result from sexual violence, and acts of GBV can occur during the course of a pregnancy, with direct effects on the fetus. Intimate partner violence during pregnancy has been associated with poor maternal weight gain, infection, stillbirth, pelvic fracture, placental abruption, fetal injury, preterm birth, and low birth weight (American College of Obstetricians and Gynecologists 2012). Furthermore, murder of pregnant women is a leading cause of maternal death (American College of Obstetricians and Gynecologists 2012). Pregnancies occurring as a result of violence—coercion, contraceptive manipulation, or sexual violence—can be a challenging issue for women, children, and families. Gaining a better understanding of the needs of children born from sexual-violence-related pregnancies has become a growing focus in research and programming. In general, the approach to unplanned pregnancies resulting from violence varies depending on the cultural and legal contexts. As a health-care provider, it is critical to be knowledgeable about existing family planning services in the local community in order to provide referrals and recommendations.

Table 10.1 Health consequences of intimate-partner violence

Physical	Sexual and reproductive	Psychological and behavioral	Fatal consequences
Abdominal and thoracic injuries	Pelvic inflammatory disease	Alcohol and drug abuse	AIDS-related mortality
Bruises and welts	Pregnancy complications	Depression and anxiety	Maternal mortality
Chronic pain syndromes	Sexual dysfunction	Eating and sleep disorders	Homicide
Reduced physical functioning and disability	Sexually transmitted infections	Post-traumatic stress disorder	Suicide
Fibromyalgia	Unsafe abortion	Psychosomatic disorders	
Gastrointestinal disorders	Undesired pregnancy	Suicidal behavior and self-harm	
Lacerations and abrasions	Trauma-related injuries	Phobias and panic disorder	

Source: Reprinted from Krug et al. (2002, 101), Table 4.6. © World Health Organization 2002.

Gender-based violence affects a woman's sense of self and her relationships within her family and her larger community. Stigma has been reported among survivors of GBV, including cultural stigma, internalized stigma, and anticipated stigma. It is hypothesized that stigma may hinder help-seeking behaviors following GBV (Overstreet and Quinn 2013). In addition, family and marital relations become strained when there is violence against women. For example, a study of female survivors of sexual assault in rural eastern Democratic Republic of Congo revealed that survivors are at increased risk for family rejection and mental-health disorders (Kohli et al. 2014; Kelly et al. 2011). Stigma and rejection following sexual violence can lead to complex physical, psychosocial, behavioral, and economic consequences.

Researchers have also investigated social dyads, particularly the mother-child relationship, in the context of violence. One study showed that mothers who endured intimate-partner violence and experienced clinical internalized problems (anxiety, depression, withdrawn affect, and somatic complaints) were seven times more likely to have children with similar complaints compared with mothers who did not experience intimate-partner violence (McFarlane et al. 2014). Additionally, survivors of violence who reported clinical externalized problems (aggression, rule breaking, and intrusive behaviors) were nearly five times more likely to have children with similar problems (McFarlane et al. 2014).

The true social and economic costs of GBV are challenging to estimate. According to the United States Department of Health and Human Services, over 5 million women aged eighteen and older experience intimate partner violence, resulting in approximately 2 million injuries, of which 550,000 require medical attention (National Center for Injury Prevention and Control 2003). Survivors of intimate-partner violence lose nearly 8 million days of work, the equivalent of approximately 32,000 full-time jobs (National Center for Injury Prevention and Control 2003). The overall yearly cost of intimate-partner violence has been estimated at nearly $6 billion dollars. Direct costs of medical care for injuries and psychosocial consequences account for the majority of costs (National Center for Injury Prevention and Control 2003). Indirect costs such as lost productivity, strained relationships, psychological stress, and compromised quality of life are difficult to quantify but remain important consequences of GBV. These figures are generated from data relevant to the United States; there are limited comparative data for the true costs of GBV on a global level.

TREATMENT AND GUIDELINES FOR CARE

While the cornerstone of abolishing violence against women is eliminating gender inequality, primary prevention of violence is critical. While many political organizations, nongovernmental organizations, health-care providers, and advocates for women strive to attain gender equality, this goal requires normative change that permeates global legal and social institutions that are historically slow to change. Health-care providers, such as obstetricians and gynecologists, occupy a critical position in (1) advancing primary prevention of violence through education and awareness, (2) addressing secondary prevention through universal screening in healthcare settings, and (3) completing tertiary prevention through providing a comprehensive assessment of injuries and appropriate referrals if violence is disclosed.

While working in a clinical capacity, take the time to prepare the clinical setting and staff to respond appropriately to cases of GBV. Various guidelines are available (Chamberlain and Levenson 2012; Inter-Agency Working Group on Reproductive Health in Crises 2012), and they share several common features. The World Health Organization and the United

Nation High Commissioner for Refugees (2004) have made practical suggestions for the clinical setting:

- Have a written policy on GBV in the clinical setting.
- Train staff to screen, manage, and refer cases of GBV.
- Provide privacy for conducting interviews and physical exams.
- Have educational resources available in the appropriate language and at the literacy level of the population served.
- Develop a referral pathway and collaborate with partnering organizations to build and strengthen referral capacity.
- Understand the local legal and cultural context of violence.
- Follow clinical protocols and standards.

Universal screening for violence in a safe environment is critical for identifying women at risk and providing appropriate awareness about the subject; however, it is important to balance the benefits and potential risks of universal screening. After assuring the patient regarding confidentiality, verbal screening questions or written questionnaires can be administered in a private clinic setting. Depending on the cultural context, women may be accompanied by their intimate partner, spouse, or a family member. Dialogue with local colleagues can provide further insight into how to best perform a medical and psychosocial assessment while respecting certain cultural norms. Some proposed screening questions, such as, "Are you afraid of your partner or anyone else?" and "Have you felt threatened in any way by your partner or anyone else?," should be asked when the woman is alone. The American College of Obstetricians and Gynecologists (2012) has issued a committee opinion on intimate-partner violence that includes sample scripts (Chamberlain and Levenson 2012). (Table 10.2.)

If violence is disclosed, the key goals are to acknowledge the woman's experience and willingness to share her experience, assess her immediate safety, evaluate patterns of violence, address acute injuries, and provide appropriate counseling and referrals. Owing to the substantial psychological sequelae of experiencing violence, the World Health Organization (WHO 2003) has put forth some suggestions for responding to the emotional needs of women who are survivors of GBV (Table 10.3). During the encounter, it is also helpful to share the local community and legal resources available to women who have endured violence. It is important to know the legal precedents around violence against women and which authorities (hospitals, clinics, or police) may be advocates for survivors of violence.

Table 10.2   Sample intimate-partner violence screening questions

Framing statement	"We've started talking to all of our patients about safe and healthy relationships because it can have such a large impact on your health."
Confidentiality	"Before we get started, I want you to know that everything here is confidential, meaning that I won't talk to anyone else about what is said unless you tell me that . . . [insert the laws of your local context about what is necessary to disclose]."
General sample questions	"Has your current partner ever threatened you or made you feel afraid?" (Threatened to hurt you or your children if you did or did not do something, controlled who you talked to or where you went, or gone into rages.) "Has your partner ever hit, choked, or physically hurt you?" ("Hurt" includes being hit, slapped, kicked, bitten, pushed, or shoved.)
Sample questions for women of reproductive age	"Has your partner ever forced you to do something sexually that you did not want to do, or refused your request to use condoms?" "Does your partner support your decision about when or if you want to become pregnant?" "Has your partner ever tampered with your birth control or tried to get you pregnant when you didn't want to be?"
Sample questions for women with disabilities	"Has your partner prevented you from using a wheelchair, cane, respirator, or other assistive device?" "Has your partner refused to help you with an important personal need such as taking your medicine, getting to the bathroom, getting out of bed, bathing, getting dressed, getting food or drink, or threatened not to help you with these personal needs?"

Source: Reprinted from American College of Obstetricians and Gynecologists (2012), Box 1. © 2012 by American College of Obstetricians and Gynecologists.

In responding to sexual violence, a complete gynecologic exam and assessment should be performed, including testing for pregnancy and screening for sexually transmitted infections (HIV, syphilis, hepatitis B and C, gonorrhea, chlamydia). Where diagnostic tests for infections are not widely available, it is appropriate to consider empiric treatment or syndromic management (WHO 2001) of sexually transmitted infections. Emergency contraception should be given if available, ideally within 24 hours and up to 120 hours after the sexual assault. In the event of a pregnancy resulting from sexual violence, it is important to be familiar with the local abortion laws and awareness of clinical services for comprehensive abortion care, in addition to other clinical and social services (United

Table 10.3   Helping victims of sexual violence deal with their emotions

Emotion	Some ways to respond
Hopelessness	"You are a valuable person."
Despair	Focus on the strategies and resourcefulness that the person used to survive.
Powerlessness and loss of control	"You have choices and options today in how to proceed."
Flashbacks	"These will resolve with the healing process."
Disturbed sleep	"This will resolve with the healing process."
Denial	"I'm taking what you have told me seriously. I will be here if you need help in the future."
Guilt and self-blame	"You are not to blame for what happened to you. The person who assaulted you is responsible for the violence."
Shame	"There is no loss of honor in being assaulted. You are an honorable person."
Fear	"You are safe here. That must have been very frightening for you."
Numbness	"This is a common reaction to severe trauma. You will feel again. All in good time."
Mood swings	"These are common and should resolve with the healing process."
Anger	"You sound very angry. This is a legitimate feeling given what you have experienced. There are ways to express your anger safely."
Anxiety	"These symptoms can get better with certain stress management techniques." Offer to explain these techniques.
Helplessness	"It sounds as if you are feeling helpless. We are here to help you."

Source: Reprinted with minor modifications from WHO (2003, 33), Table 5. © World Health Organization 2003.

Nations Population Fund 2012). There are countries with laws that will allow for termination of a pregnancy conceived from rape, even if abortion is considered illegal for other reasons in that particular country. Depending on the prevalence of HIV in the community, postexposure prophylaxis should be considered according to local ministry of health guidelines. Appropriate vaccinations, such as hepatitis and tetanus, should be considered, if available, and according to the recommended schedule of administration. Throughout these sensitive encounters, a woman's privacy and safety take precedence, and it is necessary to consider her risk for recurrent violence when referring her for clinical and judicial services. See Table 10.4 for recommendations in low-resource settings.

Documenting the account of the assault and the injuries sustained is critical in countries where a legal or judicial infrastructure exists to protect

Table 10.4   Minimum resources required for treatment of rape survivors in a
clinical setting

---

1. Protocol   Available
 Written medical protocol in language of provider[a]
2. Personnel   Available
 Trained (local) health care professionals (on call twenty-four
   hours a day)[a]
 For female survivors, a female health-care provider who speaks
   the same language; if not possible, a female health worker (or
   companion) in the room during the examination[a]
3. Furniture and setting   Available
 Room (private, quiet, accessible, with access to a toilet or latrine)[a]
 Examination table[a]
 Light, preferably fixed (so as not to threaten children by flashlight)[a]
 Magnifying glass (or colposcope)
 Access to an autoclave to sterilize equipment[a]
 Access to laboratory facilities, a microscope, and a trained
   technician
 Weighing scales and height chart for children
4. Rape kit supplies for collection of forensic evidence   Available
 Speculum (preferably plastic, disposable, only adult sizes)[a]
 Comb for collecting foreign matter in pubic hair
 Syringes and needles (butterfly for children) or tubes for col-
   lecting blood
 Glass slides for preparing wet or dry mounts (for sperm)
 Cotton-tipped swabs, applicators, and gauze compresses for
   collecting samples
 Paper sheet for collecting debris as the survivor undresses
 Tape measure for measuring the size of bruises, lacerations, and
   so on[a]
 Paper bags for collection of evidence[a]
 Paper tape for sealing and labeling containers and bags[a]
 Supplies for universal precautions (gloves, box for safe disposal of
   contaminated and sharp materials, soap)[a]
 Resuscitation equipment[a]
 Sterile medical instruments (kit) for repair of tears, suture
   material[a]
 Needles, syringes[a]
 Cover (gown, cloth, sheet) to cover the survivor during the
   examination[a]
 Spare items of clothing to replace those that are torn or taken for
   evidence
 Sanitary supplies (pads or local cloths)[a]
 Pregnancy tests
 Pregnancy calculator disk to determine the age of a pregnancy
5. Drugs   Available
 For treatment of STIs as per country protocol[a]
 For postexposure prophylaxis (PEP) of HIV transmission
 Emergency contraceptive pills or copper-bearing intrauterine
   device (IUD) (or both)[a]

Table 10.4   (continued)

Tetanus toxoid, tetanus immunoglobulin	
Hepatitis B vaccine	
For pain relief (for example, paracetamol/tylenol)[a]	
Anxiolytic (for example, diazepam)	
Sedative for children (for example, diazepam)	
Local anaesthetic for suturing[a]	
Antibiotics for wound care[a]	
6. Administrative supplies	Available
Medical chart with pictograms[a]	
Forms for recording post-rape care	
Consent forms[a]	
Information pamphlets for post-rape care (for survivor)[a]	
Safe, locked filing space to keep records confidential	

Source: Reprinted with minor modifications from World Health Organization and United Nations High Commissioner for Refugees (2004), pp. 7–8. © World Health Organization/ United Nations High Commissioner for Refugees, 2004.

a. Minimum requirements for examination and treatment of a rape survivor.

women against violence. The World Health Organization (WHO 2003) has published a care protocol that includes an initial assessment with informed consent, a medical history, a comprehensive physical exam with documentation of injuries, collection of medical specimens for diagnostic purposes, collection and transportation of forensic specimens for legal purposes, therapeutic treatment for injuries, arranging follow-up care, and developing a medico-legal report. When documenting the injury, it is important to note the age of the injury, the mechanism by which the injury was produced, the circumstances in which the injury was sustained, and the consequences of the injury (World Health Organization 2003). When working internationally, it is essential to consult local health authorities, partnering organizations, law enforcement agencies, and judicial experts to identify the most relevant documentation and legal processes for survivors of GBV.

In general, the response to GBV requires coordination—among programs, organizations, and community leaders—and adherence to an ethical code of conduct. In humanitarian settings, there are guidelines for responding to GBV with specific recommendations that correlate to the phase of the emergency. For example, the Minimum Initial Services Package for Reproductive Health in Crisis Situations offers training, guidelines, and supplies for responding to GBV (Women's Refugee Commission 2011). However, the key to providing comprehensive services to survivors is collaboration among numerous local, governmental, and international partners to provide appropriate clinical, psychosocial, and legal services.

In addition to clinical protocols and services, ethical guidelines have been created for conducting research on GBV in international settings (2007).

While working in international settings, the role of a health-care provider often extends beyond the direct clinical role. It is important to have not only an understanding of the clinical protocols and resources for addressing GBV but also a multidisciplinary framework in which to think broadly about addressing GBV. As an example, GBV increased following the earthquake in Haiti, and a multidisciplinary approach was required to accomplish the following:

- Provide support to GBV survivors (that is, ensure access to GBV services, provide training to identify and refer cases, work in partnership with organizations to provide legal assistance, improve preparedness and prevention capacity).
- Strengthen security mechanisms (that is, support preventive security measures, build capacity of police force, increase female representation in law enforcement, support local agencies that offer protection and prevention programs, protect displaced women and girls).
- Improve legislation and capacity (that is, strengthen legal protection for women, enforce existing legislation, promote multisectorial coordination, build capacity of local organizations).
- Create economic opportunities (that is, provide sustainable economic solutions, vocational training, and livelihood projects to vulnerable or marginalized groups and link women to capital).
- Raise awareness (that is, partner to create community-based programs, train female mediators, promote new social norms, supportive innovative responses, and protection strategies). (United States Department of State 2012)

In general, as part of developing a multidisciplinary approach to GBV, the Henry J. Kaiser Family Foundation (2012) suggests a framework that supports gender equality in global-health programming and could include the following elements:

- Ensure equitable access to essential health services (facility and community levels).
- Increase the participation of women and girls in health program implementation.

- Monitor, prevent, and respond to GBV.
- Empower girls by strengthening social networks, educational opportunities, and economic assets.
- Engage men and boys as clients, supportive partners, and role models for equality.
- Promote policies and laws that will improve gender equality.
- Address social, economic, legal, and cultural determinants of health (multisectorial approach).
- Encourage community-based approaches and engagement of community leaders.
- Build the capacity of individuals as health-care providers and decision makers.
- Strengthen the capacity of institutions to set gender-equitable policies and guidelines.

CONCLUSION

Gender-based violence occupies a critical place on the global-health agenda, as it is rooted in the gender inequality that remains pervasive throughout family units, social and cultural norms, and legal frameworks. Health-care providers can serve as advocates for women who have experienced GBV by promoting education outreach about violence and healthy relationships, providing universal screening for violence in a confidential and compassionate environment, assessing and treating acute and chronic injuries resulting from GBV, participating in policy and advocacy work through nongovernmental organizations and professional societies domestically and abroad, and identifying and supporting local champions of gender equality in the community.

USEFUL RESOURCES

The list below is not meant to be comprehensive. Rather, it is an attempt to identify some potential organizations and websites that contain further information about addressing gender inequality and gender-based violence.

National (United States)

Futures without Violence: www.futureswithoutviolence.org.
National Coalition against Domestic Violence: www.ncadv.org
National Network to End Domestic Violence: www.nnedv.org
National Resource Center on Domestic Violence: www.nrcdv.org

National Sexual Violence Resource Center: http://www.nsvrc.org

Office on Violence against Women (United States Department of Justice): http://www.ovw.usdoj.gov
Prevent Connect: http://www.preventconnect.org

International

Futures without Violence: http://www.futureswithoutviolence.org/
GBV Prevention Network: http://preventgbvafrica.org/
Gender-Based Violence Area of Responsibility: http://gbvaor.net/
Humanitarian Practice Network: http://www.odihpn.org/hpn-resources/network-papers/preventing-and-responding-to-gender-based-violence-in-humanitarian-crises
InterAction: http://www.interaction.org/work/gender-equality
Inter-Agency Field Manual on Reproductive Health in Humanitarian Settings: http://www.who.int/reproductivehealth/publications/emergencies/field_manual/en/
Inter-Agency Standing Committee, *Guidelines for Gender-Based Violence Interventions in Emergency Settings*: http://www.who.int/hac/network/interagency/news/ias_gender_based_violence/en/
International Women's Development Agency: https://www.iwda.org.au/
Minimum Initial Service Package (MISP) for Reproductive Health in Crisis Situations: www.who.int/disasters/repo/7345.doc
Sexual Violence Research Initiative: http://www.svri.org
UNiTE: http://endviolence.un.org/who_undp.shtml.
United Nations Population Fund: http://www.unfpa.org/gender/violence.htm.
World Health Organization and the United Nations High Commissioner for Refugees, *Clinical Management of Rape Survivors* (2004): http://www.unfpa.org/publications/clinical-management-rape-survivors
World Health Organization, Ethical and Safety Recommendations for Researching, Documenting, and Monitoring Sexual Violence in Emergencies (2007): http://www.who.int/gender/documents/OMS_Ethics&Safety10Aug07.pdf
World Health Organization, "Gender, Equity, and Human Rights": http://www.who.int/gender/violence/gbv/en/

REFERENCES

Abrahams, N., K. Devries, C. Watts, C. Pallitto, M. Petzold, S. Shamu, and C. Garcia-Moreno. 2014. Worldwide prevalence of non-partner sexual violence: A systematic review. *Lancet* 383:1648–1654. doi:10.1016/s0140-6736(13)62243-6.

American College of Obstetricians and Gynecologists. 2012. Intimate partner violence. Committee Opinion 518. *Obstetrics and Gynecology* 119 (2 pt. 1): 412–417.

Amowitz, L. L., C. Reis, K. H. Lyons, B. Vann, B. Mansaray, A. M. Akinsulure-Smith, L. Taylor, and V. Iacopino. 2002. Prevalence of war-related sexual violence and other human rights abuses among internally displaced persons in Sierra Leone. *JAMA* 287:513–521.

Chamberlain, L., and R. Levenson. 2012. "Addressing Intimate Partner Violence, Reproductive and Sexual Coercion: A Guide for Obstetric, Gynecologic, and Reproductive Health Care Settings." Futures without Violence. San Francisco, CA: Futures Without Violence and American College of Obstetricians and Gynecologists. Accessed June 5, 2016. https://www.acog.org/-/media /Departments/Violence-Against-Women/Reproguidelines.pdf.

Crowell, N. A., and A. W. Burgess, eds. 1996. *Understanding Violence against Women.* Washington, D.C.: National Academy Press.

Deering, K. N., A. Amin, J. Shoveller, A. Nesbitt, C. Garcia-Moreno, P. Duff, E. Argento, and K. Shannon. 2014. A systematic review of the correlates of violence against sex workers. *Am J Public Health* 104 (5): e42–54. doi:10.2105/ ajph.2014.301909.

Devries, K. M., J. Y. Mak, C. Garcia-Moreno, M. Petzold, J. C. Child, G. Falder, S. Lim, et al. 2013. Global health: The global prevalence of intimate partner violence against women. *Science* 340:1527–1528. doi:10.1126/science.1240937.

European Institute for Gender Equality. n.d. *What Is Gender-Based Violence?* European Institute for Gender Equality. Accessed May 26, 2016. http://eige.europa.eu /content/what-is-gender-based-violence.

Heise, L., M. Ellsberg, M., and M. Gottemoeller. 1999. *Ending Violence against Women.* Vol. Population Information Program, Center for Communications Programs. Baltimore: Johns Hopkins University School of Public Health.

Henry J. Kaiser Family Foundation. 2012. *The U.S. Global Health Initiative.* Accessed June 5, 2016. http://kff.org/global-health-policy/fact-sheet/the-u-s-global -health-initiative/.

Inter-Agency Standing Committee. 2015. "Guidelines on Gender-Based Violence Interventions in Humanitarian Settings." Accessed June 5, 2016. http:// gbvguidelines.org/wp-content/uploads/2015/09/2015-IASC-Gender-based -Violence-Guidelines_lo-res.pdf.

Inter-Agency Working Group on Reproductive Health in Crises. 2012. "Inter-agency Field Manual on Reproductive Health in Humanitarian Settings: 2010." Accessed June 5, 2016. http://www.who.int/reproductivehealth/publications /emergencies/field_manual_rh_humanitarian_settings.pdf?ua=1.

Jewkes, R., E. Fulu, T. Roselli, and C. Garcia-Moreno. 2013. Prevalence of and factors associated with non-partner rape perpetration: Findings from the UN

Multi-country Cross-sectional Study on Men and Violence in Asia and the Pacific." *Lancet Global Health* 1 (4): e208–e218.

Johnson, K., J. Scott, B. Rughita, M. Kisielewski, J. Asher, R. Ong, and L. Lawry. 2010. Association of sexual violence and human rights violations with physical and mental health in territories of the Eastern Democratic Republic of the Congo." *JAMA* 304:553–562. doi:10.1001/jama.2010.1086.

Kelly, J., J. Kabanga, W. Cragin, L. Alcayna-Stevens, S. Haider, and M. J. Vanrooyen. 2011. "If your husband doesn't humiliate you, other people won't": Gendered attitudes towards sexual violence in eastern Democratic Republic of Congo. *Global Public Health* 7 (3): 285–298. doi:10.1080/17441692.2011.585344.

Kohli, A., N. A. Perrin, R. M. Mpanano, L. C. Mullany, C. M. Murhula, A. K. Binkurhorhwa, A. B. Mirindi, et al. 2014. Risk for family rejection and associated mental health outcomes among conflict-affected adult women living in rural Eastern Democratic Republic of the Congo. *Health Care Women Int* 35 (7–9): 789–807. doi:10.1080/07399332.2014.903953. Epub 2014 May 16.

Krug, E. G., L. L. Dahlberg, J. A. Mercy, A. B. Zwi, and R. Lozano, eds. 2002. *World Report on Violence and Health*. Geneva: World Health Organization.

McFarlane, J., L. Symes, B. K. Binder, J. Maddoux, and R. Paulson. 2014. Maternal-child dyads of functioning: The intergenerational impact of violence against women on children. *Matern Child Health J*. 18 (9): 2236–2243. doi:10.1007/s10995-014-1473-4.

National Center for Injury Prevention and Control. 2003. *Costs of Intimate Partner Violence against Women in the United States*. Atlanta: Centers for Disease Control and Prevention.

OECD (Organisation for Economic Co-Operation and Development) Development Assistance Committee. 1998. *Guidelines for Gender Equality and Women's Empowerment in Development Co-Operation, Development Co-operation Guidelines Series*. Paris: OECD. Accessed June 5, 2016. http://www.oecd.org/dac/gender-development/28313843.pdf.

Overstreet, N. M., and D. M. Quinn. 2013. The intimate partner violence stigmatization model and barriers to help-seeking. *Basic Appl Soc Psych* 35 (1): 109–122. doi:10.1080/01973533.2012.746599.

Palermo, T., J. Bleck, and A. Peterman. 2014. Tip of the iceberg: Reporting and gender-based violence in developing countries. *Am J Epidemiol* 179 (5): 602–612. doi:10.1093/aje/kwt295.

Stark, L., and A. Ager. 2011. A systematic review of prevalence studies of gender-based violence in complex emergencies. *Trauma Violence Abuse* 12 (3): 127–134. doi:10.1177/1524838011404252.

Stockl, H., K. Devries, A. Rotstein, N. Abrahams, J. Campbell, C. Watts, and C. G. Moreno. 2013. The global prevalence of intimate partner homicide: A systematic review. *Lancet* 382:859–865. doi:10.1016/s0140-6736(13)61030-2.

United Nations. 1993. *Declaration on the Elimination of Violence against Women*. A/RES 48/104. 85th plenary meeting, United Nations General Assembly. Geneva: United Nations.

———. 1995. *Beijing Declaration and Platform for Action*. Fourth World Conference on Women, United Nations Entity for Gender Equality and the Empowerment of Women. Geneva: United Nations. Accessed May 26, 2016. http://www.un.org /womenwatch/daw/beijing/platform/violence.htm.

———. 2008. *Security Council Resolution 1820*. Geneva: United Nations.

———. 2013. *The Millennium Development Goals Report 2013*. Geneva: United Nations.

———. 2016. *Transforming Our World: The 2030 Agenda for Sustainable Development*. Accessed May 27, 2016. https://sustainabledevelopment.un.org/post2015 /transformingourworld.

United Nations Population Fund. 2005. "Frequently Asked Questions about Gender Equality." Accessed May 26, 2016. http://www.unfpa.org/resources/frequently -asked-questions-about-gender-equality.

———. 2012. "By Choice, Not by Chance: Family Planning, Human Rights and Development." "State of World Population 2012." Accessed May 26, 2016. http://www.unfpa.org/publications/state-world-population-2012.

United States Agency for International Development (USAID). 2012. "United States Strategy to Prevent and Respond to Gender-Based Violence Globally." Washington, D.C.: USAID.

United States Department of State. 2012. *State Department Fact Sheet on Gender-Based Violence in Haiti*. Accessed May 26, 2016. http://iipdigital.usembassy.gov/st /english/texttrans/2012/11/20121126139127.html#axzz33gNN5yPA.

UN Women. n.d. "Facts and Figures: Ending Violence against Women: A pandemic in diverse forms." Last update February 2016. http:// http://www.unwomen. org/en/what-we-do/ending-violence-against-women/facts-and-figures.

WHO (World Health Organization). 2001. *Guidelines for the Management of Sexually Transmitted Infections*. Geneva: World Health Organization.

———. 2003. *Guidelines for Medico-Legal Care for Victims of Sexual Violence*. Geneva: World Health Organization.

———. 2007. *Ethical and Safety Recommendations for Researching, Documenting and Monitoring Sexual Violence in Emergencies*. Geneva: World Health Organization.

Women's Refugee Commission. 2011. *Minimum Initial Service Package for Reproductive Health in Crisis Situations: A Distance Learning Module*. New York: Inter-Agency Working Group on Reproductive Health in Crises. Women's Refugee Commission. Accessed May 26, 2016. https://www.womensrefugeecommission.org/srh /emergency-response/misp

World Health Organization and United Nations High Commissioner for Refugees. 2004. *Clinical Management of Rape Survivors: Developing Protocols for Use with Refugees and Internally Displaced Persons*. Geneva: World Health Organization and United Nations High Commissioner for Refugees.

11

Female Genital Cutting

Nawal M. Nour

More than 200 million women across the world have undergone female genital cutting (FGC). This practice persists in parts of Africa and Asia across religious groups, ethnicities, and cultures and for various reasons: to mark a rite of passage, preserve chastity, and ensure marriageability; to follow perceived religious traditions, to improve hygiene and fertility, and to improve men's sexual pleasure. While immediate complications are quite serious and include hemorrhage, infection, sepsis, and death, longer-term repercussions also encompass pain, scarring, urinary tract problems, and poor obstetric and neonatal outcomes. There are national and international efforts to eliminate this practice, including a December 2012 resolution by the United Nations General Assembly. To provide culturally and linguistically competent care to populations of women with who have experienced FGC, we must educate ourselves regarding its history, cultural factors, medical complications, and methods for surgical reconstruction.

If you will be traveling to a country where FGC is an established practice, educate yourself about the local customs and procedures used. This information will help you prepare in the event that you see a large number of patients who have been cut. Do your homework first, including familiarizing yourself with local or international organizations who work in the field of FGC. It is important to realize that each organization has its own approach and messaging; therefore you will be well served to "go with the local flow." In addition, take time to get to know the law of the country, whether there are systems in place for reporting FGC (including the medicalization of the procedure), the ongoing progress of such reporting, and whether any cases have been tried. However, your immediate focus should be on recognizing the types of FGC and providing appropriate care for both immediate and short- and long-term complications.

DEFINITIONS AND NOMENCLATURE

Nearly twenty years ago, the World Health Organization defined female genital cutting as "all procedures involving partial or total removal of the external female genitalia or other injury to the female genital organs whether for cultural or other non-therapeutic reasons." This encompasses touching, nicking, pricking, or burning the genitals (WHO 1997, 7).

Not only does this practice take several forms, but simply referring to the practice has also been complicated. Originally, *female circumcision* was the common term. But as the practice received more international attention, "circumcision" was felt to understate what was being done. If the procedure were exactly analogous to the removal of a boy's foreskin, only the girl's prepuce would be involved. The word *mutilation* was adopted to reflect the degree of damage done by cutting off much more of the female genitalia. However, "mutilation" was criticized as reflecting a Western cultural judgment of the practice. Though most women with experience of FGC would not describe themselves as mutilated and would reject that term (along with the discrimination likely to accompany it), some African and international organizations have settled on *female genital mutilation* for political and economic reasons. Another alternative, *female genital surgery*, is generally felt to be too clinical and also incorrectly implies medical justification for a practice that has been consistently rejected by medical professionals around the world. The more neutral *female genital cutting* allows for clinicians to ask their patients when they were "cut" rather than "mutilated"; it is the term that is used throughout this chapter.

EPIDEMIOLOGY

The United Nations Children's Emergency Fund (UNICEF) estimated in 2015 that female cutting has been performed on over 200 million women and girls in the 30 countries in Africa, the Middle East, and Asia (UNICEF 2016). Encouragingly, FGC is becoming less frequent; this is reflected in the UNICEF report's finding of a prevalence of 54% in women aged forty-five to forty-nine years but a dramatically lower 36% among girls aged fifteen to nineteen years (Cappa et al. 2013).

CLASSIFICATION

Female genital cutting has been classified by the World Health Organization into four types. Type I (sunna) is removal of the prepuce and clitoridectomy (partial or total). Type II encompasses clitoridectomy and excision (partial or total) of the labia minora. In type III (also known as pharaonic cutting or infibulation), part or all of the external genitalia are removed (with or without clitoridectomy), labia minora and labia majora are excised, and infibulation is performed. This joins the raw edges of remnant tissue in the midline and leaves a small opening for urine and menses. Type IV, the mildest form, covers any other alteration of the genitalia by burning, pricking, stretching, scraping, or piercing (WHO 2016).

Table 11.1 gives descriptions of four types of female genital cutting. The specific types tend to be practiced consistently throughout a region. For example, type I is predominant in Ethiopia and Eritrea, while type II is most common in Sierra Leone, Gambia, and Guinea. Women in Somalia, northern Sudan, Djibouti, and southern Egypt generally undergo infibulation (type III), the most extensive practice. Figure 11.1 illustrates the three types of cutting.

Table 11.1 WHO classifications of female genital cutting

Type	Other names	Description
I	Clitoridectomy, sunna	Partial or total removal of the clitoris and, in very rare cases, only the prepuce.
II	Excision	Partial or total removal of the clitoris and the labia minora, with or without excision of the labia majora
III	Infibulation, pharaonic	Narrowing of the vaginal opening through the creation of a covering seal. The seal is formed by cutting and repositioning the inner, or outer, labia, with or without removal of the clitoris.
IV		All other harmful procedures to the female genitalia for non-medical purposes, for example, pricking, piercing, incising, scraping and cauterizing the genital area.

Source: Reprinted with minor modifications from WHO (2016), © World Health Organization 2016.

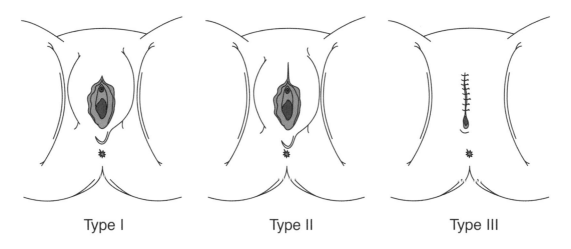

FIGURE 11.1. WHO classification of female genital cutting, by type.

HISTORICAL BACKGROUND

Contrary to some popular misconceptions, female genital cutting appears to predate Islam (WHO 2016). However, though it is unrelated to Islam and not performed by the majority of believers, some Muslims have embraced the practice. Neither the Qur'an nor the Hadith (the Muslim holy book and the collected sayings of the Prophet Mohammed, respectively) proposes FGC. In fact, the tradition survives regionally among Christians, Muslims, Jews, and others; it also crosses all socioeconomic barriers and transcends urbanization. In fact, though we know little of the origins of this practice, it may have actually begun in ancient Egypt, ancient Greece, pre-Islamic Arabia, and ancient Ethiopia.

GLOBAL IMPACT

The secrecy surrounding FGC makes prevalence difficult to estimate; for example, the practice occurs underground in the many African countries that have made the procedure illegal. The countries in which over 85% of the women are believed to be cut include Djibouti, Egypt, Eritrea, Guinea, Mali, Sierra Leone, Somalia, and Sudan. However, in Cameroon, Ghana, Niger, Togo, and Uganda, fewer than 5% have undergone the practice. Female genital cutting is also practiced in parts of the Middle East (Iraq, United

Arab Emirates, and Yemen), Asia (Malaysia, Indonesia, Pakistan), and a small region in India. It has been encouraging to see a sharp decline in female genital cutting in a number of countries including Kenya, Tanzania, Egypt, Iraq, and Nigeria (ACOG 2008).

THE PRACTICE OF FEMALE GENITAL CUTTING

Girls most often undergo FGC between the ages of six and twelve, but girls in some areas can be cut at birth, menarche, or before marriage. Female genital cutting is sometimes performed in a celebratory atmosphere accompanied by food, music, and gifts, as girls are gathered to celebrate their coming of age. Other girls are cut at home, very privately.

Most of the women who carry out these procedures are midwives, traditional birth attendants, or "circumcisers" with no medical training. They rarely use anesthesia, antibiotics, or sterile techniques, and their instruments may be razors, scissors, knives, clippers, or hot objects. Making matters worse, the tools can be dull, rusty, or old and are not sterilized between uses, even when several girls are being cut together. After the procedure, sutures, thread, or thorns may be used to close wounds, with the aid of various concoctions incorporating oils, dough, sugar, eggs, honey, or tree sap. The amount of tissue removed determines postoperative care; some girls who have experienced type I can be mobile the following day. However, girls who undergo type III frequently have their legs tied around their thighs, knees, and ankles and are confined to bed for approximately a week.

In the urban clinical setting, some nurses and physicians now perform genital cutting using anesthesia and antiseptics. This "medicalization" of the practice has sparked a fierce international debate on the ethics of legitimizing this procedure. In 1994, the International Federation of Gynecology and Obstetrics (FIGO) General Assembly resolved that obstetricians and gynecologists "oppose any attempt to medicalize the procedure or to allow its performance under any circumstances, in health establishments or by health professionals" (International Federation of Gynecology and Obstetrics 1994, 2). The FIGO assembly specified that health professionals must avoid any practice that adversely affects a woman's sexuality while legitimizing FGC and fostering its perpetuation. The World Health Organization has added its own concerns regarding medicalization, "strongly urg[ing] health professionals not to perform such procedures" (WHO 2014, 3).

THE REASONS BEHIND THE TRADITION

The persistence of female genital cutting depends on a variety of psycho-sexual, sociocultural, and religious rationales. Even women with some direct involvement in the practice have conflicting attitudes. For example, while a mother may hate seeing her daughter undergo this painful procedure, she may firmly believe that it is necessary to ensure the girl's future.

One of the strongest driving forces is parental concern over their daughter's marriageability. In many of the communities in which FGC survives, a woman's main goal (in fact, her career) is to marry and have children. Therefore, parents show their love for a daughter by attempting to present her as both attractive and virginal. Some inside the culture would say that opting against cutting would condemn a girl to terrible isolation and poverty. Essentially, loving parents make sure their daughters are cut.

Another part of protecting a girl's marriageability is ensuring her chastity and virginity. Some of these societies believe that because women are such highly sexual beings, cutting is one way to preserve their virginity. Girls in some regions eagerly await womanhood, even if the rite of passage from childhood is a painful one. Since the girls are offered clothes, food, and presents after the procedure, delightful anticipation more than balances any trepidation they might feel.

A woman who has undergone FGC is considered not only clean and pure but also more beautiful. Some women who have been infibulated describe their scar as beautiful because it differs dramatically from the genitals of uncut women, with their folds of labia, hair, and association with possible unpleasant odor. One of the more common justifications for FGC is that without it, women are dirty and smelly; uncut girls can be subject to being called filthy, prostitutes, and other derogatory terms.

Another source of justification for genital cutting is folklore regarding the dangers posed by the clitoris. There is a belief that the clitoris is actually toxic, capable of killing a baby who comes in contact with it. Another theory is that fertility—such a critical issue in these women's lives—will be improved by removing the clitoris. One other persistent belief is that if allowed to remain, the clitoris will start to resemble a penis or even grow until it touches the ground. Of course though neither contention has any factual basis, both are terrible and frightening for a girl to contemplate, given the emphasis in these communities on genital beauty.

It is worth restating that FGC is performed among communities of Christians, Muslims, Jews, and other religions as well. Some Muslims mistakenly believe that having their daughters cut is a virtuous act; that FGC is "sunna" (a good deed sanctioned by the Phophet Muhammad). Confusingly, some imams agree with this idea; others strongly discourage the practice.

Another strong influence in perpetuating FGC is the contention that it improves a man's sexual experience, reflecting the cross-cultural insistence on "the tighter the better." It is instructive to keep in mind that this practice is not without its Western adherents. Well into the twentieth century, Western obstetricians sought to tighten the introitus after an episiotomy using the "father stitch." After multiple vaginal births, some women are now seeking surgery to craft "designer vaginas." However, studies suggest that in addition to the many negative aspects of infibulation, some men actually prefer uninfibulated women (Cook, Dickens, and Fathalla 2002). Because it can take months of painful attempts at intercourse for a man to successfully penetrate an infibulated woman, the procedure actually decreases sexual pleasure.

IMMEDIATE HEALTH COMPLICATIONS

Not surprisingly, the immediate complications of type I female genital cutting are less severe than those of type III. If the dorsal artery of the clitoris or the labial branches of the pudendal artery are ligated, hemorrhage and anemia are common (4 to 19% of cases), exposing the girl to the risk of hypotension, hypovolemic shock, and mortality from uncontrolled bleeding (Herieka and Dhar 2003). Table 11.2 gives a comprehensive listing of immediate complications resulting from FGC.

Type III genital cutting also poses a greater risk of infection; the lack of sterile conditions and instruments, combined with restriction of the girl's movements for a week and the absence of daily wound cleansing, prevent drainage and foster bacterial growth. Studies have confirmed the incidence of fever (22%), acute cellulites (15%), abscesses, tetanus (2%), gangrene, and septic shock (2%) following type III cutting. Oliguria is also very common,

Table 11.2 Immediate complications

Bleeding	Infection	Urinary issues	Fractures
Hemorrhage	Cellulitis	Oliguria	Clavicle
Anemia	Abscess	Dehydration	Femur
Hypotension	Fever	Urethral injury	Humerus
Oliguria	Tetanus	Urethral edema	
Shock	Gangrene	Urinary retention	
Death	Septic shock		
	Poor healing		
	Pelvic inflammatory disease		

Source: Reprinted from Nour (2004), Table 1. © 2004 by Lippincott Williams & Wilkins.

given the deliberate nonhydration before the procedure and urinary retention that is a reflex when urine touches the infibulated scar. Reflecting the lack of anatomical knowledge on the part of the practitioner, the more serious risks include lacerations of the urethra, bladder, vagina, and rectum during the infibulation procedure. Since the terrified and struggling girl must often be held down, other injuries include fractured bones such as the clavicle, femur, or humerus (Herieka and Dhar 2003).

LONG-TERM COMPLICATIONS

Although long-term complications will not affect the majority of cut women, those who have had type III cutting are forced to live with at least one of the following complaints: urinary incontinence, scarring, infertility, and sexual dysfunction or pain (Herieka and Dhar 2003). Table 11.3 lists the forms these complaints take. A large study has indicated that FGC puts women at elevated risk of adverse obstetric outcomes, including cesarean deliveries, postpartum hemorrhage, episiotomy, prolonged hospital stay, the necessity for infant resuscitation, stillbirth, and even neonatal death. Such risks grow with the severity of the cutting (Banks et al. 2006). Infibulated women run the risk of menorrhagia and dysmenorrhea (65%), chronic vaginal infections (26%), chronic urinary-tract infections, neuromas, and sebaceous cysts and abscesses; less common problems include hematocolpos and hematometria as well as keloids (Herieka and Dhar 2003). When an infibulated woman's scar is opened, imbedded foreign bodies and urinary calculi have been found (Nour 2006).

Table 11.3   Long-term complications

Pain	Scarring	Urinary	Infertility and sexuality
Dysmenorrhea	Fibrosis	Urethral strictures	**Physical barriers**
Menorrhagia	Keloids	Meatal obstruction	Vaginal stenosis
Hematocolpos	Partial fusion	Meatitis	Infibulated scar
Hematometria	Complete fusion	Urinary crystals	**Psychological barriers**
Foreign bodies	Abscess	Chronic urinary-tract infection	Dyspareunia
Neuromas	Inclusion/ sebaceous cyst		Apareunia
Dyspareunia			
Vaginismus			
Chronic vaginal infections			

Source: Reprinted from Nour (2004), Table 2. © 2004 by Lippincott Williams & Wilkins.

Despite the belief that FGC makes a woman more fertile, both anatomic and psychological issues raise infertility rates among women with type III FGC to 25 to 30% (Nour 2004). Though the infibulated scar will eventually stretch, this can take months; a couple can easily become discouraged after many failed attempts at penetration. Women are likely to experience dyspareunia and vaginismus, while men may be led to doubt their potency. Both partners are clearly at risk for developing a detrimental psychological association between sex and pain. More and more studies find that men prefer noninfibulated women; some husbands state that the likelihood of hurting their wives in this way depresses them (Herieka and Dhar 2003).

In examining the effects of female genital cutting on women's sexuality, one study compared uncut women and women with type II and III FGC; intact women reported greater sexual desire and arousal, more orgasms, and better sexual satisfaction (Nour 2006). In an interview study of 432 infibulated women, 70% experienced dyspareunia and 78% did not find sexual intercourse enjoyable (Thabet and Thabet 2003).

However, one research study found that some women whose genitals had been cut experienced coital orgasms (Chalmers and Hashi 2000), and two other studies comparing cut and uncut women found no association between FGC and frequency of coitus (Lightfoot-Klein and Shaw 1991; Stewart, Morison, and White 2002). Women subjected to FGC reported that other areas such as their breasts came to play a greater role in sex. In addition, cut women also were more likely than uncut women to initiate coitus (Stewart, Morison, and White 2002). Though it may be that cut women find alternative routes to sexual arousal, satisfaction, and orgasm, the contradictory findings in these studies clearly indicate the need for more research.

In fact, the frequency of infertility appears to correlate with the anatomical extent of female genital cutting (Almroth et al. 2005). Introital and vaginal stenosis create a physical barrier; thus, couples may attempt coitus for months before completing penetration (Nour, Michels, and Bryant 2006). Failure and persistent dyspareunia can progress to apareunia (Almroth et al. 2005). Infertility may also be related to tubal damage from ascending infection related to FGC.

Because of the sensitive nature of the topic, the long-term effects of FGC on sexual satisfaction have been difficult to quantify (Andersson et al. 2012). One set of researchers found that women with type III cutting (infibulation) were significantly compromised in terms of libido, arousal, and orgasm compared with women who had the type I procedure (Thabet and Thabet 2003).

A WHO study group compared obstetrical outcomes of women with and without FGC (n=7,171 no cutting, 6,856 type 1, 7,771 type II, and 6,595 type III) (Banks et al. 2006). Types II and III (but not type I) of female genital cutting were associated with significantly higher risk of cesarean delivery, postpartum bleeding, and extended postpartum hospitalization. The infants of cut women were at significantly higher risk of needing resuscitation and of dying while still in the hospital compared with the babies of women who had not been cut (these risks were greater in women who had experiences type III cutting than those with type II). Compared with intact women, nulliparous and parous women subjected to any type of genital cutting were at higher risk of needing episiotomy and of sustaining perineal tears.

TREATMENT AND GUIDELINES FOR CARE

To improve or even avoid long-term complications of type III female genital cutting, defibulation is performed. The optimal time is before a woman's first sexual experience, both to avoid trauma and negative associations and to increase fertility. One study found that nearly half of infibulated women who were later defibulated still had an intact clitoris (Nour, Michels, and Bryant 2006).

Defibulation is surgical division of the infibulated scar to expose the urethra and vaginal introitus. In Somalia and parts of Djibouti, women are defibulated by midwives or traditional birth attendants immediately after marriage to facilitate coitus. However, in other areas such as northern Sudan and southern Egypt, defibulation is left to the husband, whose multiple attempts at penetration eventually dilate the neo-introitus.

Some infibulated women may request defibulation from health providers; they may be pregnant or planning pregnancy, or they may be suffering from apareunia, dyspareunia, dysmenorrhea, or difficulty urinating (ACOG 2008). In fact, health providers should suggest the procedure to women who are newly married, pregnant, or who present with common complications from infibulation, such as chronic vaginitis or urinary-tract infections, dysmenorrhea, or dyspareunia. Defibulation is a day procedure that any gynecologist can perform. To expose the urethra and vagina, an anterior incision is made into the infibulated scar and a subcuticular stitch is taken on each raw edge of the neo-labias. Every care should be taken to avoid injuring the clitoris, which may remain intact beneath the scar. Rates of complications are low with defibulation, and satisfaction rates are high (WHO 2016; Okonofu et al. 2002; Nour, Michels, and Bryant 2006).

Defibulation or reconstruction after genital cutting is generally associated with positive outcomes. One prospective study of 2,938 women with type II or III genital cutting who underwent mobilization of the clitoral stump reported complications in only 5% of patients. There was either no change or reduced sexual pain and increased clitoral pleasure among 97 percent of the women who underwent a one-year post-op evaluation (N=866) (Foldes, Cuzin, and Andro 2012). A much smaller series of thirty-two defibulated women reported that all of the women and their husbands were satisfied with the outcome (Nour, Michels, and Bryant 2006).

The optimum time to defibulate a woman is before first coitus (to prevent dyspareunia) or before pregnancy (to prevent obstetric complications). However, the optimal time for a specific woman may not be when it is medically most beneficial. Since one of the reasons for genital cutting is performed to protect a woman's virginity, some women may choose to delay defibulation until after they marry and have proved their virginal status.

Defibulation can safely be performed during pregnancy—though effective counseling may require several conversations at prenatal visits before a woman finally consents (ACOG 2008). Toward this goal, it is crucial to inform a patient that her infibulated scar poses serious risks to safe delivery, which include infection, bleeding, further scar formation, and even preterm labor. The benefits of—and changes that follow—defibulation should also be reviewed, for example, the increase in a woman's urine stream will make voiding feel different.

Both obstetrical and fetal risks are decreased by performing defibulation during the second trimester with regional anesthesia; general anesthesia is also an alternative. However, local anesthesia should be avoided, as it could precipitate flashbacks to the original cutting for some women.

The infibulated scar obstructs both the vaginal introitus and urethra; it can be excised through the following steps (AGOG 2008):

- Begin regional or general analgesics and long-acting local anesthetics.
- Assess the scar's length by inserting a Kelly clamp under it.
- Determine whether the clitoris remains intact beneath the scar by palpating anteriorly (Figure 11.2).
- Along the scar place two Allis clamps (Figure 11.3).
- Using Mayo scissors, make an anterior incision between the clamps, making sure to avoid injuring a buried clitoris (Figure 11.4).
- It is not necessary to incise too anteriorly toward the clitoral region, as the object is to gain an easy view of the introitus and urethra.
- On both sides place 4-0 subcuticular running sutures (Figure 11.5).

The patient should be instructed to take sitz baths twice each day; after each bath lidocaine cream (2%) can be applied. Postoperative pain control with opioid analgesics is usually necessary for only one or two days (Nour, Michels, and Bryant 2006). The literature also describes a method for carbon-dioxide laser surgery (Penna et al. 2002).

REINFIBULATION

Immediately after giving birth, some women will request reinfibulation. This should be discouraged as strongly as possible, as it simply recreates

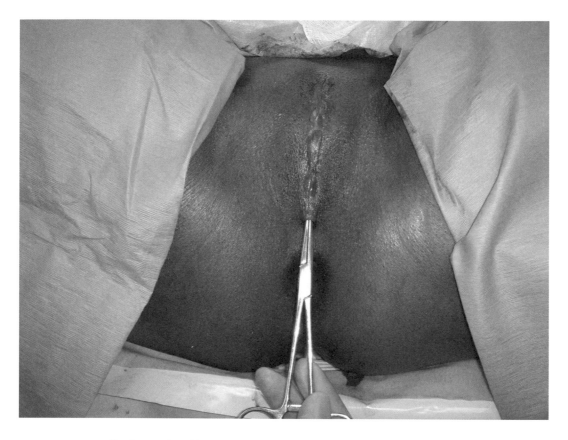

FIGURE 11.2. Kelly clamp placed beneath the infibulated scar.

all the risks of the long-term complications outlined above. However, because a woman infibulated as a girl may always feel uncomfortable in this new state, her request for reinfibulation should be respected. In March 1997 the United States passed a law making it a federal crime to carry out any medically unnecessary surgery on the genitalia of a girl under the age of eighteen. However, because reinfibulation was not included, it can be performed legally (using running absorbable sutures) if the young woman strongly insists (Nour 2004). Laws vary between countries. Familiarize yourself with these laws before you travel.

As stated elsewhere in this chapter, if a woman is pregnant and in labor, defibulation is beneficial for her own health and that of her baby. The ultimate goal is to avoid reinfibulation. However, if lengthy counseling does not persuade your patient, and she insists on reinfibulation, whether to proceed must depend on your own level of comfort.

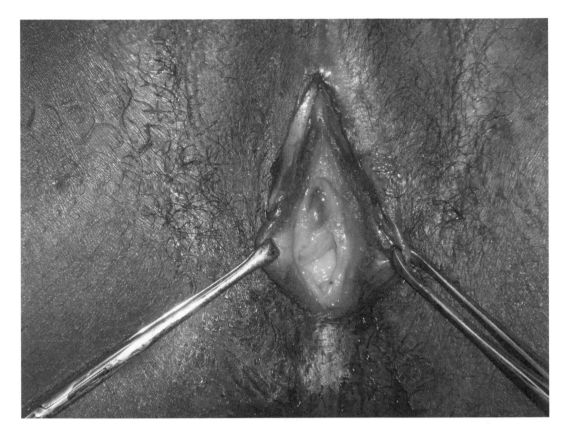

FIGURE 11.3. Incision performed anteriorly.

CONCLUSION

Clearly, female genital cutting is a complex issue—an emotionally charged health and human rights issue with serious consequences for a woman's psychological, sexual, and medical well-being. In addition, its cultural underpinnings evoke strong attitudes and entrenched beliefs from all involved. When we as health providers care for women who have been subjected to genital cutting, we must first try to understand why the practice survives, then offer the best possible care, informed by both linguistic and cultural competence. Naturally, such women feel judged and condemned when a health-care practitioner who examines them seems shocked or repulsed. Anticipating a caregiver's disapproval or simple unfamiliarity, cut women often feel forced into the awkward and inappropriate role of

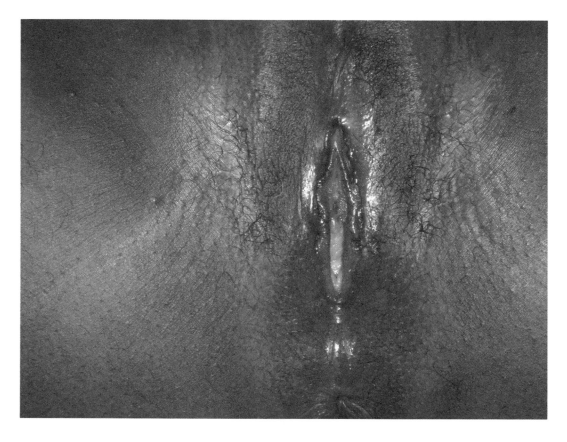

FIGURE 11.4. Subcuticular closures, buried clitoris is visible.

educating providers. Instead, if we educate ourselves about the traditions and cultural meaning behind FGC, we can relieve our patients of this educational burden and return our focus to their appropriate care. The diversity of cut women encompasses different languages, countries, cultures, religions, and socioeconomic backgrounds. Thus as health providers we are obliged to treat each woman individually, not only with respect and sensitivity but also with the best care we can offer.

Fortunately, both grassroots and international efforts are beginning to chip away at the persistence of FGC, causing the practice to be abandoned in both villages and cities. Not only individuals but entire communities are being engaged by an astonishing variety of entities—community organizations, media, policy makers, religious leaders, and international nongovernmental organizations—in an examination of the human rights violations, the religious misconceptions, the immediate health risks to

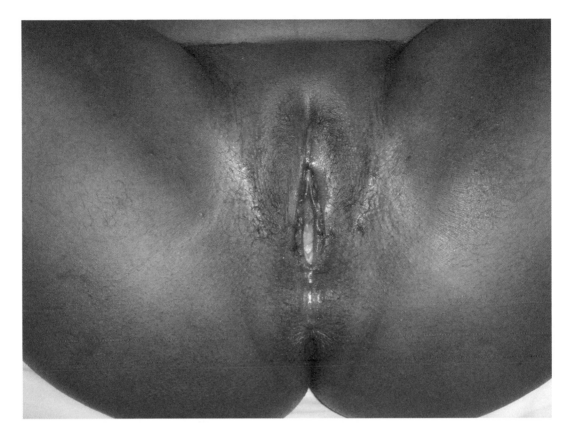

FIGURE 11.5. Labia minora reconstructed with intact clitoris.

the girl, and the long-term impact on girls' and women's lives of female genital cutting in all its forms. The consistent message of the harmful nature of FGC has brought discussion of the practice into the public sphere. These shifts in attitude and increased openness provide real hope that we will see an end to cutting in our lifetime.

REFERENCES

ACOG (American College of Obstetricians and Gynecologists). 2008. *Female Genital Cutting: Clinical Management of Circumcised Women*. 2nd ed. Washington, DC: ACOG.

Almroth, L., S. Elmusharaf, N. El Hadi, A. Obeid, M. A. El Sheikh, S. M. Elfadil, and S. Bergström. 2005. Primary infertility after genital mutilation in girlhood in Sudan: A case-control study. *Lancet* 366:385.

Andersson, S. H., J. Rymer, D. W. Joyce, C. Momoh, and C. M. Gayle. 2012. Sexual quality of life in women who have undergone female genital mutilation: A case-control study. *BJOG* 119:1606.

Banks, E., O. Meirik, T. Farley, O. Akande, H. Bathija, and M. Ali. 2006. Female genital mutilation and obstetric outcome: WHO collaborative prospective study in six African countries. *Lancet* 367:1835–1841.

Cappa, C., F. Moneti, T. Wardlaw, and S. Bissell. 2013. Elimination of female genital mutilation/cutting. *Lancet* 382:1080.

Chalmers, B., and K. O. Hashi. 2000. 432 Somali women's birth experiences in Canada after early female genital mutilation. *Birth* 27:227–234.

Cook, R. J., B. M. Dickens, and M. F. Fathalla. 2002. Female genital cutting (mutilation/circumcision): Ethical and legal dimensions. *Int J Gynaecol Obstet* 79:281–287.

Foldes, P., B. Cuzin, and A. Andro. 2012. Reconstructive surgery after female genital mutilation: A prospective cohort study. *Lancet* 380: 134–141.

Herieka, E., and J. Dhar. 2003. Female genital mutilation in the Sudan: Survey of the attitude of Khartoum University students toward this practice. *Sex Transm Infect* 79:220–223.

International Federation of Gynecology and Obstetrics (FIGO). 1994. Resolution on Female Genital Mutilation. FIGO General Assembly, Montreal, Canada. London: FIGO. Accessed June 5, 2016. http://www.figo.org/sites/default/files /uploads/OurWork/1994%20Resolution%20on%20Female%20Genital%20 Mutilation.pdf.

Lightfoot-Klein, H., and E. Shaw. 1991. Special needs of ritually circumcised women patients. *J Obstet Gynecol Neonatal Nurs* 20:102–107.

Nour, N. M. 2004. Female genital cutting: Clinical and cultural guidelines. *Obstet Gynecol Surv* 59:272–279.

———. 2006. Urinary calculus associated with female genital cutting. *Obstet Gynecol* 107:521–523.

Nour, N., K. Michels, and A. Bryant. 2006. Defibulation to treat female genital cutting: Effect on health and sexual function. *Obstet Gynecol* 108:55–60.

Okonofu, F., U. Larsen, F. Orosaye, R. C. Snow, and T. E. Slanger. 2002. The association between female genital cutting and correlates of sexual and gynaecololgical morbidity in Edo State Nigeria. *BJOG* 109:1089–1096.

Penna, C., M. G. Fallani, M. Fambrini, E. Zipoli, and M. Marchionni. 2002. Type III female genital mutilation: Clinical implications and treatment by carbon dioxide laser surgery. *Am J Obstet Gynecol* 187:1550.

Stewart, H., L. Morison, and R. White R. 2002. Determinants of coital frequency among married women in Central African Republic: The role of female genital cutting. *J Biosoc Sci.* 34:525–539.

Thabet, S. M., and A. S. Thabet. 2003. Defective sexuality and female circumcision: The cause and the possible management. *J Obstet Gynaecol Res* 29:12–19.

UNICEF (United Nations Children's Emergency Fund). 2013. *Female Genital Mutilation/Cutting: A Statistical Overview and Exploration of the Dynamics of Change.* New York: UNICEF. http://www.unicef.org/media/files/FGCM_Lo_res.pdf.

——. 2016. *Female Genital Mutilation/Cutting: A Global Concern.* New York: UNICEF. http://www.unicef.org/media/files/FGMC_2016_brochure_final_UNICEF_SPREAD.pdf.

WHO (World Health Organization). 1997. *Female Genital Mutilation.* A joint WHO/UNICEF/UNFPA statement. Geneva: World Health Organization.

——. 2014. *Female Genital Mutilation Fact Sheet.* Department of Reproductive Health and Research. Geneva: World Health Organization.

——. 2016. "Female Genital Mutilation." WHO Fact Sheet 241. http://www.who.int/mediacentre/factsheets/fs241/en/.

12

Ob-Gyn Surgery and Blood Supply in Resource-Poor Areas

Although surgery has not been a focus of global health efforts until relatively recently, it is now broadly accepted that access to quality surgical care is essential for the improvement of health-care and health outcomes. The World Health Organization (WHO 2009) estimates that conditions treatable by surgery account for 11% of the global burden of disease and furthermore that "inadequate surgical knowledge" contributes up to 20% of young adult deaths in resource-poor settings.

A 2015 article by the *Lancet* Commission on Global Surgery (Meara et al. 2015) sets out the following five "key messages":

(1) of the 7.3 billion people alive in 2015, 5 billion lack access to surgical and anesthesia care that is both safe and affordable;

(2) only 6% of surgical procedures take place in the poorest countries, which contain a third of the world's population, in addition to another 143 million surgical procedures required in these areas to avoid disability and save lives;

(3) fully one quarter of people who seek surgical care will face "financial catastrophe," a burden that falls most heavily on the world's poor;

(4) improving safe and affordable access to surgical and anesthetic services in low-income areas not only is lifesaving and economically feasible but actually promotes economic growth; and

(5) it will be impossible to achieve the United Nation's post-2015 Sustainable Development Goals if we do not make sure that

"surgical and anesthesia care is available, accessible, safe, timely, and affordable."

As health systems strengthen, so too, it is hoped, will good surgical care, as surgery requires a trained workforce (surgeons, nurses, anesthetists), an uninterrupted cold chain for supplies, and facilities with running water and functioning electricity. As an obstetrician-gynecologist providing surgical services in resource-poor settings, you will often be faced with systems missing some of these elements at least part of the time. You need to be acutely aware of your abilities, limitations, and how you might adapt to provide excellent care for all women who need it.

Women access surgical care for the same reasons as men (for example, trauma, appendicitis) as well as obstetric and gynecologic purposes, and they receive a large percentage of the surgical procedures performed worldwide. Obstetric and gynecologic surgery in low-resource settings may vary technically from the same procedures performed in higher-resource settings, but it must still follow the same general principles of good surgical care. Practitioners in low-resource settings must thoughtfully consider the same basic phases of a procedure—preoperative, operative, and postoperative—to optimize patient outcomes. The difference in practice between low-resource and high-resource settings is less likely the surgical technique itself than the decision making surrounding who is an appropriate candidate for surgery, what type of surgery is undertaken, and how to manage perioperative care. Most important, just as you consider the basic principles of medical ethics at home, that is, respect for autonomy, beneficence, nonmaleficence, and justice, you must do so abroad, understanding the challenge that maintaining each principle may bring.

This chapter begins by presenting the variables you will encounter as an ob-gyn working in the field in a resource-poor setting and discussing how they will most likely differ from both your training and your practice at home. It outlines preoperative care and decision making and intraoperative care with specific emphasis on blood loss and resuscitation, issues unique to postoperative care. It then ends with a short series of cases to illustrate basic guidelines for treatment and care as well as useful tricks in managing frequently encountered conditions.

COUNTRY-SPECIFIC LEGAL CONCERNS

Licensure

Before working abroad, it is critical to educate yourself in regard to legal considerations in the particular country, region, and area in which you will be working. Medical licensing is a good place to start. Most countries, via their respective ministries of health, require that physicians have an in-country license to practice medicine and operate. The licensure process may be facilitated by host-country sponsors (such as the hospital, clinic, or group you are working with) and may include only a temporary or limited license. In addition, you should research the need for malpractice insurance while abroad or find out whether your home malpractice insurance will cover you while away.

Law versus Local Practice

Understanding both the legal and cultural practices of a specific site is critical to providing good patient care. There are risks associated with ignoring one consideration for the other. For example, while it may be local practice to accept blood donations from a family member, it may actually be illegal; operating outside of legal boundaries can be dangerous to yourself as well as your patient. Or in the reverse situation, a woman may legally be able to consent to sterilization, but culturally her husband might also be asked to consent; ignoring the social and cultural norms of a site can have devastating consequences for the patient.

Specific attention should be paid to the legal status of abortion, as pregnancy termination is illegal in many countries. In other countries, it may be permitted only in certain circumstances (for example if the mother's life is in danger, or the pregnancy was the result of a rape) or legal only up to a specific gestational age (twelve weeks is the most common). Cultural and religious considerations need to be taken into account as well, as views about pregnancy termination can differ from patient to patient within the same legal framework. Central and South America, Africa, and the Middle East currently have the highest number of countries where abortion is illegal or otherwise restricted (Center for Reproductive Rights 2016).

Contraception is another area in which policies may vary from clinic to clinic—for example, a hospital may receive funding from religious organizations that do not support the use of intrauterine devices or more broadly do not allow for the prescription of birth control. Our role as providers often requires us to be educators and advocates for women's health, which will at times be at odds with the system in which we are working. However, to effect positive change, the legal, social, and cultural expectations surrounding health care, specifically as they relate to women's health, need to be considered before working in a given site.

Informed Consent

As mentioned earlier, working to uphold the four basic principles of medical ethics (autonomy, beneficence, nonmaleficence, and justice) can be challenging in resource-poor settings. To take just one example, autonomy means that patients have a right to accept or decline any given treatment. To ensure that patients are making the best possible decisions for themselves, we need to attend to a vital component of autonomy in health care: informed consent. However, what constitutes informed consent and how it is obtained may differ dramatically from community to community. For example, some cultures expect decision making to be a family process, while others center more on the individual. Furthermore, language barriers and high rates of illiteracy can make the process of obtaining consent more challenging. A committee opinion issue by the American Congress of Obstetrics and Gynecology (2010) suggests that having a "conversation [with the patient] will help make an informed and voluntary decision about accepting or declining therapy in a manner that reflects her values." It is important to understand how patient consent is defined and formalized. For example, the consent for a cesarean section may be a small slip of paper with a few lines indicating that "the doctor has determined you need a surgical procedure" and a place for the patient to leave an "X," which serves as her signature, acknowledging she understands and agrees to the procedure proposed. There are also instances when consent may not be routinely obtained, or conversely where you will need to obtain at least verbal consent, though you may not be used to doing so. For example, in many low-resource areas, women are not accustomed to undergoing pelvic exams or to the use of a speculum; this is particularly true where the Pap smear is not a routine procedure. The pelvic exam procedure should be carefully explained and consented to beforehand, and a chaperone provided if appropriate.

THE CLINICAL SETTING

Whether you find yourself working in a hospital or a freestanding clinic, it is important to prepare in terms of expectations regarding staff, infrastructure, instruments, and supplies. It is imperative to be open minded and willing to adapt to the situation; nothing will limit your effectiveness more than acting like a know-it-all foreigner. Be observant of your surroundings and ask your local colleagues what they routinely do in a given situation, as that is the best way to learn new tricks. At the same time, you are presumably working at a particular site for the specific knowledge and skills you bring, and being able to impart those in a respectful manner is essential to improving patient care. It is important to understand why things are done a specific way; sometimes it may be a lack of education, but often it is lack of resources or staff.

Nevertheless, while observing and respecting local practice is important, we should still strive to improve surgical outcomes, and implementing structural changes can have a large impact. A study of adverse events in eight low- and middle-income countries suggested that 75% of adverse events could be prevented with implementation of simple protocols such as the World Health Organization's Safe Surgery checklist (Wilson et al. 2012). Local providers are often so overburdened with clinical responsibilities that there may be little time for quality review and improvement initiatives. Additionally, knowing when to advocate for change—and what change to advocate for—is important and varies depending on the situation.

For example, episiotomy is still routine practice for delivery of nulliparous women in many places around the globe. While we no longer practice routine episiotomy in the United States, given its association with increased perineal pain and higher-order lacerations, it would be important to understand why the practice continues before implementing change. In many places, where midwives are delivering babies without continuous fetal monitoring, a small episiotomy may shorten the second stage and result in the birth of a more vigorous infant. Some providers also feel that repairing a small episiotomy, when there is poor lighting and only one suture available, is easier than a second-degree laceration, which may have ill-defined edges and be more challenging to bring back together in an anatomically correct manner. Applying our own practice—which is based on studies of postpartum pain and dyspareunia and does not take into account fetal outcomes—is not appropriate in this situation until we have a better understanding of the context in which the deliveries occur.

STAFF

Many Hats to Wear

Obstetric-gynecologic surgeons working in low-resource areas for the first time are likely to find themselves called upon to play other important roles—for which they may or may not be prepared: anesthesiologist, nurse, lab tech, social worker, counselor, or advocate. For that reason, it is crucial to understand how the care team functions in your area and to ensure that the host site has appropriate expectations of your needs and abilities. You want to make sure that you have not misrepresented your own training and abilities, as you may be called on to perform procedures you are not comfortable doing or cannot do without your usual equipment (such as a laparoscope or a suction machine).

Assistance

First, will you have any backup, or will you be the only ob-gyn—or even the only medical doctor—at the hospital or clinic? Of course, this will determine how many patients you can handle over a given period of time and the level of care you can offer.

Make sure you determine whether there are dedicated anesthesiologists, whether and how nursing is arranged, and who will care for the patient postoperatively, and confirm that there will be appropriate care of the patient when she returns home. In many resource-limited settings the patient is expected to provide her own meals (typically brought in by a family member), linens, and general toiletries. Thus making sure a patient will have appropriate care and nutrition postoperatively is necessary.

Before proceeding with any surgery, ensure that you have an assistant who can monitor the patient throughout the case. For example, you may be required to do dilation and curettage under local anesthesia with some intravenous or intramuscular analgesia, and you should have an assistant who can monitor the patient's respiratory status. In the case of a high-risk labor, another pair of hands can make all the difference if you are suddenly dealing with two crisis-level patients (mother and baby) instead of one.

Patients usually vastly outnumber medical staff in low-resource settings. Therefore it may be necessary to specifically clarify which nurse, medical assistant, or family member will help with the direct management of a particular patient. On busy surgical wards where the responsibility for bathing the patient and emptying the bladder catheter falls on the family, engaging the family can help reduce the burden of work. For example, asking a family member to mark the urometer, record the number of times the bag has been emptied, or describe the patient's bleeding can ultimately help with recording vital signs. For obstetric care, it can be valuable to have a family member ready to hold and warm a baby if you do not have an assistant.

INFRASTRUCTURE

Lighting

In case of wiring limitations or inconsistent power supply, lighting in the operating room may be problematic. Consider bringing with you energy-efficient headlamps such as those used by bikers and hikers—and some means to recharge them. Headlamps are also particularly useful for perineal repairs.

Lab Work

You may be faced with limited access to local tests and analysis; or it may take so long to send samples out and get results back that you will need to make diagnostic and treatment decisions without benefit of that information. Understanding how tests are performed and whether there are ways to modify them is useful—for example, urine hCG tests can also work with a drop of blood if urine is not available (Fromm et al. 2012); a red-top tube can serve in lieu of coagulation studies—if blood clots within ten minutes, coagulation levels can be presumed normal. Some tests may even be easier to perform there than at home—for example, malaria smears or rapid tests for HIV. A quick tour of the lab and a chat with the lab technician (if there is one) will be enlightening.

Instruments

As in any surgical situation, it is crucial to be familiar with the instruments you have available—and to find alternatives if instruments are out of commission or altogether missing. For example, manual vacuum aspirators are excellent alternatives to sharp curettage and can also avoid the need for an electronically powered suction machine. Be familiar with their parts, cleaning, and setup, especially as parts from one kit end up as parts of another (see case example below).

Supplies

Where resources are scarce, supplies are likely to be available inconsistently, perishable items may have expired, and many things you consider necessities may be unavailable altogether (see Figure 12.1). You will need to make sure all necessary supplies are in place before a particular procedure; don't make any assumptions. Basic surgical practices such as checklists, counting, and adopting procedures like the Mayo stand setup will help avoid surprises. Another example of preventive measures is making sure your sutures have not expired.

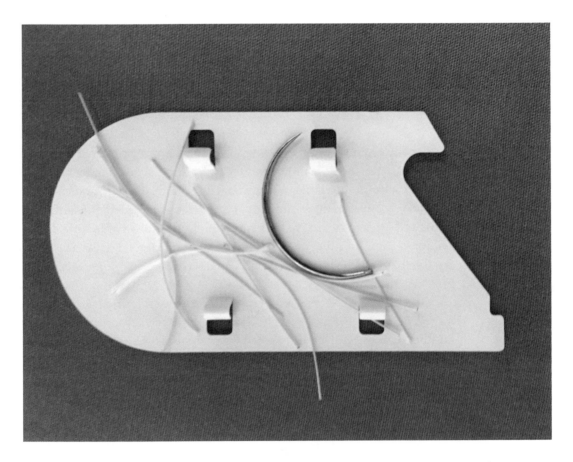

FIGURE 12.1. Contents of a newly opened pack of sutures, with disintegrating pieces inside.

Table 12.1 Suture types and characteristics

Suture	Common name	50% tensile strength, days
Natural		
Plain catgut		5
Chromic catgut		10–14
Cotton		300+
Linen		300+
Silk		300+
Synthetic		
Polyglycolic acid	Dexon, Surgicryl, Polysorb	21
Polyglactin 910	Vicryl	21
	Vicryl rapide	5
Polydioxenone	PDS (monofilament)	40–60
Polyglyconate	Maxon	40
Poliglecaprone 25	Monocryl (monofilament)	7–14
Polyamide	Nylon	300+
Polyester	Mersilene	300+
Polybutester	Novafil	300+
Polypropylene	Prolene	300+
Stainless steel	Staples	300+

Data sources: Syneture information sheet on Maxon and Maxon CV absorbable sutures (n.d.); Ethicon wound closure manual (n.d.).

For any given procedure you may need to pick from a limited selection of sutures; therefore it is important to understand suture characteristics: braided versus monofilament, length of time for absorption, and the type of needle it comes on (for example, cutting versus tapered). For example, it would be better to close skin with interrupted nonabsorbable suture (like nylon) on a small-caliber needle and remove the sutures in a few days after the skin has healed than to close with a larger-caliber or more reactive suture such as chromic.

General principles to keep in mind are that synthetic sutures are absorbed via hydrolysis and provoke less inflammatory response than natural-fiber sutures, which are absorbed via proteolysis. The larger caliber the suture, the more foreign material will be left in an incision, and braided sutures are more likely to be associated with infection than monofilaments. Table 12.1 lists commonly used sutures and their length of time to absorption. For needle selection, a tapered needle is appropriate for most soft tissue, while a conventional cutting needle will be easier to use on tougher tissue, such as the dermis.

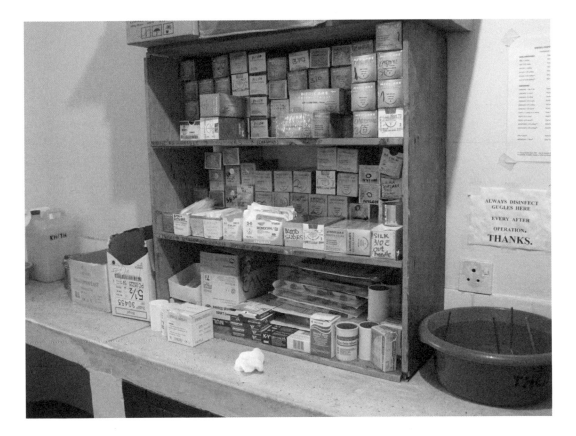

FIGURE 12.2. An actual suture supply room.

Personal Protection

Items such as goggles, masks, and even gloves may not be plentiful enough to throw out; it may be local practice to autoclave or otherwise sterilize and reuse them. Figure 12.2 shows an area where used "disposable" goggles are placed for washing and subsequent reuse. It is not uncommon to find gloves washed, repowdered, and drying in the sun as a solution to an item in high demand but short supply. You may also be responsible for protecting yourself against contaminated sharps and disposing of them safely. Empty cooking oil jars or other thick plastic containers that have screw-on tops can suffice; ensure they are properly labeled and not disposed of in areas where children or others might explore the garbage and harm themselves.

Drugs

Pharmaceuticals such as antibiotics and analgesics may be in short supply or available only intermittently. In addition, you may have limited options in terms of anesthesia; this obviously varies from site to site. Because of their scarcity and expense, narcotics are rarely used for outpatient pain management in low-resource settings. Familiarize yourself with what drugs are available locally and their common names (for example, outside of the United States acetaminophen is more commonly referred to as paracetamol; diclofenac may be more readily available than ibuprofen; Jadelle or Norplant-2 may be available in lieu of Nexplanon). While we rarely need to worry about cold chains and supply back home, disruptions in medication availability may influence your practice abroad. For example, the supply of birth control pills or Depo-Provera may fluctuate, altering your contraceptive counseling. Narcotics are rarely available outside of the hospital; postoperatively, patients are routinely sent home with a small supply of acetaminophen or ibuprofen for pain control.

Warming

Like drugs and lab tests, other basics of patient care cannot be taken for granted. For example, one fundamental is to keep patients warm and dry. Where dedicated body warmers are not available but there is electricity, a simple light may provide significant warmth. A plastic garbage bag under a patient can be used to clear blood or other fluids so a patient is not lying on a cold, wet surface. In the absence of clean blankets, a reflective Mylar wrap like that offered after marathons can be an effective means of warming a patient.

THE PATIENT

Your patient population will differ significantly from women you have cared for in resource-rich areas; thus it is critical to understand the patient's relationship to the health-care setting. Because patients in low-resource areas frequently live far from medical care (several hours by bus or on foot), they must take on cost to present to care (transport costs and hospital fees as well as lost wages or working hours). Women in these areas are likely to have delayed seeking care; therefore the presenting condition may have progressed significantly beyond what you are used to seeing. In addition, comorbidities such as poor baseline nutrition or HIV infection may alter standard recovery and healing.

Deciding on Surgery

The low-resource setting also differs from your training and current practice in terms of decision making regarding who goes to surgery in the first place. Women who would normally be medically managed in other settings may need surgery for more definitive management or a diagnostic procedure. Therefore it is important to think about follow-up requirements and potential complications. If it took this patient a day and a half to get to the hospital, would it be better to go ahead with a procedure that will avoid any need for her to return, rather than recommend expectant management? (Such a case is illustrated below.)

Costs to Patients

In many low-resource areas, all medical costs—including lab tests and even supplies, like the number of gloves used—are paid for directly by the patient and her family. For this reason, careful consideration should be given to limiting tests to the absolute minimum necessary.

Preconceptions

Finally, it is critical to remember that the patients you are caring for may have preconceptions, both positive and negative, about foreign doctors. On the one hand, there may be a lack of trust or a belief that procedures are performed for your own financial benefit or as an experiment. On the other hand, patients may believe you are capable of performing miracles; it is important to be honest and set realistic expectations.

BLOOD ISSUES AND BLOOD SUPPLY

Anemia

Per usual care, clinical assessment of a patient before surgery should include medical and surgical history for best preoperative management. Baseline anemia, from malnutrition or from infectious diseases such as malaria and HIV, should be accounted for when considering procedures with the potential for large blood loss as well as when caring for pregnant patients.

Physical exam should include assessment of the conjunctiva, oral mucosa, and nail beds for signs of pallor as well as a careful cardiac exam to listen for possible murmurs. Preoperative treatment of malaria, HIV, and vitamin deficiency is recommended if the time course allows for it.

Obstetric Hemorrhage

Postpartum hemorrhage normally occurs close to the time of delivery, and in resource-limited settings this may leave one provider managing two patients (the mother and the newborn) as well as an emergency. Therefore it is critical to have an assistant for delivery. The assistant is a critical pair of extra hands and should ideally be someone who can retrieve and administer medications. Knowing a priori what medications are available and how they are administered is also crucial. For example, an oxytocin dosage is likely ten units intramuscularly; methergine (methylergonovine), which is usually given in the United States as 0.2 mg intramuscularly, may be stocked as ergonovine, which is dosed for 0.25 milligrams and is commonly given as an intravenous injection (though intramuscularly is still the preferred route). Conversely, your site may have access to misoprostol and be accustomed to using it in small doses for induction of labor but not be used to giving it in larger doses (600 to 1,000 micrograms) or via other routes (rectal or buccal).

It is also important to remember that many women, especially those who live in malaria-endemic regions, have a baseline anemia, have not been well hydrated during labor, and will not tolerate a large-volume blood loss well. Therefore it is important to act quickly. If you do not have access to blood transfusion or surgical interventions, keep in mind the basic principles of trauma care while you plan to transport the patient. For example, keep the patient warm, elevate the feet above the heart, and apply a nonpneumatic antishock garment or otherwise wrap the patient to limit blood loss if feasible. These measures can improve patient outcome (Miller et al. 2013).

Assessing Blood Loss

It is often difficult to establish a clear idea of blood loss when it is being absorbed by sheets, cloths, or towels. In the absence of an under-buttocks drape designed to catch blood, a garbage bag may be placed under the patient and funneled into a small trash can or bucket; this will help give a clear idea of how much blood has actually been lost. In the case of large blood loss in the operating room, having someone keep track of the suction canister and check beneath the patient for concealed blood loss is also useful (see Chapter 2).

BLOOD SUPPLY AND TRANSFUSION

Before operating it is important to understand the site's capacity for blood transfusion. In particular, what blood products are available to you, how frequently they are restocked, and how well they are screened for infectious diseases or typed and cross-matched.

Per World Health Organization guidelines, a national blood-banking system should be regulated and maintained by each country's ministry of health. Minimum criteria for a functioning system require that blood be donated voluntarily (donors receive no monetary compensation) and be screened for ABO and Rh compatibility as well as for hepatitis B and C, HIV, syphilis, and malaria (in endemic countries). However, despite efforts to strengthen national blood banks, an adequate and safe blood supply is not always readily available, especially in resource-limited settings. Additionally, lack of adequate test kits or trained staff and disruptions in the cold chain can allow virally or bacterially contaminated blood into the blood-banking system, both of which pose infectious as well as transfusion-reaction risks (WHO 2009). Despite these challenges, blood transfusions remain a lifesaving procedure and are critical in many obstetric and gynecologic emergencies such as obstetric hemorrhage and ruptured ectopic pregnancies. In fact, in low-income countries, the majority of transfusions are given to women suffering from pregnancy-related complications, and the ability to give a transfusion is considered one of the eight necessary components of comprehensive emergency obstetric care.

While most countries do have specific laws and regulations regarding transfusion, products in government-run blood banks (which in a district hospital may consist of a single refrigerator) are often replaced only sporadically. Aside from the unreliable availability of blood, the other key difference you will encounter will be the use of whole blood as opposed to component therapy (that is, plasma, cryoprecipitate, platelets, or red cells).

In high-income countries, 91% of the blood supply is divided into components; because this is the case in only 31% of low-income countries, most transfusions therefore are of whole blood (WHO 2011). One advantage of transfusion of whole blood in massive hemorrhage is that it does not promote dilution coagulopathy, and though whole blood has a shorter shelf life, it also has more active clotting factors. Whole blood also has the advantage that it is not pooled from several donors (as component products are) and therefore carries less infectious and inflammatory risk. Disadvantages include the fact that patients are unnecessarily exposed to components they may not need (that is, platelets, plasma) as well as to white blood cells.

Ironically, while most hospitals in low-resource settings do not have large blood banks, data also suggest that a high percentage of transfusions given in resource-poor settings are not clinically indicated, or may have been replaced by a simpler, safer treatment (WHO 2008). In addition, while family members may offer to donate blood, this is often discouraged and may be illegal. Therefore it is critical to understand the site-specific laws and regulations surrounding blood product donation and storage, usually obtainable from the site's medical director. Alternatives to autologous blood transfusion (both preventative and therapeutic) should be well understood in these situations. Table 12.2 gives the components and characteristics of blood.

While a unit of whole blood has a Hct of 38 to 50%, platelets 150K to 400K, 100% of coagulation factors, and 1,000 milligrams of fibrinogen), the combination of one unit packed red cells plus one unit platelets plus one unit FFP plus one unit cryoprecipitate would have Hct 29%, platelets 80K, coagulation factors at 65% of initial concentration, and 1,000 mg fibrinogen (Armond and Hess 2003).

AUTOLOGOUS BLOOD TRANSFUSION

An alternative to donor (allogenic) blood transfusion is autotransfusion, and in specific cases in which blood is found within the patient's peritoneal cavity (such as in a ruptured ectopic pregnancy or a ruptured hemorrhagic cyst), this technique may be lifesaving.

Autotransfusions are relatively easy to perform. The blood is collected from the abdominal cavity with a scooping device; this may be something as simple as a sterile metal cup, a soup ladle, or a device specifically designed for the procedure such as the Tanguieta funnel (Priuli et al. 2009). Once the blood is removed, clot and debris are filtered (in Figure 12.3, pouring it through gauze into a sterile bottle), and then the blood is prepared for reinfusion, either by injecting it into bags prepared in advance with citrate-phosphate-dextrose-adenine (CPDA) anticoagulant solution or by putting heparin into sterile tubing and retransfusing the blood from the sterile bottles directly back to the patient. Of note, successful autotransfusion has been described in cases of ruptured ectopic pregnancy as well, despite prior beliefs that pregnancy tissue could create an anaphylactic reaction (Schantz-Dunn and Nour 2011).

ANTICIPATING LARGE-VOLUME BLOOD LOSS

Perioperative Hemodilution

When bleeding has not occurred but is anticipated, preoperative autologous blood donation or perioperative hemodilution may be used. For preoperative donation, the patient donates one to two units of blood for storage in a blood bank a few weeks before the planned procedure (of course, this assumes a functioning blood bank). It should be confirmed that the patient's baseline hematocrit and functional status will tolerate the donation. Another approach is perioperative hemodilution, in which the patient receives crystalloid hydration in exchange for an equal amount of autologous blood. This lowers the patient's hematocrit, so blood loss during the procedure has a lower total volume of red blood cells, allowing for the donated blood to be retransfused at the end of the procedure, thereby restoring the hematocrit.

Myomectomies

Several methods to limit blood loss during myomectomies have proved efficacious, including administration of vaginal misoprostol, injection of a solution containing vasopressin, and use of a pericervical tourniquet (Kongnyuy and Wiysonge 2014). If the medications are not available, many sterile items can be used as a tourniquet: a Penrose drain, a Foley catheter, a sterile glove, or even a suture—either tied or clamped in place around the uterus—to compress the uterine arteries.

Table 12.2 Blood products: Indications and characteristics

Blood component	Indication	What is it made of?	How long does it last?	What effect does it have?	Downside
Packed red blood cells	Increases oxygen-carrying capacity; typically indicated if hemoglobin is less than 6gm/dL.	Red blood cells, concentrated to hematocrit of 70 to 80%, in 200 to 300cc of volume if CPDA used; if other storage solution, Hct may be 55 to 65%.	Lasts forty-two days if stored just above freezing.	Raises hematocrit by 3%, hemoglobin by 1gm/dL.	Platelets and neutrophils ruined.
Platelets	Indicated if platelets less than 50,000/cc^3 or 50 to 100,000 in patients requiring surgery.	Pooled platelets from separate centrifuged units of whole blood (usually six donors) in 50 to 70 cc of plasma.	Five days with proper storage (including continuous agitation, temperature 1 to 6°C).	One "six-pack" will raise platelet count approximately 40,000.	Difficult to store, rarely available in resource-poor settings; pooled donors.
Fresh-frozen plasma	Correction of DIC (INR greater than 1.5).	Separating and freezing plasma collected from whole blood within six hours of donation.	Up to one year by freezing at –18°C. Once thawed, kept refrigerated and used within twenty four hours.	One unit FFP = coagulation factors in one unit whole blood.	ABO-compatible plasma should be used (no need to Rh type).

Cryoprecipitate	For use in coagulopathy.	Cold-insoluble precipitate from thawed FFP, refrozen. Contains most of the Factor VIII, fibrinogen, Factor XIII, VWF, fibronectin.	Twelve months at −25°C or below. Once thawed, use within six hours; half life of fibrinogen is three to five days.	One unit approximately = two units of whole-blood derived cryoprecipitate. One unit = 200 mg fibrinogen, often dispensed as one bag of five units, increases fibrinogen 1,000 mg.	ABO-compatible (Rh typing not necessary).
Whole blood	In developed countries used for pediatric, military, trauma, or massive blood loss. More routine in resource-poor settings.	Considered "fresh" if not older than forty-eight hours; typically 500 mL.	Stored at −2 to 6°C. Lasts for twenty-one days.	• Hct: 38 to 50% (depending on donor). • Plt: 150K to 400K • Coagulation factor concentration 100% • 1,000 mg Fibrinogen	Depending on indication, exposure to unnecessary components, WBCs.

Data sources: Silvergleid (2014); Arya et al. (2011).

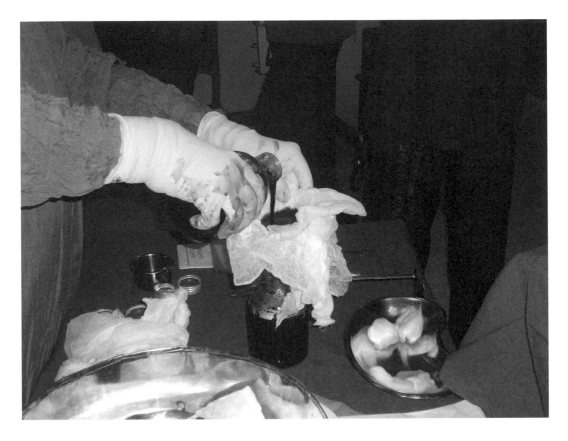

FIGURE 12.3. Peritoneal blood being prepared for autotransfusion.

Future Developments

Future developments in blood product replacement, it is hoped, will include a less expensive form of powdered fibrinogen concentrate, a heat-stable product that can be critical in cases of obstetric hemorrhage when hypofibrinogenemia contributes to coagulopathy. Other products that may come into use in resource-limited settings include tranexamic acid (TXA), an inexpensive antifibrinolytic agent shown to reduce blood loss and the need for transfusion. The WOMAN trial is a large multicenter randomized control trial evaluating the efficacy of TXA in postpartum hemorrhage that has enrolled over 20,000 women (London School of Hygiene and Tropical Medicine n.d.).

TREATMENT AND CARE GUIDELINES

In this section, case examples are used to highlight specific diagnostic skills and surgical techniques that are particularly useful in resource-limited settings. Note: All the specific cases have been taken from the author's personal experience, and patient identifiers have been removed. Photographs are used with prior consent of the patient.

Case: Pelvic Pain

This case is used to illustrate careful selection of diagnostic tools as well as consideration of management options as they relate to low-resource settings.

History and Physical Examination

A twenty-three-year-old nulliparous woman presents to an outpatient clinic with pelvic pain and vaginal spotting. She is unsure of her last menstrual period and reports no other medical problems or prior surgeries. Her physical exam is notable for a blood pressure of 110/65, pulse of 80. She appears mildly uncomfortable with moderate tenderness to abdominal palpation, no rebound or guarding.

Commentary. Further elucidation of her history and presentation may be useful, such as sexual history or use of contraception, but the interviewer should ensure that this is performed in a culturally competent as well as a confidential manner. Often this is not possible, and therefore care should be used even in determining how detailed a clinical history to take or how much of the physical exam to perform.

Work-Up

The patient had a positive urine human chorionic gonadotropin (hCG) test. A bedside ultrasound with an abdominal probe did not identify a gestational sac within the uterus. A small amount of free fluid was seen in the posterior cul-de-sac.

Commentary. Because pregnancy is first on the differential, an hCG test is necessary. Often this is available via urine assay instead of serum assay and therefore will detect levels around 30 to 80 IUs per liter, depending on the sensitivity of the test. For women who may be in the implantation phase of pregnancy, a low hCG may show up as a negative urine hCG. Ultrasound would also be extremely useful (see note above regarding ultrasound skills). In a higher-resource setting, this patient would likely have also had a blood count sent as well as a blood type and screen. Before sending either, we must first consider whether either of those results would change our management. If this patient were hemodynamically unstable and needed a blood transfusion, a hemoglobin level as well as the blood type and screen would be useful. Testing for Rhesus antigen is often unnecessary on its own, as Rho(D) immune globulin is rarely available.

Management

The patient was observed for four hours, during which time her abdominal pain was consistent, and she was no longer comfortably ambulating. The patient was designated "nothing by mouth" and prepared for an exploratory laparotomy. Preparation included gaining the patient's consent (discussed above) and informing the operating room staff to ensure availability of a room, equipment, and an anesthetist. After general anesthesia, the patient underwent a minilaparotomy (Pfannensteil), revealing a small amount of blood in the cul-de-sac and an ectopic pregnancy in process of tubal abortion on the right side. A right salpingectomy was performed (using clamps and 0-polyglactin ties). The patient tolerated the procedure well.

Commentary. Management options for this patient, who was presumed to have an ectopic pregnancy, included observation and expectant management, further diagnostic measures such as posterior cul-de-sac sampling, or an exploratory laparotomy. In this hospital methotrexate was not an option for medical management of ectopic pregnancy, and laparoscopic surgery was also unavailable. The patient had traveled very far to seek care, which along with the suspicion of ectopic pregnancy ruled out expectant management. A posterior cul-de-sac sampling, in which a long needle (such as a spinal needle) is inserted into the posterior cul-de-sac via the posterior vaginal fornix, can be used to confirm blood in the pelvis. However, here clinical suspicion negated further diagnostic measures. Had we found something other than an ectopic pregnancy (that is, early pregnancy or miscarriage) or a very small ectopic in which the side of the pregnancy could not be determined, an exploratory laparotomy would have led to unnecessary anesthesia risk, cost, and surgical morbidity.

Outcome

The patient tolerated the procedure well and was discharged home on postoperative day 2 with ten tablets of acetaminophen and ten tablets of ibuprofen for pain management. She was also counseled on contraceptive options and future fertility.

Commentary. An opportunity was missed to screen (or presumptively treat) for sexually transmitted infections, such as chlamydia, which may have been a risk factor for tubal disease and the ectopic pregnancy.

Case: Pelvic Mass

This case is used to illustrate operative technique and preparation, suture selection, and autotransfusion.

History and Physical

A twenty-one-year-old woman presents with a week-long history of worsening pelvic pain, which began in her left lower quadrant and has progressed to the entire abdomen. She has not been eating or drinking well. She has never been pregnant, and her last menstrual period was three weeks before admission. She is afebrile, hypotensive, with a blood pressure of 70/40 and a pulse of 120. Her exam is notable for a distended abdomen, with a palpable mass just above the umbilicus, diffuse tenderness to palpation, rebound, and voluntary guarding.

Commentary. Because this patient appears unstable, management to help stabilize her vital signs should not be delayed while considering which diagnostics are necessary.

Work-Up

While an intravenous line was placed and saline infused, the patient was positioned in mild Trendelenburg to improve her blood pressure. A bedside ultrasound shows a mass, possibly adnexal, and moderate complex free fluid. A blood sample was taken to check for pregnancy, hemoglobin level, and type and to screen. The hemoglobin level returned at 5.2, and the hCG was negative. The patient consented to go to the operating room for an exploratory laparotomy.

Commentary. The patient was hemodynamically unstable with complex free fluid in the pelvis. The differential included a hemorrhagic cyst/mass, a tubo-ovarian abscess, a ruptured ectopic pregnancy, or a gastrointestinal source. Of note, because this patient was not able to urinate on admission, a few drops of her whole blood were added to the urine hCG test to achieve a result. Several studies have supported using a few drops of whole blood in lieu of urine if urine is not immediately available to a rapid hCG interpretation (Fromm et al. 2011).

Though additional imaging was not available, the patient's vital signs warrant urgent surgical intervention. However, it is still imperative to ensure adequate anesthesia support and ideally back-up surgical support in the event of unexpected findings.

Management

The patient underwent general anesthesia and a vertical exploratory laparotomy, which revealed a ruptured, hemorrhagic, torsed left ovary, measuring approximately fifteen by fifteen centimeters (Figure 12.4). There was a large amount of hemoperitoneum. Given the conclusion that the patient's initial vital signs were secondary to hemorrhage and the low starting hemoglobin, the blood was retained for an autotransfusion, and the patient was given back a liter of her own blood.

Commentary. Of note, autotransfusion has been successfully described in cases of ruptured ectopic pregnancy despite prior beliefs that pregnancy tissue could create an anaphylactic reaction (Schantz-Dunn and Nour 2011).

The patient underwent a left salpingoophorectomy, as it seemed to be the most expeditious way to stop further blood loss. On inspection of the ovary, there were some areas with nodular components, possibly consistent with a dermoid. The hypothesis was that the dermoid had led to the ovarian torsion, which ultimately caused rupture and hemorrhage. The decision was made to send the specimen to another city for pathology, given that it might assist with further patient counseling; however, four weeks later the results were still pending.

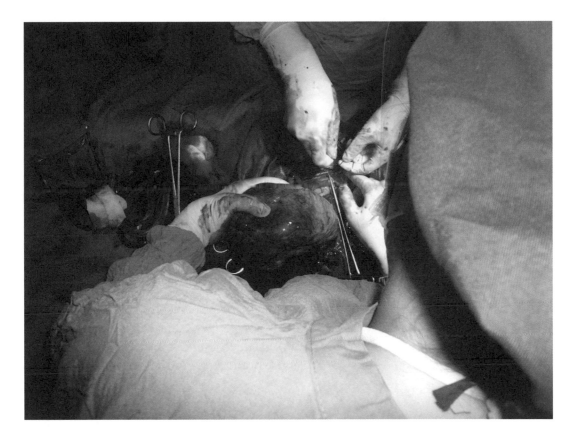

FIGURE 12.4. Patient's ovary.

Outcome

The patient did well postoperatively. Her hemoglobin level the following day was 2.9, and she received one additional unit of whole blood from the blood bank. She recovered in the hospital for seven days. On discharge her hemoglobin had improved to 3.6, and she was discharged home in stable condition.

Commentary. As noted earlier in the chapter, this case illustrates how long patients often wait before presentation with pain, which must be kept in mind when making management decisions. Additionally, that this young woman did very well with a hemoglobin level of 3.6 suggests chronic anemia; this is discussed above.

Case: Vaginal Bleeding and Early Pregnancy

This case is used to illustrate use of a manual vacuum aspirator.

History and Physical

A thirty-four-year-old gravida 4, para 2 (history of two full-term vaginal deliveries, a subsequent neonatal demise, and a prior miscarriage) presents at twelve weeks' gestation as calculated by her last menstrual period with vaginal spotting. Her physical exam is notable for a blood pressure of 100/60, pulse 72, risk ratio 18. Her abdomen is soft, nontender, and her pelvic exam reveals a mildly tender, eight-week-size uterus, dark blood in the vaginal vault, and a one-centimeter dilated cervical os.

Commentary. The presentation is highly suspicious for a missed abortion, and the dilated cervical os implies incomplete miscarriage. However, fetal demise needs to be confirmed before any intervention (see sections above on country-specific pregnancy termination laws as well as local practice in confirming pregnancy demise prior to proceeding).

Work-Up

Bedside ultrasound with abdominal probe demonstrates a gestational sac with a crown-rump length (CRL) of eight centimeters and no fetal cardiac activity.

Commentary. It is helpful to have on hand a table correlating CRL with weeks' gestation. Otherwise the rule of thumb is that after five weeks, add one millimeter per week. For diagnosis of missed abortion, there should be an empty gestational sac of at least twenty-five millimeters or an embryo of at least seven millimeters with no cardiac activity (Doubilet et al. 2013).

Management

The patient was offered expectant management or a dilatation and evacuation, and she opted for the latter. She gave consent for the procedure, an IV line was started, and she then received a dose of diazepam intramuscularly and morphine intravenously for pain control as well as doxycycline for antibiotic prophylaxis. The procedure was carried out using a reusable, autoclavable manual vacuum aspirator. Bedside ultrasound confirmed complete evacuation of the uterine cavity. Total blood loss was approximately fifty cubic centimeters, and the patient tolerated the procedure well.

Commentary. Although we typically offer women three options for management of a missed abortion smaller than nine-week-size (expectant, medical, or surgical), it is important to know what is available as well as feasible in the center where you are practicing. In this instance, medical management of missed abortions with misoprostol is not common practice, and though it can be offered, you must first make certain that the patient can stay in the hospital for at least forty-eight hours to ensure passage of the pregnancy and no heavy bleeding. The World Health Organization recommends 800 micrograms misoprostol vaginally or 600 micrograms sublingally for a missed abortion or 600 micrograms orally for an incomplete abortion. A repeat dose of 800 micrograms can be given in twenty-four hours if there is no passage of tissue. In this case, the patient had traveled a long distance to the hospital, so a dilation and evacuation made the most sense: it has a higher success rate and less risk of postprocedure bleeding, which could require her to return to the hospital.

To operate a manual vacuum aspirator (see the section on infrastructure above), the double barrels are depressed and the plunger pulled out to create suction that will be activated inside the uterus when the barrels are released (instructions can be found online, and it is possible to practice with a cup of water, or even a papaya). Figure 12.5 shows a manual vacuum aspirator distributed by International Pregnancy Advisory Services. If a manual vacuum aspirator or suction machine is unavailable, dilation and evacuations are often performed with sharp curettage alone. In the latter case, if misoprostol is available it can be given buccally or rectally to help minimize blood loss. That approach has also been used successfully for second-trimester abortions (Castleman et al. 2006).

Knowing which narcotics and anxiolytics are available for pain management is also important before proceeding—as well as ensuring that you have an assistant who can monitor the patient's respiratory status throughout the case. Although a paracervical block can also be offered, spinal needles are not always readily available, and the procedure poses the additional risk of a needle stick. It can be added if intravenous sedation seems insufficient.

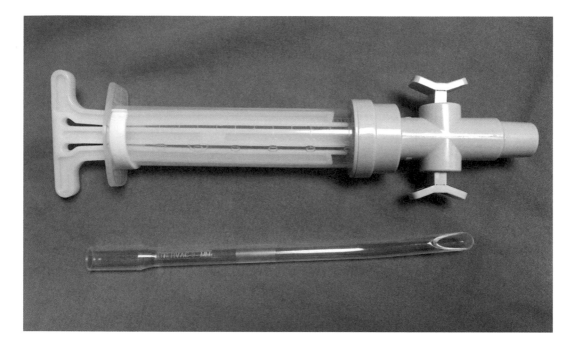

FIGURE 12.5. Double-barrel manual vacuum aspirator and a nine millimeter curved curette.

These manual vacuum aspirators are easy to assemble and disassemble. They are reusable and steam autoclavable at 121°C (250°F). They can be processed by standard cold methods such as Cidex and Sporox II. More information can be found at www.womancareglobal.org.

Outcome

The patient did well postprocedure with minimal vaginal bleeding and pain. She went home the same evening with no pain medication and three additional days of antibiotics.

Commentary. Missed abortions can be another opportunity to discuss contraception management as well as future prenatal care, depending on what the patient is considering.

Case: Obstetric Hemorrhage

This case illustrates the need for creativity and innovation in managing acute emergencies.

History and Physical

A thirty-eight-year-old woman, para 5, had successfully completed a spontaneous vaginal delivery. The placenta was delivered, and while her laceration was repaired, she began to have brisk vaginal bleeding. The stitch was tied off and a manual exam revealed a small amount of blood clot in the lower uterine segment, which was removed. Bimanual massage was performed, but the uterus remained atonic and the bleeding continued. The birth assistant was notified that help was needed.

Commentary. Obstetric hemorrhage normally occurs close to the time of delivery, and in resource-limited settings this may leave one provider managing two patients (the mother and the newborn) as well as an emergency. It is therefore critical to have an assistant, who serves not only as a critical extra pair of hands but also a way to alert others to the need for additional help.

Work-Up

The working diagnosis was uterine atony given the boggy uterus, though the placenta was intact. Assistance was requested to examine the vagina and the cervix further to rule out any additional lacerations. The patient's history was reviewed with the assistant, and it was confirmed that she had no signs of infection or hypertensive disorder. She received intermittent preventative treatment for malaria during this pregnancy.

Commentary. Multiparity is a risk factor for uterine atony. Active management of the third stage of labor can be useful in reducing blood loss, but timely administration of oxytocin or misoprostol can be difficult if there is only one provider at the birth. As stated above, the likelihood of baseline anemia makes it even more important to act quickly to restore blood volume.

Management

Ten units of intramuscular oxytocin was administered, and an under-buttocks drape (made of a garbage bag, funneled into a small trash can) allowed us to estimate blood loss at 700 milliliters. Intra-uterine tamponade was performed using a condom-catheter set-up (Figure 12.6). The condom was filled with 500 milliliters of saline, and the catheter was clamped off. The patient was given 0.25 milligrams

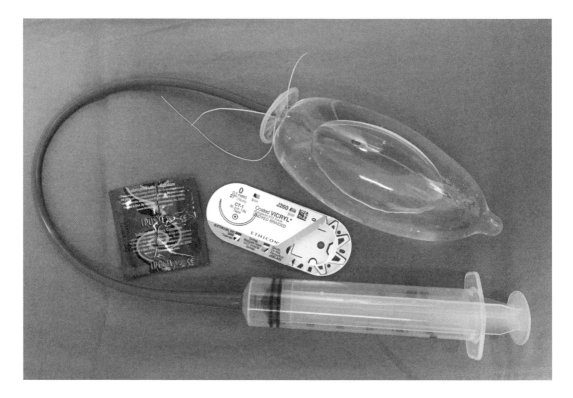

FIGURE 12.6. Condom catheter created with a condom tied around a red rubber catheter with a 0-vicryl, a 60 cubic centimeter syringe, and saline. The balloon has a total of 180 cubic centimeters. The end can be clamped or folded against itself and tied off.

ergometrine delivered intramuscularly to help contract the uterus. The vaginal laceration was again inspected and two additional stitches were placed. The patient was given an additional liter of intravenous fluid and placed under a warming wrap and light to maintain her core temperature.

Commentary. Intrauterine tamponade can also be achieved with a variety of other methods including a Bakri balloon, Foley balloons, or gauze packing. Tamponade has shown to be successful more than 90% of time and may avoid further management such as a hysterectomy or blood transfusion—especially critical when these are not readily available (Georgiou 2009). One author has suggested using three condoms together to give strength to the balloon and to thread a detached catheter into the uterus before insertion of the balloon to allow for outflow (Simaika 2010). There is no evidence that using misoprostol in addition to oxytocin provides additional benefit in cases of uterine atony (Mousa et al. 2014), though it is not unreasonable to try it as a third medication in this case, given the likelihood that some medications may be expired or have lost their effectiveness.

Outcome

The bleeding slowed with the intrauterine tamponade. The balloon was removed in twelve hours, and the patient remained stable. Within two hours of delivery she initiated breast-feeding, which also helped keep the uterus contracted.

Commentary. Every site will have different items available for use in an emergency. Remembering basic principles and then applying creative solutions can improve outcomes.

CONCLUSION

Offering women in low-resource areas safe, high-quality surgical care will certainly require that you apply all the training and experience you received in higher-resource settings. But the differences in equipment, staffing, facilities, and materials you are likely to find will also call upon your adaptability and deepest creativity. The guidelines and suggestions presented here regarding aspects of care both inside and outside the operating room (and before and after surgery) as well as a brief discussion of issues surrounding blood supply should become useful additions to your toolkit during this important work.

As health systems strengthen, so too will good surgical care, as surgery requires a trained workforce (surgeons, nurses, anesthetists), an uninterrupted cold chain for supplies, and facilities with running water and functioning electricity. As an obstetrician-gynecologist providing surgical services in resource-poor settings, you will often be faced with systems that are missing some of these elements at least part of the time. You need to be acutely aware of your abilities and limitations and how you might adapt to provide excellent care for all women who need it.

USEFUL RESOURCES

Ethicon Wound Closure Manual. Somerville, NJ: Ethicon, Inc., 2005. http://surgery.
uthscsa.edu/pediatric/training/woundclosuremanual.pdf.

Online "global surgery" modules can be accessed at http://www.uniteforsight.org
/global-health-surgery/.

World Health Organization: Surgical Care at the District Hospital, 2003.
http://www.who.int/surgery/publications/en/SCDH.pdf.

REFERENCES

American College of Obstetricians and Gynecologists. 2010. Ethical considerations
for performing gynecologic surgery in low-resource settings abroad. Committee
on Ethics and Committee on Global Women's Health, Committee Opinion 466.
Obstet Gynecol 116:793–799. http://www.acog.org/Resources-And-Publications
/Committee-Opinions/Committee-on-Ethics/Ethical-Considerations-for
-Performing-Gynecologic-Surgery-in-Low-Resource-Settings-Abroad.

Armand, R., and J. R. Hess. 2003. Treating coagulopathy in trauma patients. *Transfus
Med Rev* 17 (3): 223–231.

Arya R. C., G. Wander, and P. J. Gupta. 2011. Blood component therapy: Which,
when and how much. *Anaesthesiol Clin Pharmacol* 27 (2): 278–284.
doi:10.4103/0970-9185.81849.

Castleman, L. D., K. T. Oanh, A. G. Hyman, le T. Thuy, and P. D. Blumenthal. 2006.
Introduction of the dilation and evacuation procedure for second-trimester
abortion in Vietnam using manual vacuum aspiration and buccal misoprostol.
Contraception 74 (3): 272–276.

Center for Reproductive Rights. 2016. *World Abortion Laws 2016.* New York: Center for
Reproductive Rights. Accessed June 5, 2016. http://worldabortionlaws.com/map/.

Doubilet, P. M., C. B. Benson, T. Bourne, M. Blaivas; Society of Radiologists in
Ultrasound Multispecialty Panel on Early First Trimester Diagnosis of
Miscarriage and Exclusion of a Viable Intrauterine Pregnancy, K. T. Barn-
hart, B. R. Benacerraf, et al. 2013. Diagnostic criteria for nonviable pregnancy
early in the first trimester. *N Engl J Med* 369:1443–1451.

Ethicon, Inc. n.d. Ethicon wound closure manual. Somerville, NJ: Ethicon, Inc.
Accessed June 5, 2016. http://surgery.uthscsa.edu/pediatric/training/woundclo
suremanual.pdf.

Fromm, C., A. Likourezos, L. Haines, A. N. Khan, J. Williams, and J. Berezow. 2012.
Substituting whole blood for urine in a bedside pregnancy test. *J Emerg Med*
43:478–482.

Georgiou, C. 2009. Balloon tamponade in the management of postpartum haemorrhage: A review. *BJOG* 116:748–757.

Howe, K. L., A. O. Malomo, and M. A. Bernstein. 2013. Ethical challenges in international surgical education, for visitors and hosts. *World Neurosurg* 80 (6): 751–758.

Kongnyuy, E. J., and C. S. Wiysonge. 2014. Interventions to reduce haemorrhage during myomectomy for fibroids. *Cochrane Database Syst Rev* 15 (8): CD005355.

London School of Hygiene and Tropical Medicine. n.d. World Maternal Antifibrinolytic (Woman) Trial. Accessed June 5, 2016. http://womantrial.lshtm.ac.uk/.

Meara J. G., A. J. Leather, L. Hagander, B. C. Alkire, N. Alonso, E. A. Ameh, S. W. Bickler, et al. 2015. Global Surgery 2030: Evidence and solutions for achieving health, welfare, and economic development. *Surgery* 158 (1): 3–6. doi:10.1016/j.surg.2015.04.011. Epub May 16, 2015. https://iths.pure.elsevier.com/en/publications/global-surgery-2030-evidence-and-solutions-for-achieving-health-w-3

Miller, S., D. F. Burgel, A. M. El Ayadi, L. Gibbons, E. A. Butrick, T. Magwali, G. Mkumba, et al. 2013. Non-pneumatic anti-shock garment (NASG), a first-aid device to decrease mortality from obstetric hemorrhage: A cluster randomized trial. *PLoS One* 8 (10): e76477.

Mousa, H. A., J. Blum, G. Abou El Senoun, H. Shakur, and Z. Alfirevic. 2014. Treatment for primary postpartum haemorrhage. *Cochrane Database Syst Rev*, no. 2: CD003249.

Priuli, G., R. Darate, R. X. Perrin, J. Lankoande, and N. Drouet, et al. 2009. Multi-centre experience with a simple blood salvage technique in patients with ruptured ectopic pregnancy in sub-Sahelian West Africa. *Vox Sang*, no. 97: 317–323.

Schantz-Dunn, J., and N. M. Nour. 2011. The use of blood in obstetrics and gynecology in the developing world. *Rev Obstet Gynecol* 4 (2): 86–91.

Silvergleid, A. 2014. Clinical Use of Plasma Components. *UpToDate*. February 14. http://www.uptodate.com/contents/clinical-use-of-plasma-components.

Simaika, Y. S. 2010. The "trio" condom catheter: A modification of the condom catheter in the management of postpartum haemorrhage. *BJOG* 117: 372.

Weiser, T. G., S. E. Regenbogen, K. D. Thompson, A. B. Haynes, S. R. Lipsitz, W. R. Berry, and A. A. Gawande. 2008. An estimation of the global volume of surgery: A modelling strategy based on available data. *Lancet* 372:139–144.

Wilson, R. M., P. Michael, S. Olsen, R. W. Gibberd, C. Vincent, R. El-Assady, O. Rasslan, et al. 2012. Patient safety in developing countries: Retrospective estimation of scale and nature of harm to patients in hospital. *BMJ* 344:e832.

WHO (World Health Organization). 2006. *Blood Transfusion Safety*. Geneva: WHO. Accessed August 14, 2014. http://www.who.int/bloodsafety/en/Blood_Transfusion_Safety.pdf.

———. 2009. *WHO Guidelines for Safe Surgery 2009: Safe Surgery Saves Lives*. Geneva: WHO. Accessed August 15, 2014. http://whqlibdoc.who.int/publications/2009/9789241598552_eng.pdf.

———. 2011. *Summary Report 2011*. Geneva: WHO, June. Accessed March 15, 2014. http://www.who.int/bloodsafety/global_database/GDBS_Summary_Report_2011.pdf?ua=1.

PART FOUR

Teamwork Challenges

13

Obstetric Anesthesia in Low-Resource Settings

DINESH KUMAR JAGANNATHAN AND
BHAVANI SHANKAR KODALI

The World Health Organization (WHO) estimates that nearly 287,000 women worldwide died in 2010 from pregnancy-related causes (WHO 2015). Compared with 1990, this represents a 47% reduction in maternal mortality globally. However, 99% of these deaths still occurred in the developing world, and the majority were considered preventable. In low-resource areas, the most common causes of preventable death during pregnancy and delivery include bleeding, hypertensive disorders of pregnancy, and infection. High fertility rates and adolescent pregnancies, along with unsafe abortion practices, contribute significantly to mortality and morbidity. Coexisting conditions like HIV, tuberculosis, malaria, and pre-existing heart disease that are prevalent in many low-resource countries contribute directly or indirectly to maternal death. The cornerstone of policies and programs initiated by WHO and other international entities like the United Nations Population Fund (UNFPA) to reduce maternal mortality involve ready access to quality obstetric and anesthesia care. This goal is envisioned as being reached primarily by establishing basic and comprehensive emergency obstetric-care facilities, providing access to family-planning services, and promoting the presence of skilled attendants at births. Key points in obstetric anesthesia practice include the following:

- Maternal mortality remains high in resource-poor countries.
- A well-managed obstetric anesthesia service can help reduce maternal mortality.
- Identification of specific problems is the first step.

- Cost-effective and sustainable solutions are needed; innovation is the key.
- Anesthesia safety is compromised in low-resource settings owing to lack of qualified providers.
- Lack of basic resources and disposables exacerbate the problem.
- Audits and initiatives aimed at quality assurance (QA) and quality improvement (QI) can identify deficiencies and improve patient outcomes.

The huge difference in estimated maternal mortality ratio (MMR) between low-resource and higher-resource countries (239 maternal deaths per 100,000 live births vs. 12 maternal deaths per 100,000 live births) (WHO 2015) is attributable to a number of socioeconomic factors, poverty chief among them. There are strong associations among maternal death, poverty, and access to health care. Even within the same country, poor and rural populations are greatly affected by the inequitable distribution of health resources. Additional socioeconomic factors include lack of education or a sense of empowerment among women, limited transportation infrastructure, and the absence of well-equipped health-care facilities with trained medical personnel. Hence a holistic approach is needed to improve maternal health and reduce mortality and morbidity in low-resource countries; it should be tailored to the specific needs of the country and available resources (see Chapter 2).

Historically, anesthesiologists have led the field of patient safety in higher-resource areas (Gaba 2000). Trends in anesthesia-related mortality and morbidity, especially in the obstetric population, attest to this fact (Ngan Kee 2005). A well-trained anesthesiologist not only provides analgesia and anesthesia for labor and cesarean delivery but also assists with maternal and neonatal resuscitation (for further information, please refer to Chapter 7 on neonatal care and resuscitation). As members of the health-care team, anesthesiologists aid in triaging patients and recommending appropriate referral. They also play a key role in management of emergencies and critical care. However, the improved outcomes associated with anesthesia services have coincided with technological advances, increased monitoring, structured training, continual attention to QA and QI, and a robust regulatory framework—all unique to countries with more abundant resources.

Translating these advances to low-resource settings is a challenge. Inadequately trained personnel can significantly worsen anesthesia-related mortality and morbidity, and the lack of basic or essential supplies and equipment can contribute to unsafe anesthetic practices (Enohumah and Imarengiaye 2006). This is especially true for pregnant patients, for whom lack of knowledge and skills to manage complications can easily result in injury or death (see Chapter 12).

This chapter focuses on challenges and possible solutions for providing safe anesthesia care to pregnant patients in low-resource settings.

KEY PRINCIPLES: IDENTIFYING ISSUES

As a technology-based specialty, anesthesia is especially vulnerable to limitations in facilities, equipment, and supplies. However, not all low-resource countries face the same set of problems, and suggesting one-size-fits-all prescriptions without understanding the underlying issues is unrealistic. Hodges et al. (2007) administered a simple questionnaire to anesthesiologists in Uganda to help identify issues related to provision of safe anesthesia in their institutions. It is interesting to note that only 6% of respondents felt that they had the ability and resources to safely anesthetize a pregnant patient for cesarean delivery. The questionnaire identified shortages in personnel, training, infrastructure, drugs, and issues related to workload as issues affecting care. Such surveys can help national and international health authorities identify key problem areas, allocate appropriate resources, and implement strategies to provide optimum care. Alternatively, involving community leaders and members of the public who use health services can help identify the felt but unmet needs of the society. "Felt needs" refers to the aspects of health-care that the community feels are important, which is a subset of all unmet health-care needs as determined by professionals. Attending to both communities helps in allocating resources and getting active participation of the public.

SUGGESTED SOLUTIONS

The goal should be to develop integrated solutions that not only address obvious problems such as lack of personnel, training, equipment, and so forth but are also simple, culturally acceptable, and easily incorporated into the existing infrastructure. Safety should be paramount, as the new solution should neither contribute to existing problems nor create new ones. It should be cost effective, scalable to larger sections of the population, sustainable, and not dependent on foreign aid in either disposables or technical expertise. In addition, the success of any intervention depends on the involvement of policy makers and local stakeholders. Professional anesthesia societies can play a vital role in identifying problems, setting standards, educating both their professional colleagues and the public, and working with policy makers to bring about change (Chamberlain et al. 2003).

Key to successful solutions is innovation. One example is the creation in India of Lifeline Express, the first mobile-hospital train equipped with operating room and anesthesia facilities, which made excellent use of the country's existing extensive railway network. Started in 1991 by the Impact India Foundation in partnership with Indian Railways, the hospital on wheels has benefited more than 600,000 people in the remotest rural parts of the country (Impact India Foundation 2014).

In another example of a successful initiative, one of the authors of this chapter, Bhavani Shankar Kodali, while serving as consultant anesthesiologist in the government-run Queen Elizabeth Hospital in Bridgetown, Barbados, identified various issues related to anesthesia delivery in the hospital. He and his colleagues helped implement various innovative and practical solutions for the problems identified, including using oxygen concentrators, auditing and ordering disposables, repairing anesthesia monitors, and administering anesthesia without nitrous oxide (Shankar et al. 1997).

MONITORING PROGRESS

An important limiting factor in practice improvement in low-resource settings is the paucity of data. Though collection of data can increase costs, it is the only way to identify problems and determine whether a particular intervention has had the desired effect. Feedback from QA and QI audits will benefit not only individual patient care but the overall program as well. Metrics will help identify areas needing improvement (Paech and Sinha 2010). Maternal mortality was reduced by 34% in a regional hospital in Ghana following implementation of a continuous quality-improvement program (Srofenyoh et al. 2012). This project, administered by the Kybele

Foundation in partnership with Ghana Health Service, is a prime example of the success of simple, cost-effective measures in producing sustainable change.

SAFE PRACTICE OF OBSTETRIC ANESTHESIA IN LOW-RESOURCE COUNTRIES

Provider Shortages

One of the central standards established for the practice of anesthesia is the presence of a trained anesthesia provider. This standard is among those initially established by the American Society of Anesthesiologists (2011) in 1986, since modified and accepted by many professional anesthesia societies and endorsed by the World Federation of Societies of Anaesthesiologists. However, there is a critical shortage of trained anesthesiologists in low-resource countries (Dubowitz, Delefs, and McQueen 2010). Clinical officers (non physician medical providers) or their equivalents provide the backbone of anesthesia services in many countries. For example, in a survey of hospitals in Zambia, nonphysicians performed 78% of anesthesia (Jochberger et al. 2008). Although these caregivers perform admirably in difficult conditions, significant limitations of their knowledge, skills, and training can affect patient outcomes.

There are many reasons for this shortage of trained personnel. First, education opportunities and training programs for anesthesiologists in low-resource countries may be lacking or inadequate and expensive. Second, trained anesthesiologists may emigrate to other countries in search of better opportunities (Hagopian et al. 2004). Such brain drain has a huge impact on health-care delivery and translates into significant financial loss for low-resource countries, as the cost of training these specialist doctors is considerable and is usually subsidized by the home country. Third, anesthesiologists who do remain in their home country may choose to practice in more urban centers or in the private sector, which typically offer better facilities and remuneration.

India, which bears nearly 20% of the world's burden of maternal mortality, recently launched a program to put medical officers who had not been specially trained in anesthesiology through a short certification course enabling them to provide spinal or general anesthesia for cesarean delivery (Mavalankar et al. 2009). This is in accordance with the WHO strategy to increase the availability of trained providers in emergency obstetric care centers through task shifting. The World Health Organization (2008) defines task shifting as the process whereby "specific tasks are moved, where appropriate, from highly qualified health workers to health workers with shorter training and fewer qualifications in order to make more efficient use of the available human resources for health."

However, there are genuine safety concerns around nondoctor anesthetists' serving rural areas and creating a dual standard of care. However, similar measures involving the training of nonphysicians to provide care have been implemented with moderate success in low-resource areas and could serve as a viable model (Newton and Bird 2010).

Outreach programs initiated by various education institutions in higher-resource countries are an important source of anesthesia performed by trained physician and nonphysician providers in low-resource countries. Nonprofit organizations like the Kybele Foundation have set up education programs in multiple low-resource countries with the aim of improving childbirth conditions, many of which involve anesthesia training (see Figure 13.1). Those trainees are able not only to provide better care but also to teach and supervise other providers, propagating and sustaining the gains made initially. The impact of such teaching programs on practice patterns is dramatic. For example, twelve months following a two-week teaching program in eight hospitals across Croatia, the rate of utilization of regional anesthesia for cesarean delivery increased from 18 to 59% (Kopic, Sedensky, and Owen 2009).

Continued medical education is considered the cornerstone of the goal of keeping professional knowledge current in higher-resource countries. However, it is a luxury in many resource-poor countries owing to limited access to books, journals, and Internet-based educational materials. Seminars and lectures organized by donor nations or where invited delegates disseminate current knowledge and practices have tremendous impact. Currently, the increasing availability of Internet access is substantially broadening the availability of literature and videos on any subject anywhere in the world. Future strategies should take full advantage of this access to educate and to provide clinical, technological, and logistical information.

The World Federation of Societies of Anaesthesiologists has launched advanced fellowship programs in some low-resource countries with the goal of providing training in subspecialties like pediatric anesthesia,

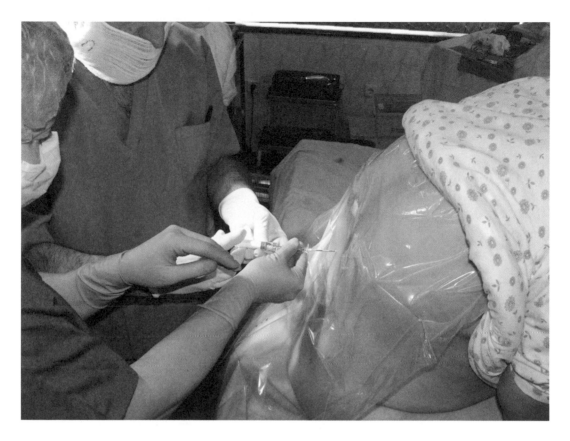

FIGURE 13.1. International training session organized by the Kybele Foundation to initiate sustainable anesthesia practice in Croatia. Training on regional spinal anesthesia placement seen here.

critical care, and pain management. It has also launched free web-based education initiatives through online publication of its "Anaesthesia Tutorial of the Week" and "Update in Anaesthesia" (Enright, Wilson, and Moyers 2007).

Developing human resources is another key to sustainable improvement in anesthesia care. However, the goal of training anesthesiologists should not stop at improving patient care at the individual level. It should proceed to create a cadre of international pioneers in the field of anesthesia who have the vision, motivation, and leadership to create sustainable change in their respective countries. That would require countries not only to provide training but also to offer incentives and ensure job satisfaction to retain its trained health-care workforce.

Table 13.1   Minimum requirements of supplies and infrastructure for provision of
             obstetric anesthesia

Oxygen source, either a cylinder or oxygen concentrator
Suction source with tubing and airway suction catheters
Self-inflating bag (Ambu) with mask for positive pressure ventilation
Airway equipment—laryngoscope with assorted blades, masks, oral airway, endotra-
   cheal tubes with stylets, bougie, qualitative CO_2 detectors
Blood pressure (automatic or manual), pulse oximeter, EKG monitors
Intravenous fluid, tubing, catheters, syringes, and needles
Essential drugs—ephedrine, dextrose, furosemide, hydralazine, diazepam, ket-
   amine, suxamethonium, thiopentol, bupivacaine 0.5% hyperbaric.
Wedge or other means to allow rapid effective left uterine displacement
Cardiac arrest equipment including a defibrillator and drugs emergency like
   epinephrine and atropine
Anesthetic machine equipped for initiating and maintaining anesthesia and tilting
   operating table
Disposables—Sterile gloves, Betadine solution, spinal needles

---

Source: Adapted from WHO (2005).

Anesthesia Equipment, Disposables, and Drugs

There must be minimum requirements of infrastructure and supplies for provision of safe obstetric anesthesia care, as modified from WHO's *Guide to Infrastructure and Supplies at Various Levels of Health Care Facilities: Emergency and Essential Surgical and Anaesthesia Procedures* (WHO 2005). A list of minimum requirements of supplies is presented in Table 13.1.

Irrespective of the settings, such basic infrastructure, sterile disposables, and resuscitation equipment must be available in every anesthetizing location. Equipment must also be periodically inspected and serviced. This is essential to ensuring the safety of patients, and no compromise should be entertained in establishing and maintaining such minimum basic standards (Figure 13.2).

Many low-resource countries are dependent on donated equipment and disposables for maintaining and providing anesthesia services. However, there are significant problems associated with unsolicited donations. The equipment may not be needed in that particular country or may not work under those environmental conditions; there may be inadequate training in use of the equipment; and there may be a lack of maintenance facilities or local source of spare parts (Gatrad, Gatrad, and Gatrad 2007). There is also significant concern around donated materials about the risk of infection created by reuse of single-use disposables, deg-

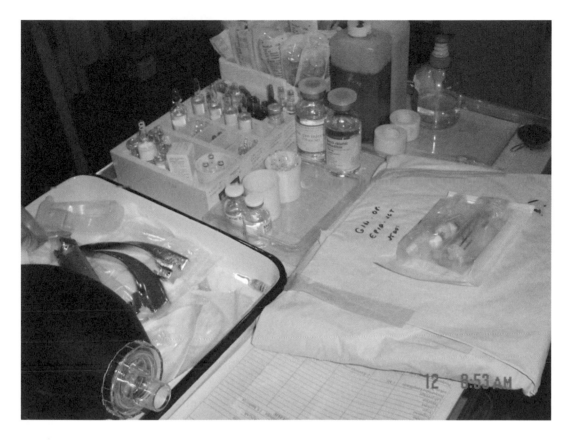

FIGURE 13.2. Resuscitation equipment and essential drugs must be consistently available.

radation of material resulting in breakage, and so on. In addition, there are substantial ethical issues regarding use of date-expired disposables. In an effort to promote safe donation practices, WHO has published guidelines for health-care equipment donations that can help avoid these pitfalls while allowing vital medical supplies to reach low-resource areas.

Oxygen Supply

Oxygen is considered an essential medication and is needed not only for administration of safe anesthesia but also in the management of many obstetric and neonatal emergencies such as acute hemorrhagic shock, pulmonary edema, and neonatal resuscitation. A report by Belle at al. (2010) indicated that only 44% of the 231 health centers, district hospitals, and provincial or general hospitals surveyed in twelve African countries had

Table 13.2   Comparison between oxygen cylinders and concentrators

	Oxygen cylinders	Oxygen concentrators
Power source requirement	No.	Yes. Need backup generators or battery source.
Transport requirement	Yes; frequent replenishment of exhausted tanks.	No.
Exhaustible supply	Yes. Exact length of supply depends on flow rates, duration of use, system leaks.	No. Continuous supply as long as power remains uninterrupted.
Maintenance	Minimal.	Moderate. Both preventative maintenance and intermittent repairs; spare parts are needed.
Reliability	Excellent, if supply chain adequate.	Self-sustained source, if no equipment malfunction.
Oxygen purity	Up to 99%	90–95%

Source: Adapted from Howie et al. (2009).

access to oxygen on a continuous basis. Unreliable power supply, poor transportation facilities, and equipment malfunction all contribute to this shortage. There are two main viable sources of oxygen in hospitals in low-resource settings: oxygen in cylinders and oxygen produced from oxygen concentrators. Table 13.2 summarizes the advantages and disadvantages of both options.

Depending of local infrastructure and resources, either of these options can be utilized. Additional point-of-care oxygen supply requires piping, adapters, pressure regulators, and oxygen masks or cannulas, which can add to expense.

In the absence of a reliable oxygen supply, many anesthesia providers in low-resource settings prefer to use ketamine-based intravenous sedation or general anesthesia with spontaneous breathing. Hence promoting and establishing a reliable supply of oxygen is a prerequisite for safe obstetric anesthesia care. Simple measures like daily estimating of oxygen levels in the tanks and anticipating the need for renewed supply can go a long way in preventing supply failure.

Anesthesia Machines

The anesthesia machine has evolved from a simple apparatus for delivery of anesthetic gases and supplemental oxygen to a complex workstation with sophisticated delivery systems, ventilator settings, and integrated monitoring equipment. Incorporated into these workstations are many safety features such as oxygen sensors, disconnection alarms, fail-safe mechanisms, high- and low-pressure alarms, an so on. Additional safety features such as color-coding for cylinders, hoses, pin index, and diametric index safety systems have reduced incidents of cross-connection of medical gases. A recent review of the Closed Claims Project database of the American Society of Anesthesiologists showed that patient injuries related to gas delivery have decreased dramatically since the 1990s compared with the preceding two decades (Mehta et al. 2013). However, translating these safety advantages to low-resource settings is a challenge. It is essential that low-cost, robust, and safe anesthesia equipment be made available in low-income countries. These anesthesia machines should be able to function without compressed gases or a reliable supply of electricity (McCormick and Eltringham 2007).

Currently there are two commercial machines designed specifically for low-resource conditions: Glostavent and the Universal Anesthesia Machine. These machines have been found safe and easy to use in a variety of countries and adhere to the standards prescribed by the World Federation of Societies of Anaesthesiologists' safety committee on anesthesia equipment for low- and low-middle income countries. These machines use oxygen concentrators instead of an external oxygen source. As a part of the concentrator process, compressed air is created and used to drive the bellows. If electricity fails, a backup battery maintains operation. In case of prolonged power failure or oxygen supply failure, room air is used for ventilation, preventing delivery of a hypoxic mixture, and the backup hand-held bellows can provide positive-pressure ventilation. Low-resistance draw-over vaporizers provide anesthetic gases and are easy to use and maintain. These machines are relatively inexpensive, and local personnel can be trained in their maintenance.

Traditionally, anesthesia based on nitrous oxide and oxygen was favored owing to the reduced need for potent inhaled anesthetics. As early as 1987, one of the authors of this book, Bhavani Shankar Kodali, and his colleagues reported that the air-oxygen combination costs less than half as much as nitrous oxide-oxygen for general anesthesia (Mosely et al. 1987). An additional advantage of the air-oxygen combination is its inherent safety, which makes it impossible for a hypoxic mixture to be given to patients, making it ideal for application in low-resource countries.

Monitors

Pulse oximetry has been declared by WHO as essential for patients undergoing anesthesia and surgery and has been endorsed by various national and international guidelines and standards. However, it is estimated that nearly 77,000 facilities worldwide where anesthesia is provided for surgery do not use pulse oximeters (Funk et al. 2010). The World Health Organization launched the international collaborative effort, the Global Pulse Oximetry Project, to supply pulse oximeters at low cost and encourage their use. The charitable organization Lifebox has been crucial in developing and distributing low-cost pulse oximeters.

Capnography is also a valuable monitor of adequacy of ventilation and confirmation of endotracheal intubation and should be promoted as aggressively as oximetry in an effort to reduce anesthesia-related respiratory complications in settings including obstetric anesthesia care (Kodali 2013).

Blood pressure monitoring at least every five minutes is mandatory following initiation of anesthesia, whether spinal or general. Efforts to maintain adequate placental perfusion through left uterine displacement as well as administration of fluids and vasopressors are important. Additionally, early detection and management of such pathological states as preeclampsia and hemorrhagic shock are facilitated by serial blood-pressure measurements.

Additional monitoring of inhaled anesthetic gases and patient temperature are also recommended when feasible.

Drugs

A reliable supply of drugs is essential to the safe practice of anesthesia. Close cooperation among anesthesiologists, pharmacists, and hospital administrators can help anticipate drug shortages and promote procurement. Maintaining inventory and placing orders in advance is helpful in overcoming delays. However, safe preparation, transportation, and storage are problems in some areas. In tropical countries, drugs that are reconstituted just before use, have a long shelf life, and do not require cold storage are suitable. Local manufacturing ability and subsidized procurement strategies can reduce costs.

In a low-resource country, it is advisable to become familiar with a limited number of drugs and dosages and use them consistently with a clear understanding of their pharmacokinetics, pharmacodynamics, and contraindications. Ketamine is the mainstay of anesthesia in low-resource countries owing to its analgesic and anesthetic properties along with cardiorespiratory stability. Suxamethonium is still the drug of choice for rapid-sequence intubation and is particularly useful in pregnant women. Hyperbaric bupivacaine is commonly used for spinal anesthesia for cesarean delivery, although lidocaine is used in some places. Vasopressors like ephedrine and phenylephrine along with resuscitation medications like epinephrine and atropine are necessary for management of complications and treatment of emergencies. Uterotonics like oxytocin, methergine, and misoprostol are important in reducing the risk of postpartum hemorrhage. Hypertensive disorders of pregnancy are a major cause of mortality and morbidity in low-resource areas, and drugs like hydralazine, labetalol, and magnesium are required for management of blood pressure and for seizure prophylaxis.

Ancillary Resources: Blood Bank, Laboratory, and Radiology Services

Anesthesia services cannot function optimally without adequate support from ancillary services like blood bank or appropriate referral mechanisms. Obstetric hemorrhage is one of the leading causes of direct maternal death in low-resource areas (please also refer to Chapter 12, on obstetric surgery). Delay in diagnosis, referral, and transport to health-care facilities are the main reasons for such high mortality. An example of a successful community-level strategy to reduce the severity of postpartum hemorrhage was implemented in Ghana. It included training of midwives to recognize excessive bleeding, the use of blood collection drapes, and give early oral misoprostol (Kapungu et al. 2013). However, treatment of an acutely bleeding patient may require resuscitation with fluids and blood. Hence blood banks must have adequate supplies of type-specific blood and, in case of emergencies, O-negative blood. Although blood banks are rarely under the control of anesthesiologists, it is important that these specialists be allowed to set up and manage the blood supply.

Laboratory testing is crucial in clinical decision making and management of obstetric complications such as hemorrhage. For example, platelet counts may help determine whether it is safe to administer regional analgesia or anesthesia to a pregnant patient with preeclampsia in conjunction with clinical presentation. Technological advances under development such as the portable transcutaneous hemoglobin meters could aid in supplementing laboratory testing or replacing it in remote locations.

PROTOCOL DEVELOPMENT

It is essential to develop clinical-management protocols to ensure consistency of care and patient safety. A written procedure manual or unit policy can guide all anesthesia providers in the standard use of medications and doses to help avoid drug errors. It can also help establish a minimum standard of care consistent with local regulations, thus enhancing patient safety.

Some salient features of the use of protocols are considered in the following sections.

Anesthesia for Cesarean Delivery

Anesthesia for cesarean delivery depends upon the obstetric indication for surgical intervention, presence of maternal comorbidities, urgency of the surgery, and availability of resources. Adequate preoperative evaluation with focused history and physical examination including airway examination is recommended. Obtaining informed consent after discussing various anesthesia options and associated risks is warranted.

Neuraxial Anesthesia

Neuraxial anesthesia—spinal, epidural, or combined spinal epidural—has become the mainstay of anesthesia for cesarean delivery in high-resource countries like the United States (Bucklin et al. 2005). This has in turn decreased the mortality and morbidity associated with failed intubation or ventilation (Hawkins et al. 2011). However, a single-shot spinal technique with hyperbaric bupivacaine is the method of choice for the majority of patients in low-resource countries. Addition of intrathecal opioids can be considered in appropriate settings.

Preoperative evaluation of contraindications for spinal anesthesia like hypovolemia (active bleeding), coagulopathy, infection at site of needle insertion, and so on is important and must be incorporated into any protocol. Left uterine displacement using a wedge or manual tilting should be the standard of care, and all members of the team must be aware of its importance. Adequate blood-pressure monitoring and maintenance of perfusion of the uterus is important, and fluids and vasopressors must be available to treat any spinal-induced hypotension. The ability to rapidly convert to general anesthesia for high spinal or failed block is also important.

Dedicated personnel, ideally a pediatrician, should be available for neonatal resuscitation. However, in many low-resource areas the anesthesiologist may be the most qualified person for neonatal resuscitation.

The protocol should incorporate measures to identify and treat anesthesia-related side effects and complications such as postdural puncture headache. Simple measures like promoting the use of 25-gauge noncutting spinal needles will reduce the incidence of this complication. Though rare and potentially devastating, serious complications like epidural hematoma should be identified as early as possible through follow-up of persistent block and expedited imaging. Early (within six hours) treatment to relieve spinal-cord compression is important to prevent permanent neurological deficit.

General Anesthesia

Complete history and focused physical examination are a must, and the importance of airway examination cannot be overemphasized. Using acoustic reflectometry, Kodali et al. (2008) demonstrated significant changes in pregnant patients during labor and delivery that can contribute to difficult ventilation or intubation. All pregnant patients are considered at risk for aspiration of gastric contents, and use of nonparticulate antacids thirty minutes before induction and performance of rapid-sequence intubation with cricoid pressure is recommended. Careful airway examination, appropriate positioning, adequate preoxygenation, and additional help and backup equipment during induction are important. To decrease the incidence of neonatal depression, it is advisable to minimize the time from induction to delivery by prepping the abdomen first, using 100% oxygen, and avoiding opioids until delivery. Early use of uterotonics and reduction of the amount of potent inhaled anesthetics can decrease the incidence of uterine atony and subsequent postpartum hemorrhage. Appropriate measures should be considered for safe emergence, postoperative recovery, and pain management.

Local Anesthesia

Though local anesthesia has traditionally been used to supplement inadequate neuraxial anesthesia during cesarean delivery, the use of local infiltration as a stand-alone technique is a potentially viable option in lower-resource countries where anesthesia services are not readily available. The success of local infiltrative anesthesia is dependent upon the skill of the obstetrician administering it and use of a midline incision, avoiding retractors or uterine exteriorization. Because of concerns regarding the cumulative toxicity of local anesthesia, use of 0.5% lidocaine with epinephrine and limiting the total dose to seven milligrams per kilogram are recommended.

Postoperative Pain Management

Intrathecal long-acting opioids such as extended-release morphine are the mainstay of pain management in high-resource countries. However, they may require additional monitoring for respiratory depression in the postoperative period, adding to costs (Carvalho 2008). Multimodal analgesia techniques that include local infiltration, nonsteroidal anti-inflammatory drugs, acetaminophen, and systemic opioids may be a viable option in low-resource countries. Transverse-abdominis-plane block is an accepted technique for postoperative pain management following lower abdominal surgery like cesarean delivery. Use of real-time ultrasound guidance during the block can enhance accuracy and decrease the risk of bowel perforation. However, the costs of real-time ultrasound guidance can be prohibitive, making it unfeasible in low-resource settings. A novel approach that can be easily learned and performed is surgical transverse-abdominis-plane block under direct vision by the obstetrician during closure (Owen et al. 2011).

Analgesia for Labor and Delivery

Owing to a shortage of resources and personnel, labor analgesia has been a neglected area in low-resource countries. Lack of awareness among patients and providers and cultural barriers to pain relief during delivery contribute to this situation. Among the various options for labor analgesia are neuraxial analgesia, parenteral opioids, inhaled nitrous oxide, and peripheral nerve blocks. Following are brief summaries of each of the options.

Neuraxial Analgesia

Epidural labor analgesia has been found to be safe and effective, and its use has greatly increased in high-resource countries (Howell and Chalmers

1992). The advantages of epidural labor analgesia include its ability to manage pain during both stages of labor and the ease of rapid conversion to surgical anesthesia for operative delivery. However, the need for disposables, infusion systems, and personnel to administer and monitor both the mother and fetus limit its usefulness in low-resource areas. Single-shot spinal analgesia has been explored as an alternative regional analgesia technique in the second stage of labor. Its applicability in low-resource settings was explored through a pilot program with moderate success (Owen et al. 2009). As with regional anesthesia for cesarean delivery, development of clinical management protocols will greatly enhance safety and efficacy.

Parenteral Opioids

Systemic opioids are the mainstay of labor analgesia in many low-resource countries. Pure opioid agonists such as morphine, meperidine, fentanyl, or mixed agonist-antagonists such as nalbuphine and pentazocine are commonly used. Because all opioids are to some extent lipid soluble and able to cross the placenta, they pose the risk of fetal and neonatal depression depending on dose and timing. Care should be taken in monitoring respiration and oxygenation when parturients receive parenteral opioids.

Inhaled Nitrous Oxide

Inhaled nitrous oxide can provide analgesia for labor and is popular in some countries; it does not interfere with uterine activity and provides good analgesia during the first stage of labor. However, inhaled nitrous oxide requires maternal cooperation for its efficacy, and there are concerns regarding potential environmental pollution. It also requires suitable equipment, appropriate training, and monitoring to prevent hypoxia, thereby limiting its usefulness in low-resource countries.

Nerve Blocks

Nerve blocks can be a viable option for labor analgesia in low-resource countries and can be performed by the obstetrician. Though paracervical block can be used for pain associated with cervical dilation during the first stage of labor (Palomaki, Huhtala, and Kirkinen 2005), it is rarely practiced, owing to potential complications including infection, hematoma formation, local anesthetic toxicity, fetal bradycardia, and fetal death. Because duration of block is limited, repeated injections may be needed. Similarly, pain during the second stage of labor owing to distention of the perineum can be alleviated by pudendal nerve block.

In the absence of effective labor analgesia options, prenatal education, teaching of coping mechanisms, and continuous labor support can be useful for management of labor pain (Huntley, Coon, and Ernst 2004).

Anesthesia for Gynecological Procedures

Common gynecological procedures include myomectomy, hysterectomy, postpartum sterilization, and interval sterilization. Most of these procedures can be performed safely under spinal anesthesia. Laparoscopic procedures usually require general anesthesia with controlled ventilation, although there are reports of using spinal anesthesia in select cases. The general principles of management for spinal or general anesthesia in low-resource settings have been outlined in prior sections. Minor procedures such as dilation and curettage can be performed under IV sedation supplemented with paracervical block. Ketamine continues to play a significant role in such situations, owing to its ability to provide analgesia while maintaining hemodynamics and respiration.

SUMMARY

Maternal mortality continues to be high in low-resource areas. The first step toward reducing mortality is to establish minimum safety standards of obstetric and anesthesia care. These require adequately trained staff, availability of essential equipment, disposables, drugs, and appropriate clinical protocols. Identifying areas of deficiency, implementing innovative strategies, and monitoring progress are also key in making sustainable change. Through financial and technical support and outreach programs, international health organizations and other nonprofit organizations play a crucial role in improving anesthesia services in lower-resource countries. Ultimately, local governments, with input from professional anesthesia societies, must develop holistic solutions individualized to the particular country.

REFERENCES

American Society of Anesthesiologists. 2011. "Standards, Guidelines, Statements and Other Documents: Standards for Basic Anesthetic Monitoring (effective July 1, 2011)." Accessed May 19, 2016. http://www.asahq.org/quality-and -practice-management/standards-and-guidelines.

Belle, J., H. Cohen, N. Shindo, M. Lim, A. Velazquez-Berumen, J. B. Ndihokub-wayo, and M. Cherian. 2010. Influenza preparedness in low-resource settings: A look at oxygen delivery in 12 African countries. *J Infect Dev Ctries* 4 (7): 419–424.

Bucklin, B. A., J. L. Hawkins, J. R. Anderson, and F. A. Ullrich. 2005. Obstetric anesthesia workforce survey: Twenty-year update. *Anesthesiology* 103:645–653.

Carvalho, B. 2008. Respiratory depression after neuraxial opioids in the obstetric setting. *Anesth Analg* 107:956–961.

Chamberlain, J., R. Mcdonagh, A. Lalonde, and S. Arulkumaran. 2003. The role of Professional associations in reducing maternal mortality worldwide. *Int J Gynaecol Obstet* 83:94–102.

Dubowitz, G., S. Detlefs, and K. A. McQueen. 2010. Global anesthesia work force crisis: A preliminary survey revealing shortages contributing to undesirable outcomes and unsafe practices. *World J Surg* 34:438–444.

Enohumah, K. O., and C. O. Imarengiaye. 2006. Factors associated with anaesthesia-related maternal mortality in a tertiary hospital in Nigeria. *Acta Anaesthesiol Scand* 50:206–210.

Enright, A., I. H. Wilson, and J. R. Moyers. 2007. The World Federation of Societies of Anaesthesiologists: Supporting education in the developing world. *Anaesthesia* 62 (S1): 67–71.

Funk, L. M., T. G. Weiser, W. R. Berry, S. R. Lipsitz, A. F. Merry, A. C. Enright, I. H. Wilson, G. Dziekan, and A. A. Gawande. 2010. Global operating theatre distribution and pulse oximetry supply: An estimation from reported data." *Lancet* 376:1055–1061.

Gaba, D. M. 2000. Anaesthesiology as a model for patient safety in health care. *BMJ* 320:785–788.

Gatrad, A. R., S. Gatrad, and A. Gatrad. 2007. Equipment donation to developing countries. *Anaesthesia* 62 (S1): 90–95.

Hagopian, A., M. J. Thompson, M. Fordyce, K. E. Johnson, and L. G. Hart. 2004. The migration of physicians from sub-Saharan Africa to United States of America: Measures of the African brain drain." *Hum Resour Health* 2 (1): 17.

Hawkins, J. L., J. Chang, S. K. Palmer, C. P. Gibbs, and W. M. Callaghan. 2011. Anesthesia-related maternal mortality in the United States: 1979–2002. *Obstet Gynecol* 117:69–74.

Hodges, S. C., C. Mijumbi, M. Okello, B. A. McCormick, I. A. Walker, and I. H. Wilson. 2007. Anaesthesia services in developing countries: Defining the problems. *Anaesthesia* 62:4–11.

Howell, C. J., and I. Chalmers. 1992. A review of prospectively controlled comparison of epidural with non-epidural forms of pain relief during labor. *Int J Obstet Anesth* 1:93–110.

Howie S. R., S. Hill, A. Ebonyi, G. Krishnan, O. Njie, M. Sanneh, M. Jallow, et al. 2009. Meeting oxygen needs in Africa: An options analysis from the Gambia. *Bull World Health Organ* 87 (10): 763–771.

Huntley, A. L., J. T. Coon, and E. Ernst. 2004. Complementary and alternative medicine for labor pain: A systematic review. *Am J Obstet Gynecol* 191:36–44.

Impact India Foundation. 2014. Lifeline Express. Accessed May 19, 2016.
    http://www.impactindia.org/lifeline-express.php.

Jochberger, S., F. Ismailova, W. Lederer, V. D. Mayr, G. Luckner, V. Wenzel,
    H. Ulmer, W. R. Hasibeder, and M. W. Dünser. 2008. Anesthesia and its allied
    disciplines in the developing world: A nationwide survey of the Republic of
    Zambia. *Anesth Analg* 106:942–948.

Kapungu C. T., J. Mensah-Homiah, E. Akosah, G. Asare, L. Carnahan, M. A.
    Frimpong, P. Mensah-Bonsu, S. Ohemeng-Dapaah, L. Owusu-Ansah, and
    S. E. Geller. 2013. A community-based continuum of care model for the
    prevention of postpartum hemorrhage in rural Ghana. *Int J Gynaecol Obstet*
    120:156–159.

Kodali, B. S. 2013. Capnography outside the operating rooms. *Anesthesiology*
    118:192–201.

Kodali, B. S., S. Chandrasekhar, L. N. Bulich, G. P. Topulos, and S. Datta. 2008.
    Airway changes during labor and delivery. *Anesthesiology* 108:357–362.

Kopic, D., M. Sedensky, and M. Owen. 2009. The impact of a teaching program on
    obstetric anesthesia practices in Croatia. *Int J Obstet Anesth* 18:4–9.

Mavalankar, D., K. Callahan, V. Sriram, P. Singh, and A. Desai. 2009. Where there is
    no anaesthetist-increasing capacity for emergency obstetric care in rural India:
    An evaluation of a pilot program to train general doctors. *Int J Gynecol Obstet*
    107:283–288.

McCormick., B. A., and R. J. Eltringham. 2007. Anaesthesia equipment for resource
    poor environments. *Anaesthesia* 62 (S1): 54–60.

Mehta, S. P., J. B. Eisenkraft, K. L. Posner, and K. B. Domino. 2013. Patient injuries
    from anesthesia gas delivery equipment: A closed claims update. *Anesthesiology*
    119:788–795.

Mosely, H., A. Y. Kumar, K. B. Shankar, P. S. Rao, and J. Homi. 1987. Should air-oxygen
    replace nitrous oxide-oxygen in general anaesthesia? *Anaesthesia* 42:609–612.

Newton, M., and P. Bird. 2010. Impact of parallel anesthesia and surgical provider
    training in sub-Saharan Africa: A model for a resource-poor setting. *World J
    Surg* 34:445–452.

Ngan Kee, W. D. 2005. Confidential enquiries into maternal deaths: 50 years of
    closing the loop. *Br J Anaesth* 94:413–416

Owen, D., I. Harrod, J. Ford, M. Luckas, and V. Gudimetla. 2011. The surgical
    transversus abdominis plane block: A novel approach for performing an
    established technique. *BJOG* 118:24–27.

Owen, M. D., A. J. Olufolabi, and E. Srofenyoh E. 2009. "Abstract A-49: Pilot
    Program to Introduce Spinal Labor Analgesia in a West African Hospital."
    Paper presented at the annual meeting for the Society for Obstetric Anesthesia
    and Perinatology. Washington, DC.

Paech, M., and A. Sinha. 2010. Obstetric audit and its implication for obstetric
    anaesthesia. *Best Pract Res Clin Obstet Gynaecol* 24:413–425.

Palomaki, O., H. Huhtala, and P. Kirkinen. 2005. What determines the analgesic
    effect of paracervical block? *Acta Obstet Gynecol Scand* 84:962 966.

Shankar, K. B., H. S. L. Moseley, P. S. Mushlin, R. A. Hallsworth, M. Fakoory, and
    E. R. Walrond. 1997. Anaesthesia in Barbados. *Canad J Anaesth* 44:559–568.
Srofenyoh, E., T. Ivester, C. Engmann, A. Olufolabi, L. Bookman, and M. Owen. 2012.
    Advancing obstetric and neonatal care in a regional hospital in Ghana via
    continuous quality improvement. *Int J Gynaecol Obstet* 116:17–21.
WHO (World Health Organization). 2005. *Guide to Infrastructure and Supplies at
    Various Levels of Health Care Facilities: Emergency and Essential Surgical and Anaes-
    thesia Procedures.* Geneva: World Health Organization. www.who.int/surgery
    /publications/s15983e.pdf.
——. 2008. *Task Shifting: Rational Redistribution of Tasks among Health Workforce Teams:
    Global Recommendations and Guidelines.* Geneva: World Health Organization.
    Accessed May 26, 2016. http://www.who.int/healthsystems/TTR-TaskShifting
    .pdf.
——. 2015. *Maternal Mortality.* Fact sheet No. 348. Geneva: World Health Organization.
    Accessed May 26, 2016. http://www.who.int/mediacentre/factsheets/fs348/en/.

14

Neonatal Care and Resuscitation

SADATH ALI SAYEED

A newborn is a unique potential patient, dependent on others from the moment of birth onward to survive. The ability of newborns to handle the many common insults of daily life (for example, cold temperature) is limited because most of their organ systems are in a state of physiological immaturity. The risks associated with such insults are correspondingly higher.

In low-resource settings, newborns often die quickly, quietly, and without much notice by or attention from health-care providers. Because neonatal mortality, defined as death in the first twenty-eight days of life, is such a common experience in the most socially and economically vulnerable communities, an indictment of fatalism is often ascribed to the same (Winch et al. 2005). Names are bestowed on infants in some places only after they have completed several weeks of life, demonstrating a survival fitness of sorts (Winch et al. 2005).

A biological reductionist model attributes neonatal mortality to three main (and often overlapping) clinical conditions: infection, prematurity, and intrapartum asphyxia (Lawn, Cousens, and Zupan 2005). In a high-functioning health-care delivery system, each of these problems is usually manageable. In fact, the materials and skills needed to prevent most global neonatal mortality are not sophisticated; nor need the personnel who deliver most of the care be formally medically trained (Bang et al. 2005). However, structural barriers complicate efforts to implement effective interventions both locally and at scale (Wall et al. 2009).

Because the major problems in low-resource settings are structural and systemic, one-time "trainings" of local providers in sound clinical newborn-care practice, such as basic neonatal resuscitation, are unlikely to sub-

stantially improve neonatal outcomes (Ersdal et al. 2012). Permanent solutions can emerge only if priority is placed on the improving the system
as a whole. The practitioner working in a low-resource setting must attend
to those modifiable behavioral factors that allow quality care practices—
whether delivered by family member, community health worker, nurse,
midwife, or physician—to take firm hold within an existing health-care
system (Wall et al. 2009).

EPIDEMIOLOGY

As Bhutta et al. (2010, 2032) have noted, "Progress in neonatal mortality
(first 28 days) remains slow, and in Africa almost no change was recorded.
Neonatal deaths now account for 41% of deaths in children younger than
5 years, and this mortality is linked closely to slow progress in reduction
of maternal mortality."

Because many low- and middle-income countries lack comprehensive
systems to collect vital registration data on births and deaths, the true
number in any year is unknown. Fresh stillbirths further complicate estimates of neonatal mortality, though global annual stillbirths are currently
estimated at between 2 million and 3 million (Cousens et al. 2011). Some
degree of misclassification occurs in low-resource settings, where nonreactive, nonbreathing newborns—though born alive—are frequently not intervened upon (see Chapter 3).

The current best estimate for neonatal mortality is between 3 million
and 4 million deaths annually (Lawn et al. 2009). Over 80% of these are
directly owing to severe infection, intrapartum events (loosely referred to
as birth asphyxia), or prematurity (UNICEF 2009). Low birth weight contributes to 60 to 80% of these deaths (UNICEF 2009). Roughly half of all
neonatal deaths occur in the first day of life, and around 75% occur in the
first week. Most deaths occurring after the first few days of life are caused
by infection.

Over two-thirds of global neonatal deaths (more than 2 million) occur
in ten countries in Asia and sub-Saharan Africa: India, China, Nigeria,
Pakistan, Democratic Republic of Congo, Ethiopia, Bangladesh, Afghanistan, Indonesia, and Tanzania (from highest annual number of deaths to
lowest; Lawn et al. 2009). Although China and Indonesia have neonatal
mortality rates under twenty per 1,000 live births, their large population
sizes yield high numbers of aggregated annual deaths.

Newborns are far more likely to die at home than in hospitals, in economically vulnerable communities than in more affluent areas, and in rural locations than in urban areas. In data collected from several African countries over the past several years, the neonatal mortality rate in rural areas is more than 40% higher than in urban areas and more than 60% higher for families living in the poorest economic quintiles compared with those living in the highest brackets (Lawn et al. 2009).

PATHOPHYSIOLOGY

In low-resource settings neonates die most often from disorders related to the transition from fetal to extrauterine life, infection, complications secondary to premature birth, or a combination of these. Uncorrectable congenital anomalies or genetic derangements account for a small fraction of total newborn deaths. Anatomic anomalies that are technically correctable but might require early, sophisticated surgical intervention (for example, transposition of the great vessels or tracheoesophageal atresia) remain for the most part untreatable in most low- and middle-income countries.

ASPHYXIA

It is estimated that 10 to 15% of all newborns require some form of assistance to make the successful transition to extrauterine life, and another 1 to 5% require more substantial intervention (Wall et al. 2009). Before birth, a fetus is well adapted to thrive when removed from the placental circuit, despite its exposure to low partial pressures of oxygen within the bloodstream (PO2 of 20 to 25 milligrams Hg). Fetal hemoglobin has a higher affinity for oxygen than adult hemoglobin, and fetal tissue is highly efficient at extracting it. Additionally, fetal cells resist the untoward effects of acidosis (Merrill and Ballard 2005).

During the normal birthing process, a fetus prepares itself to adapt to this new separated existence with a host of biochemical responses, highlighted by the switch from fetal to neonatal circulation. The stress of labor and delivery normally results in a surge of circulating catecholamines that promote the resorption of lung fluid, the release of surfactant, the availability of energy stores, thermoregulation, and blood flow to vital organs (Merrill and Ballard 2005). After birth, the low-resistance placenta is purposely removed from the blood circuit, and the neonate becomes dependent on its own lungs to absorb oxygen from ambient air.

The relative resistances within a newborn's own circulatory system must change to achieve adequate tissue oxygenation. Blood that formerly returned from the placenta to the fetus and bypassed the highly resistant pulmonary vasculature to shunt across a patent ductus arteriosus between the great vessels and the foramen ovale between the atria must now preferentially enter a decreasingly resistant pulmonary circuit to obtain oxygen (Merrill and Ballard 2005). In a normal transition, with well-expanded and compliant lungs, this increased blood flow returns to the left atrium, where it increases the pressure relative to the right atrium, promoting functional closure of the foramen. The ductus arteriosus simultaneously begins to undergo physiological changes that lead to its functional closure within hours after birth and its anatomical closure within weeks (Merrill and Ballard 2005).

Maternal, fetal, or other factors can disrupt this process. Any condition that prevents adequate lung expansion after birth can lead to the persistence of fetal circulation. When pulmonary vascular resistance remains high, the ductal and foramenal shunts may stay open; however, because the placenta is no longer able to supply oxygen to the tissues, a newborn is at risk for asphyxiating illness. *Asphyxia* is defined as a combination of hypoxemia, hypercapnia, and metabolic acidosis (Merrill and Ballard 2005). The acidosis worsens with progressively inadequate tissue oxygenation.

Asphyxia clinically presents in four successive, deteriorating phases: primary hyperpnea (increased respiratory effort); primary apnea (no respiratory effort); very slow, gasping respiratory effort; and finally secondary apnea. Depending on the duration and degree of asphyxia, newborns can present at birth in any one of these phases (Merrill and Ballard 2005). Regardless of the cause, asphyxia can rapidly result in death or permanent disability in the surviving newborn owing to massive end-organ cellular injury or necrosis from inadequate oxygenation.

CHALLENGES WITH INFECTION

The innate and adaptive immune systems of a newborn (regardless of gestational age) are immature. The innate system offers a rapid, species-generic response to microorganisms, and despite being operational at birth, both the complement and cellular components (for example, natural killer cells) have not yet reached full functional capacity (Williams and Cole 2005). The key cell in neonatal sepsis is the macrophage, which mediates the cytokine and inflammatory response to infection through the release of substances such as TNF-alpha and the interleukins (Williams and Cole 2005).

Polymorphonuclear neutrophils and T- and B-lymphocytes, while detectable very early in gestation, are similarly subject to specific developmental regulation and therefore unable to fully respond in cases of neonatal infection (Williams and Cole 2005). Specific immunoglobulin development only occurs after birth with exposure to common antigens in the environment. Maternal transference of IgG partially offsets this deficiency but does not begin until around twenty weeks of gestation; thus, premature neonates have lower levels than full-term infants (Williams and Cole 2005). The robustness of this maternally derived protection further depends on the mother's having high enough titers of any given specific antibody to pass them along to the fetus. As maternal IgG levels fall in the first few months of life, native IgG production increases (Williams and Cole 2005).

Early-onset bacterial sepsis can present either as distress immediately after delivery or more indolently within the first seventy-two hours of birth. In either presentation, it is presumed that the infection originates from within a colonized maternal genital tract (Polin et al. 2005). Organisms that inhabit the perineal space can ascend into the amniotic cavity through ruptured or intact membranes and cause clinical or subclinical infection in the mother. In either case, amnionitis can lead to life-threatening illness in the neonate.

The clinical presentation of early-onset sepsis is nonspecific and is shared by many other neonatal conditions. Respiratory failure and circulatory collapse are typically associated with overwhelming infection. When newborns show signs of respiratory distress immediately after birth, and surfactant deficiency or retained lung fluid is not a likely etiology, pneumonia must be considered as a result of direct inhalation of infected amniotic fluid.

Delayed presentation of sepsis often results from invasion of the neonatal bloodstream by microorganisms through compromised mucous membranes or skin surfaces (for example, umbilical cord). More common signs of neonatal bacteremia or sepsis include hypothermia or hyperthermia, mild or moderately increased work of breathing, apnea, lethargy, poor feeding, jaundice, and cyanosis.

While laboratory testing can assist in diagnosis, the clinical exam remains the mainstay for suspicion (respiratory distress, apnea, lethargy, poor feeding, hypothermia, or hyperthermia). Factors that clearly increase the risk of neonatal infection include premature birth, prolonged rupture of membranes, maternal fever, and unclean handling of the neonate after birth (cord care). The threshold for treating suspected infection based on clinical exam should be lowered when any of these factors is present.

COMPLICATIONS ASSOCIATED WITH PREMATURITY

With decreasing gestational age at birth, neonates are at increasing risk for acute pathophysiological derangements owing to multiple organ system immaturity.

Thermoregulation System

Premature neonates have high ratios of body surface area to metabolically active body mass. Depending on the degree of prematurity, their skin also lacks subcutaneous insulation and a superficial keratinized barrier. These developmental phenomena make them susceptible to much greater evaporative heat losses than adults. Neither term nor preterm infants are capable of shivering to generate heat, and preterm infants lack sufficient brown fat stores to induce nonshivering thermogenesis. Prolonged hypothermia can lead to cardiovascular and respiratory compromise.

Respiratory System

The principal cause of respiratory distress syndrome shortly after birth in very premature newborns is surfactant deficiency at the air-liquid interface of the alveoli. The incidence of respiratory distress syndrome decreases with increasing gestational age. Surfactant serves many purposes in the lung: among other things, it helps establish and maintain a functional residual capacity (gas reserve) at end expiration, reduces the work of breathing by enhancing lung compliance, facilitates the resorption of fluid from alveoli, and protects the air-lung interface from inhaled foreign material (Taeusch, Ramierez-Schrempp, and Liang 2005). High surface tension in alveoli that lack surfactant promotes microcollapse, which aggregates into lung atelectasis. If left untreated, ventilation-perfusion mismatch progresses, and right-to-left intrapulmonary shunting can result in hypoxemia.

Premature neonates born before thirty-eight weeks' gestation are also at elevated risk of apnea of prematurity, which includes the absence of air flow with breathing effort (obstructive), the absence of respiratory effort (central), or a mixed pattern. These sporadic events can lead to sudden death if not intervened upon in a timely fashion. Obstructive apnea is associated with compliant chest-wall dynamics and a relatively narrow and poorly toned upper airway passage. Central apnea is neurologically mediated and most likely the result of immature synaptic connections and incomplete myelination patterns.

Cardiovascular System

Hypotension is quite common in very premature infants and relates to the immaturity of the myocardium, which is developmentally conditioned to pump against a low-resistance placenta. A sudden increase in systemic vascular resistance after birth, coupled with increased volume load on the left ventricle, can lead to a maladaptive response, resulting in low systemic circulation. Blood pressure measurement in premature infants is not a reliable indicator of the adequacy of vital-tissue oxygenation.

GLOBAL IMPACT

Ninety-nine percent of neonatal deaths occur in low- or middle-income countries. Many of these countries have made substantial progress in reducing under-five childhood mortality after infancy through better vaccination rates and management of common communicable diseases. However, the proportion of neonatal deaths has remained static or increased.

A comprehensive analysis of the disability-adjusted life years (DALYs) of 291 diseases in twenty-one world regions as a part of the Global Burden of Disease Study revealed that neonatal disorders as a whole (including asphyxia, sepsis and infection, and prematurity and congenital disorders) represented 8.1% of all global DALYs (Murray et al. 2012). This is largely because when a neonate dies, decades of life are typically lost. Early neonatal loss often perpetuates and reinforces a shortened reproductive cycle in women living in poverty by reducing their birth intervals. This cycle further exacerbates women's poor health outcomes and prevents them from pursuing other opportunities through education or work (Canning and Schultz 2012).

NEONATAL RESUSCITATION

The primary objective in neonatal resuscitations is first to establish adequate expansion of the lungs and, if possible, a consistent native breathing pattern. Most newborns transition well after birth; with spontaneous crying, they expand their lungs, resorb lung fluid, and generate a functional residual capacity with a stable oxygen reserve. In these babies, the gas exchange necessary to complete the transition to extrauterine life proceeds seamlessly.

However, approximately one in ten newborns will need some assistance, which can include drying and stimulating, warming, or suctioning of the mouth. Approximately 1 in 100 newborns requires assistance with breathing. These statistics mean that any provider working around regular deliveries will encounter a neonate who needs immediate help to either survive or avoid some degree of morbidity (most often neurological).

A coordinated-algorithmic approach to treating newborn distress at the time of delivery can prevent death or disability. Fortunately, the skill set required to assist a neonate through most transitions is neither intellectually nor technically very demanding. Nevertheless, good resuscitation skills require routine practice as well as periodic self- and peer-assessment to ensure they do not decay over time (Wall et al. 2009).

The expert-consensus neonatal-resuscitation guideline from the International Liaison Committee on Resuscitation (ILCOR 2006) represents the standard of care applied in advanced health-care delivery systems, where access to technical expertise and equipment is readily available. The ability to perform endotracheal intubation, infuse inotropic medications, and continue neonatal intensive care are assumed when incorporating this guideline.

Simplified variations on the neonatal-resuscitation guideline have recently emerged to accommodate the global reality of low-resource conditions, where most deliveries and most newborn deaths occur (see, for example, World Health Organization 1997). These simplified algorithms are oriented toward training providers in both the formal and informal health-care sectors. The effectiveness of any particular resuscitation protocol depends on the ability to consistently implement the clinical actions at each birth, without exception (Wall et al. 2009).

An alternative to ILCOR is the Helping Babies Breathe initiative and the Golden Minute approach of the American Academy of Pediatrics, with coproducers Jhpiego and Laerdal Global Health (Norway), which many see as a simpler and less expensive method for the resuscitation of newborns. The central tenet is that within one minute after birth, a baby who is not breathing well on his or her own should be ventilated with a bag and mask. The components of Helping Babies Breathe include an evidence-based educational program, based on conclusions of the ILCOR Consensus on Science, after a scientific review by WHO; pictorially based instructional materials that are both culturally sensitive and practical for in-the-field use; a newborn simulator capable of simulating an umbilical pulse, bag-mask systems, and suction bulb that are easily sanitized (tested for use in all climates, available at cost); and a program of continuing mentorship by experts, advice on implementation, and support for ongoing improvement of outcomes and lower infant mortality.

Initial Assessment

A provider assigned to care for a neonate immediately after birth should be able to assess for signs of distress. If gestational age is uncertain, ideally the provider will also have an informed sense of the appearance of neonates at different stages of maturity. However, birth weight is an unreliable marker of maturity, especially in regions where maternal nutritional status is frequently compromised.

The lower the gestational age of a newborn, the more likely it is that resuscitation will be needed. In the first thirty seconds, the provider should focus on the work of breathing and reactivity of the newborn. The presence of a strong cry and flexed muscle tone in the extremities is the typical marker for a successful transition. In such cases, routine care consists of the provider's ensuring that the baby is dried and stays warm.

Resuscitation

If a newborn does not demonstrate a good cry or consistent breathing pattern immediately after birth, resuscitation is required. Lack of cry or responsiveness often signals primary apnea and may follow from a hypoxic event occurring before actual physical delivery. Though this absence of response or minimal responsiveness is sometimes mistaken for fresh stillbirth, it is critically important for providers to distinguish between the two conditions (Spector and Daga 2008). A few recent studies have confirmed that in low-resource settings, implementation of a resuscitation protocol typically decreases the number of stillbirths (Msemo et al. 2013). This is presumably because when providers appropriately respond to primary apnea with intervention, they are often able to elicit vital reactivity from otherwise stunned newborns.

First Steps

Resuscitation starts with positioning the baby to prepare for further interventions as needed. If a safe heating source such as a radiant warmer is available, it can be used to warm the infant. If not, the baby should be placed on a relatively flat surface that allows unimpeded access to the head and chest.

Neonates have just been born through amniotic fluid. Because there also may be oral secretions obstructing the airway, clearance either with a suction device or a clothed finger may be necessary. Vigorous, crying infants should not be suctioned, and excessive suctioning of any neonate should be avoided, as it can induce bradycardia, apnea, or cause upper-airway trauma.

The head should be positioned neutrally to allow maximal airway flow (neither extensively flexed nor extended). Once the airway has been cleared, the neonate should be simultaneously warmed, dried, and stimulated through a firm and purposeful range of tactile motions along the extremities, chest, back, and scalp. Ideally, sterile, dry clothes or towels would be used to perform this task, but any relatively clean textile will do.

Most babies who need assistance will respond to this simple intervention. It is critical for every provider of newborn care to understand this and not underestimate the effectiveness of the intervention.

After thirty seconds, if a baby has responded to basic interventions and is comfortably breathing or crying, routine care is typically all that is indicated. In resource-poor settings, further close observation may be difficult to implement. Skin-to-skin care with mothers and early initiation of breast-feeding is the best next step. If a newborn is breathing comfortably but persists in having low or poor muscular tone, more frequent observation may be indicated.

In cases of delivery through meconium-stained fluid, the standard algorithm applies. In a nonreactive, nonbreathing baby cared for in advanced-practice settings, endotracheal intubation and suctioning of the trachea are typically performed to reduce the likelihood of further aspiration of inflammatory materials into the lungs.

It is important to distinguish between vigorous stimulation of a neonate to promote native respiration and dangerous practices. When a newborn remains unresponsive, one should never escalate to violent shaking, swinging, hitting, or immersion in cold or hot water. A baby who is unresponsive to standard stimulating techniques is by definition depressed and needs assisted ventilation. There is no value in delaying this next step.

Next Steps

If standard basic resuscitation techniques have not been successful after thirty seconds, assisted ventilation is indicated, including calling for help. Assisted ventilation requires specialized equipment, typically in the form of a self-inflating bag-mask device, a tube-mask device, or in their absence, a willingness on the part of a provider to give mouth-to-mouth resuscitation. The latter should be considered within the context of local prevalence of transmissible infections such as HIV. A few studies have compared the user-friendliness of bag-mask with tube-mask devices; while strong conclusions cannot be drawn, the former enjoy a more favorable evaluation (Bang et al. 2005). Familiarity with and practice using any device or method is key to a successful resuscitation.

The goal of assisted ventilation is to push bulk volumes of air into a newborn's lungs to promote and maintain their expansion. This requires a closed system for air movement so that the path of least resistance is successively the baby's mouth, the upper airway, and then the lungs. For air to move along this path, the mask must fit appropriately over the mouth and nose, forming a tight seal, which prevents preferential escape through leaks along the edge of the face-mask interface.

Of all the skills to master in neonatal resuscitation, this is undoubtedly the hardest. Close attention must be paid to mask positioning on the face, and, even in skilled hands, tiny adjustments are routinely made as the resuscitation proceeds to ensure continued adequate ventilating technique.

An oxygen source is not required to perform assisted ventilation; thus there should be no delay in assisted ventilation to secure a supply of oxygen. If a neonate remains unresponsive despite adequate assisted ventilation with room air, or central cyanosis is observed, oxygen may be beneficial. However, ready availability of oxygen remains a limitation in many low-resource settings.

Effective ventilation is typically demonstrated by the newborn's chest rising with each delivered breath. To an untrained eye, this can be difficult to detect at first. If the chest is not rising, the seal at the face-mask interface is most likely not tight enough, and adjustments should be made. It is also possible that oral secretions are blocking the upper airway and need removal via suctioning.

A resuscitator should aim for an assisted breath rate between thirty and forty breaths per minute. It may be useful to count out loud to help establish a consistent rhythm. Increased respiratory reactivity, muscular tone, and general responsiveness of the newborn are all reassuring indications of proper technique.

Effective Ventilation and Circulatory Assessment

Most algorithms call for an evaluation of the baby's heart rate within a thirty- to sixty-second time frame after commencing a resuscitation. This skill requires familiarity with multiple anatomic locations of pulse and practice with palpation technique. Pulses often can be felt more reliably in proximal vessels such as the brachial or femoral spaces, though the radial and posterior tibial locations can also be felt. Care must be taken to palpate gently to avoid dampening out transmitted pulses.

A detected heart rate greater than 100 beats per minute signals a safe opportunity to pause in assisted ventilation and assess the baby's native effort. If the heart rate is slower or minimally palpable, or if the baby is gasping, assisted ventilation should resume, and the heart rate should be checked again after another thirty seconds. This pattern of cyclical evaluation can be continued for several minutes. If the baby continues to require assisted ventilation but is not breathing adequately on its own, every effort should be made to seek advanced care.

If the baby's heart rate is below 100 beats per minute, attention should first focus on ventilation. In the vast majority of cases, sustained bradycardia immediately after birth is a result of inadequate expansion and ventilation of the lungs.

If the heart rate stays or drops below sixty beats per minute, standard resuscitation algorithms call for cardiac massage. Just as assisted ventilation seeks to simulate natural breathing, cardiac massage is a blunt attempt to mimic the natural pumping action of the heart. With each push on the chest, the goal is to push blood through the circulatory system to vital organs. Effective cardiac massage should generate a palpable pulse.

It remains controversial and unresolved whether first-level providers should attempt chest compressions when newborns present with profound asphyxia or depression and immediate assistance or referral to higher-level care is unavailable (Wall et al. 2009). Implementation of a specific algorithm should take into account local context.

Ideally, a second provider performs cardiac massage, by one of two techniques. The first requires wrapping both hands around the torso of the baby to support the back, with placement of both thumbs along the lower third of the sternum above the xiphoid process and below the nipples. Compression should approximate one-third of the anterior to posterior chest diameter. These compressions are given in cycles of three for every breath delivered. Thus there should be 120 "events" per minute consisting of ninety chest compressions and thirty assisted breaths.

The second technique is typically employed if only one provider is performing the resuscitation. The two-finger technique requires placement of the index and middle fingertips on the sternum to deliver the same depth of compression referred to above. However, a single provider, even if highly skilled, may have difficulty performing chest compressions simultaneous with assisted ventilation.

The algorithm promulgated by the International Liaison Committee on Resuscitation also discusses the use of epinephrine and volume expansion in advanced-management settings (ILCOR 2006). These interventions require the immediate ability to obtain intravenous access, for example, through catheterization of an umbilical vessel or endotracheal intubation. In low-resource settings, it is advisable to establish consistently high-quality basic resuscitation skills among all potential providers before introducing these more advanced techniques.

Decisions Not to Initiate Resuscitation or Stop Resuscitation

Decisions not to initiate resuscitation should be sensitive to local contextual factors. The skill level of local providers must be taken into account, as should regional experience with survival at lower birth weights and gestational ages. Firm cutoffs are inadvisable, particularly since some low-birth-weight babies will be growth restricted but developmentally mature. Nevertheless, informal thresholds of 1,000 grams and approximately twenty-eight weeks' gestation remain in place in many low-resource regions (Wall et al. 2009).

It is unwise to dictate a hard-and-fast rule for discontinuing resuscitative efforts, as every case is unique, and to some degree, dependent upon the resuscitator. The International Liaison Committee on Resuscitation (ILCOR 2006) recommends discontinuing assisted ventilation after ten minutes if a baby shows no signs of life.

In advanced-practice settings in high-resource countries, success with therapeutic hypothermia in mitigating the longer-term adverse neurological impact of hypoxic injury to the brain has encouraged a willingness to resuscitate beyond fifteen minutes when any signs of life (heart rate, occasional respirations) are present (Jacobs et al. 2007). In low-resource settings, without such facilities, some experts recommend discontinuing resuscitation after ten minutes when a baby is not breathing on its own, even if a heart rate is detectable (Wall et al. 2009).

Ongoing Care after Resuscitation

Babies who respond well to basic resuscitation alone (drying, suctioning, and stimulating) typically should transition to routine care with a focus on mother-baby bonding through early and exclusive breast-feeding and skin-to-skin contact for thermoregulation.

Neonates who have needed assisted ventilation may have endured more significant periods of hypoxia and should be closely observed for at least twenty-four hours after birth. Special attention should be paid to their ability to feed and their neurological alertness.

Neonatal survivors of birth asphyxia will have varying degrees of need for ongoing monitoring and specialized management by health providers. The degree of birth asphyxia does not always or automatically correlate with the extent and duration of resuscitation. Nevertheless, any baby who has sustained hypoxemia during the peripartum period is at risk for developing encephalopathy, and an indirect indication of this can be the necessary duration of assisted ventilation.

Encephalopathy can manifest as irritability, lethargy, tone abnormalities, or seizures. Up to half of newborns with encephalopathy following asphyxia present with seizures in the first twenty-four hours of life. Phenobarbitol, if available, is generally recommended as the first-line treatment for seizures owing to its long record of use, favorable safety profile, and wide availability at low cost.

Encephalopathy must be managed at a referral center. Initially these babies are often unable to adequately feed or maintain glycemic control;

they may have ongoing respiratory difficulty and need anticonvulsant therapy.

IMPLEMENTATION AND HEALTH SYSTEMS ISSUES

The ability to dry, stimulate, and warm a baby immediately after birth should be available anywhere at any time. Adult household members, village and community health-care workers, and traditional birth attendants can all be taught these skills, and studies have demonstrated the efficacy of such training (Bang et al. 2005). Community empowerment models incorporating self-engagement, education, and action cycles are potentially powerful methods to introduce these skills (Tripathy, Nair, and Barnett 2010).

In areas where deliveries continue predominantly within homes owing to an entrenched reluctance to use health facilities (for whatever reason), there is also a need to teach community-based resuscitation (including assisted ventilation) to attendants at births. However, programs to teach assisted-ventilation skills, whether in community settings or in health facilities, must address the issues of skill retention and competency.

No one knows the number of resuscitations per year that are required for formal- and informal-sector birth attendants to maintain competency; greater supervision is required where providers encounter the need for resuscitation infrequently. Skills that are not practiced or reinforced in daily clinical work decay over a few months (Musafili et al. 2013). Conversely, there is evidence that in low-resource clinical settings, refresher trainings scheduled at three- to six-month intervals can improve skill retention (PATH 2006).

Resuscitation training as a one-time, "fly-in, fly-out" educational intervention, while often convenient for affluent trainers, should be discouraged as a model of intervention. No evidence supports the usefulness of these often short-sighted efforts without an operational plan to incorporate the skill set into an existing health delivery system, which must include specific mechanisms to supervise, reinforce, and support good clinical practices for frontline providers after the initial training (Goudar et al. 2013).

INFECTION

Bacterial sepsis or pneumonia presenting in the first seventy-two hours of newborn life typically starts during the birthing process. Neonatal tetanus is presumed to be associated with unhygienic cord or skin care, allowing for a portal of entry. The evidentiary base for several clean-birth practices remains incomplete; nevertheless, expert opinion recommends their institution where feasible (Blencowe et al. 2011). Clean birth practices may include washing of the birth attendant's hands, washing the mother's perineum before birth, using a clean birth surface, cutting the cord with a clean instrument, tying the cord with a clean thread, and applying an antimicrobial (most commonly chlorhexadine) to the cord after birth.

The diagnosis of sepsis or infection in low-resource settings remains a clinical one. Initiation of antibiotic therapy should never be delayed in a symptomatic newborn while lab results are pending. Several clinical definitions have been used, and all include fast breathing (more than sixty breaths per minute), severe chest retractions, temperature instability (either above or below normal range), lethargy or unresponsiveness, reduced interest in feeding or inability to do so, and skin pustules or cord redness (Zaidi et al. 2011). In a low-resource setting, the presence of one or more of these signs should prompt concern for sepsis and immediate antibiotic administration. Regardless of resuscitation history, newborns presenting with seizures may have meningitis and must be treated with antibiotics.

The choice of antibiotic depends on local availability. Generic penicillins, co-trimoxazole, and gentamicin have all demonstrated efficacy in low-resource settings. Ideally, antibiotics provide coverage against both gram-positive (specifically group B strep) and gram-negative organisms. Evidence suggests a favorable reduction in cause-specific neonatal mortality owing to infection when injectable antibiotics and facility-based care is instituted; however, the use of oral formulations alone is also recommended when nothing else is feasible (Zaidi et al. 2011). Though duration of therapy depends on the clinical context, it should be extended in cases of persistent symptoms. The standard of care in high-resource settings for culture-negative, clinically suspected sepsis is typically seven to ten days of therapy.

CARE OF THE LOW-BIRTH-WEIGHT AND PREMATURE NEWBORN

Especially in low-resource settings, birth weight is a poor indicator of gestational age, as stated above. Malnourishment or undernourishment of many women of reproductive age before and during pregnancy clearly results in growth restriction in infants. When accurate gestational age is in doubt, a specialized physical examination by a knowledgeable provider can help distinguish between more mature neonates who are growth restricted and those who are premature and of appropriate weight for their gestational age. The two most commonly used postnatal tools are the Ballard and Dubowitz scoring assessments. Both methods have undergone small-scale field-testing in low-resource settings and demonstrate some degree of reliability when performed by trained providers (Rosenberg et al. 2009).

The need for advanced neonatal care at a facility level depends on the individual case. In the low-resource setting, low-birth-weight babies, even those with some degree of immaturity, do not automatically need higher-level care when systematic and consistent attention to thermoregulation and adequacy of feeding can be delivered. Kangaroo-mother care should be regarded as the cornerstone of this care; however, its successful implementation at scale in most low-resource settings remains challenging (Lawn et al. 2010). The chief treatment in kangaroo-mother care is prolonged daily skin-to-skin contact between mother and newborn and typically exclusive breast-feeding. The World Health Organization has produced an excellent, freely available practical guide for implementing kangaroo-mother care (available at http://www.who.int/maternal_child_adolescent/documents/9241590351/en).

CONCLUSION

It is possible that millions of newborn deaths each year could be prevented with a dedicated effort to strengthen health systems. Often more attention is placed on the macrocomponents at a country level or in the micro-technical details of a specific treatment or intervention at the expense of the human-scale "who" and "how" of implementation. The material investments needed to reduce neonatal mortality in any specific low-resource setting are undoubtedly small. However, the systems investments are substantial and take time, consistent effort, and a willingness on the part of all local stakeholders to prioritize a change in the existing normative practices around the care of at-risk newborns.

The obstetric practitioner working in a low-resource setting should first attempt to carefully evaluate the local systems that inform and influence neonatal outcomes. Armed with a good understanding of the local factors affecting families, providers, and available resources, there is plenty of reason for optimism when deliberate approaches to improve newborn care practices are implemented.

REFERENCES

Bang, A. T., R. A. Bang, S. B. Baitule, H. M. Reddy, and M. D. Deshmukh. 2005. Management of birth asphyxia in home deliveries in rural Gadchiroli: The effect of two types of birth attendants and of resuscitating with mouth-to-mouth, tube-mask, or bag-mask. *J Perinatol* 25 (S1): S82–91.

Bang, A. T., H. M. Reddy, M. D. Deshmukh, S. B. Baitule, and R. A. Bang. 2005. Neonatal and infant mortality in the ten years (1993 to 2003) of the Gadchiroli field trial: Effect of home-based neonatal care. *J Perinatol* 25:S92–107.

Bhutta, Z., M. Chopra, H. Axelson, P. Berman, T. Boerma, J. Bryce, F. Bustreo, et al. 2010. Countdown to 2015 decade report (2000–2010): Taking stock of maternal, newborn, and childhood survival. *Lancet* 375:2032–44.

Blencowe, H., S. Cousens, L.eMullany, A. Lee, K. Kerber, S. Wall, G. L. Darmstadt, and J. E. Lawn. 2011. Clean birth and postnatal care practices to reduce neonatal deaths from sepsis and tetanus: A systematic review and Delphi estimation of mortality effect. *BioMedCentral Public Health* 11:S11.

Canning, D., and P. Schultz. 2012. The economic consequences of reproductive health and family planning. *Lancet* 380:165–171.

Cousens, S., H. Blencowe, C. Stanton, D. Chou, S. Ahmed, L. Steinhardt, A. A. Creanga, et al. 2011. National, regional, and worldwide estimates of stillbirth rates in 2009 with trends since 1995: A systematic analysis. *Lancet* 377:1319–1330.

Ersdal, H., C. Vossius, E. Bayo, M. Mduma, J. Perlman, A. Lippert, and E. Søreide. A one-day "Helping Babies Breathe" course improves simulated performance but not clinical management of neonates. *Resuscitation* 84:1422–1427.

Goudar, S., M. Somannavar, R. Clark, J. Lockyer, A. Revankar, H. M. Fidler, N. L. Sloan, S. Niermeyer, W. J. Keenan, and N. Singhal. 2013. Stillbirth and newborn mortality in India after helping babies breathe training. *Pediatrics* 131:e344–e352.

ILCOR (International Liaison Committee on Resuscitation). 2006. Consensus on science with treatment recommendations for pediatric and neonatal patients: Neonatal resuscitation. *Pediatrics* 117:e 978–988.

Jacobs, S., R. Hunt, W. Tarnow-Mordi, T. Inder, and P. Davis. 2007. Cooling for newborns with hypoxic ischaemic encephalopathy. *Cochrane Database Systematic Reviews,* no. 4: CD003311.

Lawn, J. E., S. Cousens, and J. Zupan. 2005. 4 million neonatal deaths: When? where? why? *Lancet* 365:891–900.

Lawn, J., K. Kerber, C. Enweronu-Laryea, and O. Massee Bateman. 2009. Newborn survival in low resource settings: Are we delivering? *British Journal of Obstetrics and Gynecology* 116:49–59.

Lawn, J., J. Mwansa-Kambafwile, B. Horta, F. Barros, and S. Cousens. 2010. "Kangaroo mother care" to prevent neonatal deaths due to preterm birth complications. *Int J Epidemiol* 39:i144–i154.

Merrill, J., and R. Ballard. 2005. "Resuscitation in the Delivery Room." In *Avery's Diseases of the Newborn*. 8th ed., edited by W. Taeusch, R. Ballard, and C. Gleason, 350. Philadelphia: Elsevier Saunders.

Msemo, G., A. Massawe, D. Mmbando, N. Rusibamayila, K. Manji, H. L. Kidanto, D. Mwizamuholya, P. Ringia, H. L. Ersdal, and J. Perlman. 2013. Newborn mortality and fresh stillbirth rates in Tanzania after Helping Babies Breathe training. *Pediatrics* 131:e353–e360.

Murray, C., T. Vos, R. Lazano, M. Naghavi, A. Flaxman, C. Michaud, M. Ezzati, et al. 2012. Disability-adjusted life years (DALYs) for 291 diseases and injuries in 21 regions, 1990–2010: A systematic analysis for the Global Burden of Disease Study 2010. *Lancet* 380: 2197–2223.

Musafili, A., B. Essen, C. Baribwir, A. Rukundo, and L. Persson. 2013. Evaluating Helping Babies Breathe: Training for healthcare workers at hospitals in Rwanda. *Acta Paediatrica* 102: e34–e38.

PATH (Program for Appropriate Technology in Health). 2006. *Reducing Birth Asphyxia Through the Bidan di Desa Program in Cirebon, Indonesia*. Final report to Save the Children U.S. Jakarta, Indonesia: PATH. March 15.

Polin, R. A., E. Parravicini, J. A. Regan, and H. W. Taeusch. 2005. "Bacterial Sepsis and Meningitis." In *Avery's Diseases of the Newborn*. 8th ed., edited by W. Taeusch, R. Ballard, and C. Gleason, 551–577. Philadelphia: Elsevier Saunders.

Rosenberg, R., A. Ahmed, S. Ahmed, S. Saha, M. Chowdury, R. E. Black, M. Santosham, and G. L. Darmstadt. 2009. Determining gestational age in a low-resource setting: Validity of last menstrual period. *J Health, Popul Nutr* 27:332–338.

Spector, J., and Daga S. 2008. Preventing those so-called stillbirths. *Bull World Health Organ* 86:315–316.

Taeusch, H. W., D. Ramierez-Schrempp, and I. A. Liang. 2005. "Surfactant Treatment of Respiratory Disorders." In *Avery's Diseases of the Newborn*. 8th ed., edited by W. Taeusch, R. Ballard, and C. Gleason, 670–680. Philadelphia: Elsevier Saunders.

Tripathy, P., N. Nair, S. Barnett, R. Mahapatra, J. Borghi, S. Rath, S. Rath, et al. 2010. Effect of a participatory intervention with women's groups on birth outcomes and maternal depression in Jharkhand and Orissa, India: A cluster-randomised controlled trial. *Lancet* 375:1182–92.

UNICEF (United Nations Children's Emergency Fund). 2009. *State of the World's Children, 2009*. New York: UNICEF: 2009.

Wall, S. N., A. C. C. Lee, S. Niermeyer, M. English, W. J. Keenan, W. Carlo, Z. A. Bhutta, et al. 2009. Neonatal resuscitation in low-resource set- tings: What, who, and how to overcome challenges to scale up? *Int J Gynaecol Obstet* 107:S47–S62.

Williams, C. B., and F. S. Cole. 2005. "Immunology of the Fetus and Newborn." In *Avery's Diseases of the Newborn*. 8th ed., edited by W. Taeusch, R. Ballard, and C. Gleason, 447–473. Philadelphia: Elsevier Saunders.

Winch, P. J., M. A. Alam, A. Akther, D. Afroz, N. A. Ali, A. A. Ellis, A. H. Baqui, et al. 2005. Local understandings of vulnerability and protection during the neonatal period in Sylhet district, Bangladesh: A qualitative study. *Lancet* 366:478–485.

WHO (World Health Organization). 1997. *Basic Newborn Resuscitation: A Practical Guide.* Geneva: WHO.

Zaidi, A., H. Ganatra, S. Syed, S. Cousens, A. Lee, R. Black, Z. A. Bhutta, and J. E. Lawn. 2011. Effect of case management on neonatal mortality due to sepsis and pneumonia. *BioMedCentral Public Health* 11:S13.

Contributors

ZULFIQAR AHMED BHUTTA, MD, PHD

Husein Laljee Dewraj Professor, Center for Excellence in Women and Child Health, Aga Khan University, Karachi, Pakistan; and Centre for Global Child Health, Hospital for Sick Children, Toronto, Ontario, Canada

JOHANNA DAILY, MD, MS

Departments of Medicine (Infectious Diseases) and Microbiology & Immunology, Associate Professor, Albert Einstein College of Medicine, New York, New York

JAI K. DAS, MD

Center for Excellence in Women and Child Health, Aga Khan University, Karachi, Pakistan; Pakistan Site Director for the Cochrane Collaboration; and Coordinator for the Maternal Child Link on the Global Health Network

KHADY DIOUF, MD

Division of Global Obstetric and Gynecologic Health, Department of Obstetrics and Gynecology, Brigham and Women's Hospital, Boston, Massachusetts; and Assistant Professor, Harvard Medical School, Boston, Massachusetts

DINESH KUMAR JAGANNATHAN, MD

Department of Anesthesiology, Brigham and Women's Hospital, Boston, Massachusetts; and Clinical Fellow, Harvard Medical School, Boston, Massachusetts

BHAVANI SHANKAR KODALI, MD

Associate Professor, Harvard Medical School; and Vice Chairman, Department of
Anesthesiology, Brigham and Women's Hospital, Boston, Massachusetts

ANDRE B. LALONDE, MD, FRCSC

Obstetrics, International and Humanitarian Medicine, Gynaecology,
University of Ottawa, McGill University

SUELLEN MILLER, PHD, RN, CNM, MHA

Department of Obstetrics, Gynecology & Reproductive Sciences; Director,
Safe Motherhood Program; Maternal Child Health Program,
School of Public Health, UC Berkeley

ROSE LEONARD MOLINA, MD

Division of Women's Health, Department of Medicine, Brigham and Women's
Hospital Global and Community Health Program, Boston, Massachusetts;
Department of Obstetrics and Gynecology, Beth Israel Deaconess
Medical Center, Boston, Massachusetts; Instructor,
Harvard Medical School, Boston, Massachusetts

NAWAL M. NOUR, MD, MPH

Director, Division of Global Obstetric and Gynecologic Health and African
Women's Health Center, Brigham and Women's Hospital, Boston, Massachusetts; and Associate Professor, Harvard Medical School, Boston, Massachusetts

CHRISTIN PRICE, MD

Department of Internal Medicine, Brigham and Women's Hospital, Boston,
Massachusetts; and Instructor, Harvard Medical School, Boston, Massachusetts

MARIA I. RODRIGUEZ, MD, MPH

Assistant Professor, Department of Obstetrics and Gynecology,
Oregon Health and Science University, Portland, Oregon

RENGASWAMY SANKARANARAYANAN, MD

Special Advisor on Cancer Control, Head, Screening Group, International
Agency for Research on Cancer, Lyon, France

SADATH ALI SAYEED, MD, JD

Boston Children's Hospital; Program Director, Program in Global Newborn Health and Social Change, Assistant Professor, Global Health and Social Medicine, Harvard Medical School Boston, Massachusetts

JULIANNA SCHANTZ-DUNN, MD, MPH

Division of Global Obstetric and Gynecologic Health, Department of Obstetrics and Gynecology, Brigham and Women's Hospital, Boston, Massachusetts; and Instructor, Harvard Medical School, Boston, Massachusetts

JENNIFER SCOTT, MD, MBA, MPH

Director, Global and Community Health Program, Department of Obstetrics and Gynecology, Beth Israel Deaconess Medical Center, Boston, Massachusetts; Harvard Humanitarian Initiative, Cambridge, Massachusetts; Division of Women's Health, Department of Medicine, Brigham and Women's Hospital, Boston, Massachusetts; Instructor, Harvard Medical School, Boston, Massachusetts

L. LEWIS WALL, MD, DPHIL

Selina Okin Kim Conner Professor in Arts and Sciences, Professor of Anthropology (Medical Anthropology), College of Arts and Sciences; Professor of Obstetrics and Gynecology, School of Medicine, Washington University in St. Louis; Adjunct Professor of Obstetrics and Gynecology, College of Health Sciences, Mekelle University, Mekelle, Ethiopia

BLAIR WYLIE, MD, MPH

Division of Maternal Fetal Medicine, Department of Obstetrics and Gynecology, Massachusetts General Hospital, Boston, Massachusetts; and Associate Professor, Harvard Medical School, Boston, Massachusetts

SIGAL YAWETZ, MD

Division of Infectious Disease, Department of Internal Medicine, Brigham and Women's Hospital, Boston, Massachusetts; and Assistant Professor, Harvard Medical School, Boston, Massachusetts

Illustration Credits

Figure 2.1. Reprinted from Leontine Alkema, Doris Chou, Daniel Hogan, Sanqian Zhang, Ann-Beth Moller, Alison Gemmill, Doris Ma Fat, Ties Boerma, Marleen Temmerman, Colin Mathers, and Lale Say, "Global, regional, and national levels and trends in maternal mortality between 1990 and 2015, with scenario-based projections to 2030: A systematic analysis by the UN Maternal Mortality Estimation Inter-Agency Group," *Lancet* 387: 462–474, Figure 1. © World Health Organization 2015. Published by Elsevier Ltd/Inc/BV.

Figure 2.2. Reprinted from André B. Lalonde, "Prevention and treatment of postpartum hemorrhage in low-resource settings," *International Journal of Gynecology & Obstetrics* 117 (2): 108–118, Figure 11. © 2012 International Federation of Gynecology and Obstetrics. Published by Elsevier Ireland Ltd.

Figure 2.3. Reproduced from USAID (United States Agency for International Development), Maternal and Child Health (MCH) Program, www.usaid.gov. As published in Nawal M. Nour, "An introduction to maternal mortality," *Reviews in Obstetrics & Gynecology* 1, no. 2 (Spring 2008): 77–81, Figure 1. MedReviews, LLC.

Figure 3.1. Reprinted from Joy E. Lawn, Hannah Blencowe, Robert Pattinson, Simon Cousens, Rajesh Kumar, Ibinabo Ibiebele, Jason Gardosi, Louise T. Day, Cynthia Stanton, for The Lancet's Stillbirths Series steering committee, "Stillbirths: Where? When? Why? How to make the data count?" *Lancet* 377: 1448–1463, Figure 1. © World Health Organization 2011, with permission from Elsevier.

Figure 3.2. Courtesy of Zulfiqar Ahmed Bhutta and Jai K. Das.

Figure 4.1. Photo courtesy Dr. Andrew Browning. Creative Commons Attribution 4.0 International (CC BY 4.0).

Figure 4.2. © Worldwide Fistula Fund, used by permission.

Figure 4.3. © Worldwide Fistula Fund, used by permission.

Figure 4.4. © Worldwide Fistula Fund, used by permission.

Figure 4.5. © Worldwide Fistula Fund, used by permission.

Figure 4.6. © Worldwide Fistula Fund, used by permission.

Figure 4.7. © Worldwide Fistula Fund, used by permission.

Figure 4.8. © Worldwide Fistula Fund, used by permission.

Figure 5.1. Reprinted from *Prevalence and incidence of selected sexually transmitted infections Chlamydia trachomatis, Neisseria gonorrhoeae, syphilis and Trichomonas vaginalis: Methods and results used by WHO to generate 2005 estimates,* Figures 3 and 4. © World Health Organization 2011.

Figure 5.2. Reprinted from "Guidelines for the Management of Sexually Transmitted Infections," Figure 3. © World Health Organization 2003.

Figure 5.3. Reprinted from "Guidelines for the Management of Sexually Transmitted Infections," Figure 9. © World Health Organization 2003.

Figure 5.4. Reprinted from "Guidelines for the Management of Sexually Transmitted Infections," Figure 6. © World Health Organization 2003.

Figure 7.1. Photo courtesy of Dr. Danny Milner Jr.

Figure 7.2. Photo courtesy of Johanna Daily.

Figure 7.3. Photo courtesy of Johanna Daily.

Figure 9.1. Adapted from D. Forman, F. Bray, D. H. Brewster, C. Gombe Mbakawa, B. Kohler, M. Piñeros, E. Steliarova-Foucher, R. Swaminathan, and J. Ferlay, eds., "Cancer Incidence in Five Continents, Vol. X." IARC Scientific Publication No. 164. Lyon: International Agency for Research on Cancer. © 2014 International Agency for Research on Cancer.

Figure 9.2. Adapted from M. P. Curado, B. Edwards, H. R. Shin, H. Storm, J. Ferlay, M. Heanue, and P. Boyle, eds., "Cancer Incidence in Five Continents, Vol. IX," IARC Scientific Publication No. 160. Lyon: International Agency for Research on Cancer. © 2007 International Agency for Research on Cancer. Printed in 2009.

Figure 10.1. From K. M. Devries, J. Y. T. Mak, C. García-Moreno, M. Petzold, J. C. Child, G. Falder, S. Lim, L. J. Bacchus, R. E. Engell, L. Rosenfeld, C. Pallitto, T. Vos, N. Abrahams, and C. H. Watts, "Global Health: The Global Prevalence of Intimate Partner Violence against Women," *Science* 340, Issue

6140 (June 2013): 1527–1528. © 2013 American Association for the Advancement of Science. Reprinted with permission of AAAS.

Figure 10.2. Adapted from L. Heise, "Violence against women: An integrated, ecological framework," *Violence against Women* 4, no. 3 (June 1998): 262–290. As published in L. Heise, M. Ellsberg, and M. Gottemoeller, "Ending Violence against Women," *Population Reports*, Series L, No. 11 (December 1999), Figure 1. Population Information Program, Center for Communication Programs. Baltimore: The Johns Hopkins University School of Public Health. Published in collaboration with The Center for Health and Gender Equity (CHANGE).

Figure 11.1. Courtesy of Nawal M. Nour.

Figure 11.2. Courtesy of Nawal M. Nour.

Figure 11.3. Courtesy of Nawal M. Nour.

Figure 11.4. Courtesy of Nawal M. Nour.

Figure 11.5. Courtesy of Nawal M. Nour.

Figure 12.1. Courtesy of Sharon Owusu-Darko.

Figure 12.2. Courtesy of Julianna Schantz-Dunn.

Figure 12.3. Courtesy of Julianna Schantz-Dunn. Reprinted from Julianna Schantz-Dunn and Nawal M. Nour, "The Use of Blood in Obstetrics and Gynecology in the Developing World," *Reviews in Obstetrics & Gynecology* 4, no. 2 (Summer 2011): 86–91, Figure 4. MedReviews, LLC.

Figure 12.4. Courtesy of Julianna Schantz-Dunn.

Figure 12.5. Courtesy of Julianna Schantz-Dunn.

Figure 12.6. Courtesy of Julianna Schantz-Dunn.

Figure 13.1. Courtesy of Medge Owen.

Figure 13.2. Courtesy of Medge Owen.

Acknowledgments

My parents taught me the value of education, the importance of social justice, and ultimately the underlying need to improve life in poverty-stricken areas. Growing up in Sudan and Egypt gave me a deep understanding of injustice, poverty, and disease. I remember walking through the streets of Khartoum as a child, unable to avert my gaze from the fingerless beggars who suffered from leprosy. I would quickly run past them, petrified that a fly might land on me and infect me with such a devastating fate. I also remember watching my mother enduring high fevers and praying that the malaria parasite would not take her. And I remember being gripped with fear when we heard that there was yet another car bombing in Beirut during the height of the civil war and bracing myself, hoping that my father was not in the bomb's vicinity.

I fondly recall my father, Mohamed, returning from work at the Food and Agricultural Organization after weaving through Cairo's insane traffic and telling us stories during dinner about "the poor farmer." A term my father uses frequently, "the poor farmer" referred to farmers who were struggling to plow, sow, and reap their land to feed their families. The deficit in food production was (and still is) a concern to him, but despite the mission of larger organizations that focused on receding commodity, gaps between food production and consumption, and the need for complex crops, my father always brought it back to "the poor farmer" and how to ultimately improve his life. His drive to assist the underserved, the poor, and the helpless has never flagged.

My mother, Jane, is my rock and my cheerleader. One day after I returned from school feeling utterly defeated by a teacher's demoralizing decision, my mother reminded me that life was not fair. She reminded me that despite defeats, one must forge on. A plant pathologist and teacher, my mother continuously sought to inspire us with imagery of plants persevering despite the weeds that surrounded them. At times, I wondered whether my siblings and I would survive the overgrown house plants that she nurtured in our home. But her continuous encouragement to be an instrument of change despite social and political hurdles has supported and sustained me throughout my career in women's health.

This book is dedicated to my parents for their never-ending love and support.

I am grateful that my siblings keep me grounded. My oldest sister, Johara, provides us all with a sense of calm. My brother, Tahir, finds comedy in almost everything, even a box of chocolates or a bouquet of flowers. And my sister Sarah makes us all smile with her unwavering positivity.

My ten-year-old daughter, Nejma, continuously motivates me to be a better mother and role model. After spending a few nights at a children's hospital and noticing sick bald children walking the halls, she felt the need to help. Since then, she has donated ten inches of her hair (twice) to children who have lost their hair to chemotherapy, radiation, burns, and alopecia. She is my munchkin and my inspiration!

I would not have been able to finish this book if not for Paul Guttry. He painstakingly read, edited, reread, and re-edited chapters with me. During the writing process after I suffered a retinal detachment, Paul was there to help me focus—both literally and figuratively. He was willing to meet at my home, office, and any café to move the book along. He questioned the need for certain sections in the book and challenged me on what really mattered. At times, when he sensed my fatigue, he would come up with a hysterical story or two, usually about his home renovation. These stories would ultimately revitalize me. I am utterly indebted to him and feel so fortunate that he is not squeamish when it comes to women's diseases.

Dr. Robert Barbieri, my hospital's Chairman of Obstetrics and Gynecology, has unfailingly supported my work. When I initially brought him the book proposal for review, he marked it up and returned it with encouraging words. He then smiled and said, "Now the hard work begins." I am indebted to his infinite knowledge, wisdom, and guidance.

I would also like to thank James Bell, who volunteered his time to work on graphics. Like an angel, he fell into this book out of nowhere and insisted on helping me. He rearranged images so that they would appear clear and beautiful. Without him, the graphs, tables, and photographs may have not made it in the book.

My work family sustains me on a daily basis. I am grateful to Audra Meadows, Khady Diouf, and Julianna Schantz-Dunn, my friends and colleagues, whose mission is helping underserved women locally, nationally, and globally. Betty Fenton-Diggins, RN, has worked alongside me for over twenty years, since I was an intern in residency. I am also indebted to the rest of my staff of nurses, social workers, medical assistants, and practice assistants, who keep me afloat.

Finally, I want to thank my patients, who inspire me. They have taught me to pay attention, to listen well, to remember more, and to appreciate the true meaning of compassion. Without them, I would not have grasped what it meant to live with the complications of female genital cutting. Without them, I would not have comprehended the devastation of living with an obstetric fistula. Without them, I would not have seen how physical and emotional suffering can strengthen—indeed empower— women to rise and demand better health for themselves and their families. I sincerely hope this book can help these women live longer and healthier lives.

—*Nawal M. Nour*

Index

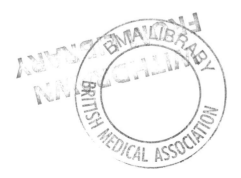